Poultry

Fourth Edition

GC Banerjee

MSc (Ag), AH and Dairy Sc., PhD (Animal Sc), Cornell University, USA

Former Professor of Animal Nutrition and
Former Dean, Postgraduate Studies
Bidhan Chandra Krishi Viswavidyalaya
Nadia, West Bengal

Revised by

L Mandal

MSc (Ag), AH PhD (Animal Nutrition)

Professor (Re-employed)
Department of Animal Science and
Former Dean, Faculty of Agriculture
Bidhan Chandra Krishi Viswavidyalaya
Nadia, West Bengal

Oxford & IBH Publishing Co. Pvt. Ltd.
New Delhi
(A Unit of CBS Publishers & Distributors Pvt Ltd)

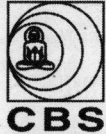

CBS

CBS Publishers & Distributors Pvt Ltd

New Delhi • Bengaluru • Chennai • Kochi • Kolkata • Mumbai
Hyderabad • Jharkhand • Nagpur • Patna • Pune • Uttarakhand

Poultry

Fourth Edition

ISBN-13: 978-81-204-1780-9
ISBN-10: 81-204-1780-1

OXFORD & IBH
New Delhi
(A *Unit* of CBS Publishers & Distributors Pvt Ltd)

CBS Publishers & Distributors Pvt Ltd
204 FIE, Patparganj Industrial Area, Delhi 110 092
E-mail: delhi@cbspd.com, cbspubs@airtelmail.in

Ph: 4934 4934   Fax: 4934 4935   Website: www.cbspd.com
                                               e-mail: publishing@cbspd.com;
                                                       publicity@cbspd.com

Branches

- **Bengaluru:** Seema House 2975, 17th Cross, K.R. Road, Banasankari 2nd Stage, Bengaluru 560 070, Karnataka
  Ph: +91-80-26771678/79   Fax: +91-80-26771680   e-mail: bangalore@cbspd.com
- **Chennai:** 7, Subbaraya Street, Shenoy Nagar, Chennai 600 030, Tamil Nadu
  Ph: +91-44-26680620, 26681266   Fax: +91-44-42032115   e-mail: chennai@cbspd.com
- **Kochi:** Ashana House, 39/1904, AM Thomas Road, Valanjambalam, Ernakulam 682 016, Kochi, Kerala
  Ph: +91-484-4059061-65,67   Fax: +91-484-4059065   e-mail: kochi@cbspd.com
- **Kolkata:** 6/B, Ground Floor, Rameswar Shaw Road, Kolkata-700014 (West Bengal), India
  Ph: +91-33-2289-1126, 2289-1127, 2289-1128   e-mail: kolkata@cbspd.com
- **Mumbai:** 83-C, Dr E Moses Road, Worli, Mumbai-400018, Maharashtra
  Ph: +91-22-24902340/41   Fax: +91-22-24902342   e-mail: mumbai@cbspd.com

Representatives

- **Hyderabad** 0-9885175004   • **Jharkhand** 0-9811541605   • **Nagpur** 0-9021734563
- **Patna** 0-9334159340   • **Pune** 0-9623451994   • **Uttarakhand** 0-9716462459

Printed at Chaman Enterprises, Daryaganj, New Delhi, India

Dedicated

To

All those related to
Poultry
In this way or that way

Preface to the Fourth Edition

It is thirty five years since the first edition of the book 'POULTRY' came out and its third edition was published in 1992. By this time the scenario of Poultry industry has changed completely. The book originally written by Late Prof. G.C. Banerjee is a unique one, and due to its unique feature this is widely accepted not only in India but also in other Asian countries. It is an exhilarating yet humble feeling that God has made use of me in spreading knowledge to the needy in this field through this book which was the creation of my reverend teacher. I am grateful to a large number of students, professional colleagues and poultry farmers who have expressed themselves about the usefulness of this book and for their suggestions for further improvement which have helped me a lot in revising and updating this book.

To cope up with the present need, information about rearing of low input technology birds, farming of Turkey, Emu, Ostrich have been incorporated. Information in detail have been provided for poultry insurance considering its importance to the poultry farmers. Topic on Management of broilers has been totally revised. Population and production data have been updated as far as possible. Disease portion along with vaccination schedule have been suitably modified.

The present form of the book thus provides educational concepts and a self study guide for students, researchers, livestock extension specialists and administrators interested in the farming of poultry. I hope like previous occasions, this time also, the book will be widely accepted by all.

I express my sincere thanks to all those who have helped me with their suggestions while revising the book. I express my thanks whole heartedly to the publishers as they have extended the time limit, beyond schedule period and supported my efforts admirably.

The book is dedicated to all classes of people related to poultry

Vijayadashami   L. Mandal
3rd October, 2014
Department of Animal Science
Bidhan Chandra Krishi Viswavidyalaya
Mohanpur-741252,Nadia
West Bengal

CONTENTS

WHAT IS POULTRY?

The term 'poultry' applies to a rather wide variety of birds of several species and it refers to them whether they are alive or dressed (slaughtered and prepared for market). The term applies to chickens, turkeys, ducks, geese, swans, guinea fowl, pigeons, pea fowl, ostriches, pheasants, quail and other game birds.

The study of birds which are not classed as poultry is known as *ornithology*.

WHY POULTRY FARMING?

1. **Requires minimum investment to start with**
   In comparison to other livestock, it requires less investment to start the farming. Persons from low income group may also start the business on a small scale.

2. **Rapid return of profit**
   Chicken starts laying when they are about 6 months of age, broiler gets ready to be marketed for poultry meat at the age between 6 to 8 weeks.

   To bring about the phenomenal increase in poultry production in short interval is relatively easy, because of the short generation interval. For example, starting with a set of grand parent, it is possible to produce 2,500 commercial pullets within 40 months which in turn can lay half a million of egg within 18 months. In terms of high quality protein, it would amount to 3 tons.

3. **Poultry convert feed to food protein efficiently**
   Among all domesticated animals broilers takes only 1.9 kg of feed protein to produce 1.0 kg of broiler protein.

4. **Poultry provides a continuous sonrce of income**
   Since they start laying at their age of six months, the farmer also starts getting return so early. Broilers pay them within 1½ to 2 months.

5. **Farming requires small space**
   Poultry requires small space with modern confinement rearing. Poultry may be produced in the backyards of cities and small towns.

6. **Stabilise farm income**
   Farmers occasionally experience crop failures due to unfavourable weather conditions when poultry raising as mixed farming will tend to stabilise farm income.

7. Poultry feeds not commonly used for human

India possesses large quantities of agro-industrial by-products which are used as feed ingredients for transformation into eggs and meat.

8. Availability of superior stocks

Some of the best breeding stocks available any where in the world is now being multiplied in this country. Number one egg producing breed i.e.. White Leghorns, strain crosses of other breeds, have been imported and are well adapted to Indian climate. Excellent White Rocks and White Cornish broiler meat strains are now available throughout the country.

9. Employment opportunities

Poultry farming offers opportunities for full-time or part-time employment -particularly for women, children or elderly people on the farm operation. Apart from direct employment on the farm, persons away from the producing center are also employed for transportation and distributions among the consumers. Factories for producing liquid egg, egg powder, dried yolk etc. may help for further employment opportunities.

10. Poultry manure used as fertiliser

Poultry manure is an extremely rich source of nitrogen and organic material. Hence it is highly regarded as a fertiliser. Poultry droppings are higher than cowdung in nitrogen, (as it also contains the secretion of the kidneys), phosphorus and potassium content. The manure either may be pure droppings of the birds or used old built-up litters which are cleaned either every year or once in every two years.

A laying hen produces about 220 gms of fresh droppings (75% moisture) every day. Average nutrient contents of various animal refuse are presented in Table 1.

Table 1 Average Nutrient Contents of Poultry Droppings Compared with other Animal Refuse

Fresh Manure	Percentage content								
	Nitrogen (N)			Phosphoric acid (P_2O_5)			Potash (K)		
Poultry manure	1.0	to	1.8	1.4	to	1.8	0.8	to	0.9
Cattle dung	0.3	to	0.4	0.1	to	0.2	0.1	to	0.3
Night soil	1.0	to	1.6	0.8	to	1.2	0.2	to	0.6
Sheep dung	0.5	to	0.7	0.4	to	0.6	0.3	to	1.0
Horse dung	0.4	to	0.5	0.3	to	0.4	0.3	to	0.4
Cattle urine	0.9	to	1.2		tr.		0.5	to	1.0
Human urine	0.6	to	1.0	0.1	to	0.2	0.2	to	0.3
Sheep urine	1.5	to	1.7		tr.		1.8	to	2.0

The built-up litter is a balanced organic fertiliser, containing 3% nitrogen, 2% phosphorus, 2% potash and humus. One tonne of litter, produced by 40 layers in a year, is equivalent to about 140 kg of ammonium sulphate, 125 kg of super-phosphate and 45 kg of potassium, without the ill effects of chemical fertilisers on the soil, when applied, without any farm yard or other organic manure.

ORIGIN

It is believed that the modern fowl probably originated from the following four wild species:

1. the Red Jungle fowl (*Gallus gallus*)
2. the Ceylon Jungle fowl (*G. lafayetti*)
3. the Grey Jungle fowl (*G. sonnerattii*)
4. the Java Jungle fowl (*G. varius*)

It is likely that of the four wild, species *G. gallus* is the main ancestor. The four species are closely related and are known to interbreed.

India and throughout mainland of Southeast Asia to the off-shore islands of Indonesia are the ancestral home of the present day domestic fowl.

Table 2 Zoological Classificaion

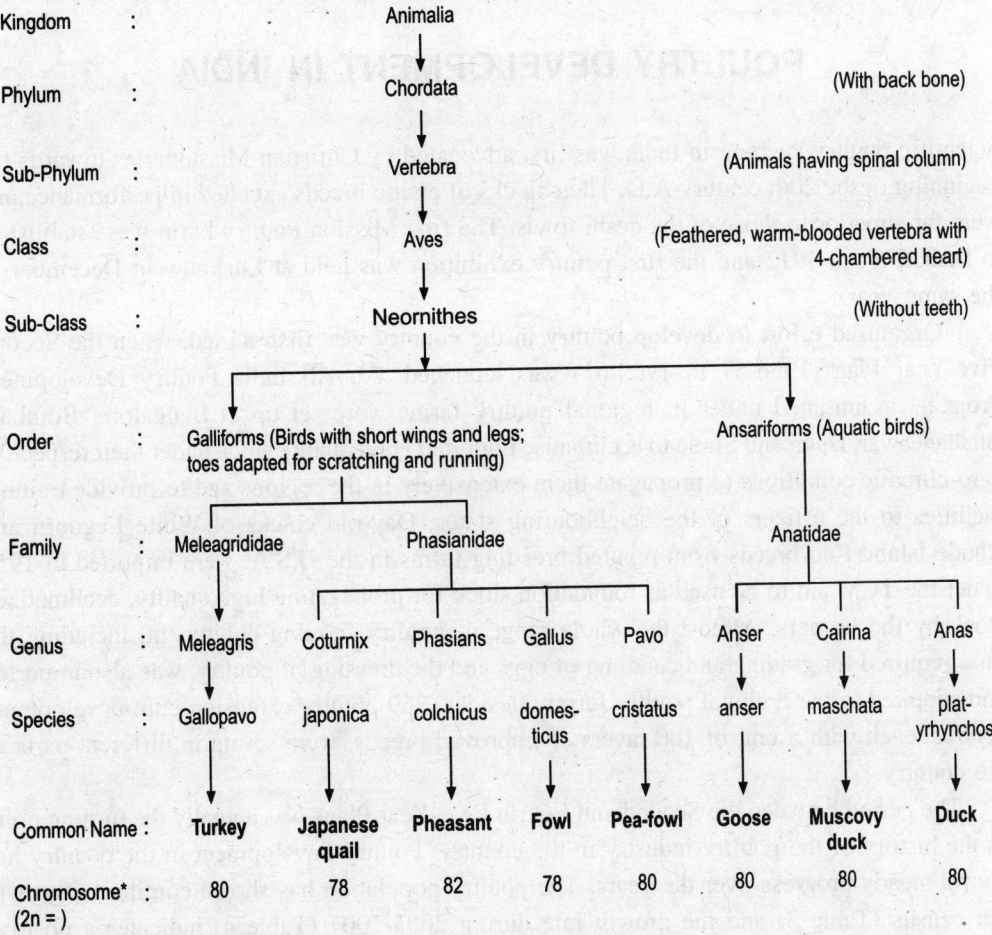

Kingdom :	Animalia	
Phylum :	Chordata	(With back bone)
Sub-Phylum :	Vertebra	(Animals having spinal column)
Class :	Aves	(Feathered, warm-blooded vertebra with 4-chambered heart)
Sub-Class :	Neornithes	(Without teeth)

	Galliforms (Birds with short wings and legs; toes adapted for scratching and running)				Ansariforms (Aquatic birds)		
Order :							
Family :	Meleagrididae	Phasianidae			Anatidae		
Genus :	Meleagris	Coturnix	Phasians	Gallus	Pavo	Anser	Cairina	Anas
Species :	Gallopavo	japonica	colchicus	domesticus	cristatus	anser	maschata	platyrhynchos
Common Name :	**Turkey**	**Japanese quail**	**Pheasant**	**Fowl**	**Pea-fowl**	**Goose**	**Muscovy duck**	**Duck**
Chromosome* (2n =)	80	78	82	78	80	80	80	80

*For avian it was once thought that the females were XO, having one fewer chromosome than the male. Recent studies, however show that the female has a very small sex chromosome, called the (w) chromosome. Thus the female is Xw (sometimes called Zw).

Domestication

Our ancient history bears witness to the fact that the people of India were quite familiar with fowl, duck, quail and turkey, about 3,200 years B. C. But the chick was considered neither a food nor an "egg machine" but something of an entertainer. Quail or cock fight provided as a source of fun.

Domesticated fowls could certainly be found in Iran by 800 B. C. and that the Persians spread them throughout Western Asia and to the shores of the Mediterranian by 600 B. C. They were common in Italy by 400 B. C. and were introduced into Northern Europe by 100 B. C. Chickens were imported into The America and Australia by the early European explorers and immigrants. To-day they are considered as vital source of animal proteins throughout the world.

POULTRY DEVELOPMENT IN INDIA

Scientific poultry keeping in India was first advocated by Christian Missionaries towards the beginning of the 20th century A.D. Their flocks of exotic breeds excelled in performance and were far superior to those of the deshi fowls. The first Mission Poultry Farm was established in Etah, U.P. in 1912 and the first poultry exhibition was held at Lucknow in December of the same year.

Organised effort to develop poultry in the country was first started, when the Second Five-Year Plan (1956-57 to 1960-61) was launched. An All India Poultry Development Project was initiated under it, regional poultry farms were set up at Bangalore, Bombay, Bhubaneswar, Delhi and Simla to acclimatise imported good quality stock under their respective agro-climatic conditions to propagate them extensively in the regions and to provide training facilities to the officers of the neighbouring states. Day-old chicks of White Leghorn and Rhode Island Red breeds from reputed breeding farms in the U.S.A. were imported in 1956 under the TCM aid to be used as foundation stock for propagating high quality, acclimatized stock by the farmers. Almost the whole range of poultry farming equipment, including the ones required for grading and candling of eggs and the dressing of poultry, was also imported and supplied to the regional poultry farms. Besides, 269 poultry extension-cum-development centres, each with a unit of 100 layers of improved breeds, were set up in different parts of the country.

The period between the Second and Fourth Five-Year Plans was actually the turning point in the history of the poultry industry in the country. Poultry development in the country has shown steady progress over the years. The poultry population has shown continuous growth per census (Table 3) and the growth rate during 2003-2007 (Table 4) indicates a positive aspect signifying greater availability of meat and eggs for human requirements.

Table 3 All India census estimates of poultry population (1951-2007) in millions

	Poultry
1951	73.50
1956	94.80
1961	114.20
1966	115.40
1972	138.50
1977	159.20
1982	207.74
1987	275.32
1992	307.07
1997	347.61
2003	489.01
2007	648.88

Table 4 Annual growth rate (%) in poultry population (1951- 2007)

	1951-56	1961-66	1972-77	1982-87	1992-97	2003-07
Poultry	5.22	0.21	2.82	5.79	2.51	7.33

Source: Livestock Census, Directorate of Economics and Statistics and Animal Husbandry Statistics Division; Department of Animal Husbandry, Dairying Fisheries, Ministry of Agriculture.

The data on statewise poultry population in India as per 18th Livestock Census is presented in Table 5.

Poultry is one of the fastest grown segments of the agricultural sector in India today. India has emerged on the world poultry map (2010-11) as the 3rd largest egg (56 billion eggs) and 5th largest poultry meat (2.6 million tons) producer. Total chicken population has registered an annual growth of 7.3% in the last decade. While annual growth rate of broiler only is 12% during 1990 to 2010-11, egg production has increased at the rate of over 6% a year leading to per capita availability of 55 eggs. Organized sector accounts for nearly 70% of the total poultry output in the country. The current strength of layers and broilers in India is estimated to be 230 million and 2300 million, respectively. Poultry processing has also gone up to 20% of total broiler production. The potential of poultry sector in employment generation and enhancing rural incomes is well-recognized. Over 7 million people are directly or indirectly engaged in poultry sector, apart from numerous small poultry keepers in rural and tribal areas of the country. The domestic broiler meat demand is expected to grow at around 15-18% while table egg demand is expected to grow at 5-7% in medium to long term. At present, poultry emerged as a very important meat supplier with significant share of 16.3% to total meat production in the country.

Continuous growth of poultry through different years is presented in Table 6. The value of poultry meat and eggs has multiplied over six fold since 1961 to Rs.16,935 crore in 2006. The growth of poultry in the past four-and-a-half decades will be evident from the fact that the annual egg production has increased from 2,881 million in 1961 to around 47,343 million

Table 5 Poultry population in India (in thousand)

States/UTs	Fowl	Duck	Total poultry*
India	617734	27643	648829
Andhra Pradesh	123036	766	123981
Arunachal Pradesh	1259	90	1348
Assam	20609	8439	29060
Bihar	10755	499	11420
Chhattisgarh	13838	127	14246
Goa	504	1	505
Gujarat	13327	18	13352
Haryana	28619	33	28785
Himachal Pradesh	725	0	810
Jammu & Kashmir	6487	190	6683
Jharkhand	10448	615	11231
Karnataka	41845	13	42068
Kerala	14219	995	15686
Madhya Pradesh	7311	59	7384
Maharashtra	64431	34	64756
Manipur	1830	559	2403
Meghalaya	3026	66	3093
Mizoram	1232	7	1239
Nagaland	2991	120	3156
Odisha	19489	594	20600
Punjab	10536	25	10685
Rajasthan	4914	27	4946
Sikkim	157	1	157
Tamil Nadu	126879	1039	128108
Tripura	2895	756	3701
Uttar Pradesh	8460	270	8754
Uttarakhand	2563	25	2602
West Bengal	73626	12160	86210
Andaman & Nicobar Islands	916	54	979
Chandigarh	129	0	129
Dadra & Nagar Haveli	169	0	170
Daman & Diu	25	0	26
Delhi	2	0	2
Lakshadweep	137	26	167
Puducherry	345	35	387

Source: 18th Indian Livestock Census 2007
* Besides fowl and duck, total number of poultry also includes other birds like turkey, quail etc.
0-Negligible

in 2006. The per capita annual availability of eggs was only 42 as compared to more than 200 eggs in many developing countries during the year 2006. The poultry production in the country has made a spectacular growth since 1961 (Table 6).

Table 6 Selected indicators of poultry development in India

Year	Egg output (million)	Per capita availability (Numbers)	Value of poultry meat and eggs at 1999-2000 prices (Rs. Million)
1961	2,881	7	27,670
1971	5,340	10	25,510
1981	10,876	16	48,650
1991	21,983	26	95,620
2001	38,729	38	142,900
2006	47,343	42	169,350
2011	63,024	53	–
2012	65,450	–	–

Source: Basic Annual Husbandry Statistics, 2012

The domestic poultry market size is estimated at more than Rs. 47,000 crore and the growth trend is likely to continue for the present decade as demand has been growing steadily on back of favourable socio-economic factors like healthy GDP growth, rising purchasing power, changing food habits, and increasing urbanization. International trade in poultry meat and table eggs accounts for about 10% and 2.5% of their global annual output, respectively. India produces close to 27 million chickens a week, of which 95% is traded alive. With modern techniques and changing from live bird to fresh chilled and frozen product market, India is constantly on the rise. The poultry sector in India is transforming from a backyard activity to large scale integrated poultry farming with wide spread adoption of modern technology.

Tamil Nadu and Andhra Pradesh are the leading states with a share of 32 and 18% in total eggs produced respectively. While Haryana, Punjab, West Bengal, Maharashtra and Karnataka each contributes 5-6%. Average egg yield of an improved layer is 305 eggs/annum, which is more than thrice the yield of an indigenous layer. Clearly, there is considerable scope for increasing egg production in substitution of indigenous layers with the improved layers or recent evolved dual purpose strains suitable under small scale and backyard systems.

The Central Poultry Development Organisations (CPDOs) at Chandigarh, Bhubaneswar, Mumbai and Hesserghata have developed high egg producing hybrid strains and the Chandigarh farm has evolved fast growing broiler strains and these farms are now supplying parent stock to hatcheries and hybrid chicks to farmers.

The CPDO, Southern region of Hesserghata is now supplying day old ducklings of high egg producing Khaki Campbell breed of ducks to various states and Union Territories. Diversification with other species like turkeys, guinea-fowl and Japanese quail is also undertaken. In the CPDOs, training is also imparted to the farmers to upgrade their technical skills. Besides, CPDO, Hesserghata is also imparting trainer's trainings to in-service personnel from within the country as well as overseas.

The Central Poultry Performance Testing Centre (CPPTC), located at Gurgaon is entrusted with responsibility of testing the performance of layer and broiler varieties. This centre gives valuable information relating to different genetic stock available in the country.

The Central Avian Research Institute, Izatnagar is also imparting training to the officers of the states, Union Territories, teachers of the Agricultural Universities and persons engaged in various specialised poultry fields.

The Regional Feed Analytical Laboratory, Chandigarh and Bhubaneswar provide feed analytical facilities to the farmers and feed manufacturers.

The Indian Council of Agricultural Research (ICAR) in New Delhi has sponsored various research projects on poultry breeding and poultry nutrition in a number of Research Institutes including State Agricultural Universities of the country.

The National Agricultural Co-operative Marketing Federation of India Ltd. (NAFED) handles marketing of eggs at national and regional levels.

Presently, the *deshi* bird under free range system yields on an average 60 eggs per year, while the low input technology birds like Gramapriya developed by PD on Poultry, Hyderabad and the modern hybrid is capable of laying 200-230 and 305 eggs respectively. This gap represents the scope of further improvement.

PRESENT STATUS OF INDIAN POULTRY

The present human population in the country is about 1210.19 million which is 17.5% of the world population and it is increasing in number by 1.9%. But the increase in crop productivity is only 1.7%. Though grains will remain the basic ingredients of world food supply, yet the demand for more animal protein will increase in future. There seems to be limited opportunities for increasing meat production (protein availability) from sheep, goat and beef cattle with existing slaughter rate and existing availability of fodder and pastures. The solution seems to remain with the poultry industry. Poultry is accepted universally as an economic converter of agricultural products and by products into a nutritionally balanced supplement fulfilling human requirements.

Poultry farming in India has registered a phenomenal growth during the past two and a half decades. From a gross annual value of production of less than Rs.40 crores in 1960, when commercial poultry farming first started it crossed Rs.1,000 crores in 1985 and Rs.1,400 crores in 1989 and 49,000 crores in 2011.

Today India ranks 3rd in world egg production and 5th largest poultry meat producer in the world. However, there is a large gap between the availability and requirements of poultry products. In light of ICMR recommendations against the requirements of 180 eggs and 11 kg poultry meat per person per year the present per capita availability is only 55 and 2.2 kg poultry meat per year by 2010 (FAO, USDA) which is far below the developed countries, leaving a big scope for further expansion by many folds.

The progress made in poultry industry has contributed significantly in improving in quality of nutrition available to millions of people. It is estimated that increasing consumption of one egg per year in India will create an additional 25,000 jobs. Over 6.5 million jobs are likely to be generated, if the target of 180 eggs and 11 kg of poultry meat per person per year is achieved.

The production of eggs, which was around 180 to 200 per bird per year has now reached an average range of 305 eggs for an improved layer. The broiler growth, which was considered as 1 kg, live weight in 8 weeks period has reached the stage of 1.75 kg per bird with 5-6 weeks. The growth of this industry during Seventh Five Year Plan has been envisaged at a very high rate.

Thus, through the concerted efforts of the Government of India and various other agencies, the poultry industry has grown tremendously. All these gains have been confined largely to the commercial sector and no significant increase in the egg and poultry output took place in the backyard sector. The initiative and vigour with which the private sector has come forward to popularize commercial poultry farming is encouraging. This tremendous growth in poultry sector has been possible mainly through the activity in the following areas.

(i) Development of high yielding layer and broiler breeds.
(ii) Improved health cover
(iii) Giving the poultry farmer the freedom to determine prices.
(iv) Increased awareness of the nutritive value of poultry products as well as enhanced purchasing power.
(v) Financing of Poultry Schemes.
(vi) Education and Training in Poultry Science in India.
(vii) Recent Advances in Poultry Nutrition.
(viii) Insurance of Poultry

(i) Development of high yielding layer and broiler breeds

Some notable achievements of the poultry breeding research undertaken in the country have been an evolution of a few commercial layers and broiler stocks which can be proud of and say are our own.

Layers: These include ILI-80, HH-260, BH-78 and MY-Chix White egg layers released from Central Avian Research Institute (CARI) at Izatnagar; Central Poultry Breeding Farms (CPBF). Hessarghata and Bangalore and State Poultry Breeding Farm, Government of Karnataka respectively. Another tinted egg layer was also released from Central Poultry Breeding Farm, Bhubaneswar under the name Bhubaneswar Rhoda White.

At Venkateshwara Research and Breeding Farm, a joint venture with the ISA Breeders Inc. of the U.S., a new genetically superior layer breed was developed in early eighties. The Babcock breed produces upto 295 eggs a year at a lower feed consumption level than that of ordinary birds.

The Indian Council of Agricultural Research has evolved the following two improved layers.

(1) ILM-90 Hen housed egg production of more than 260 eggs upto 500 days of age with egg weight of more than 52 grams at 40 weeks of age.
(2) ILR-90 Hen housed egg production of above 245 eggs upto 500 days of age with more than 52 grams egg weight at 40 weeks of age.

Some of the improved layers used presently are Starcross - 288; Starcross-579, BV-300 etc.

Apart from these, Project Directorate on Poultry Hyderabad has developed two synthetic varieties named Vanaraja (dual purpose) and Gramapriya (layer) which can be reared in rural areas following backyard system.

Broilers: These include IBL-80, B-77, IBB-83, CA-42 and CH-47 commercial broilers released from Punjab Agricultural University, Ludhiana; CARI, Izatnagar; University of Agriculture Sciences, Bangalore and CPBF, Chandigarh respectively.

Another Venkateshwara Hatcheries Private Ltd. (VHPL) group company the Venco Research and Breeding Farm, a joint venture with Cobb Vantress Inc. of the U.S., developed and released the Ven Cobb broiler breed in early eighties.

Some of the improved broilers used presently are Hubbard, Anak-2000, Kasila, Caribro-91, Pearlbro-Samrat etc.

(ii) Improved health cover

As far as health cover is concerned, India has over 250 disease diagnostic laboratories and more than 20,000 veterinary hospitals. The facilities are mostly utilized for healthcare of large animals. The manpower in veterinary organisation is inadequately trained in poultry health care. The diagnostic facilities are also lacking in the hospitals. The supply of pharmaceuticals and biological products are satisfactory. Vaccine production in private sector is doing very well to meet the need and also export to various other countries.

(iii) Giving the poultry farmer the freedom to determine prices

Until the early Eighties, prices for eggs and poultry were dictated by traders and middlemen and were often un-remunerative. In 1981, egg prices crashed to such a level where 40 per cent of the farms were on the brink of closure.

If this situation has not been brought under control, the poultry sector would have stagnated at very low levels of production. The 1981 crisis resulted in the setting up of the National Egg Coordination Committee (NECC) originally by poultry farmers from four States with the intention of making the poultry farmer the arbiter in pricing. Over the years, NECC has been able to do just that prices of eggs are now fixed by the producers and are kept at levels that are remunerative to the producers and acceptable to consumers.

Still the eggs and meat marketing are handled by a few middleman and they control the market price without any regard to market economic forces. As a result, lion's share of profit is taken away and neither the producers nor the consumers are benefitted. The central Government through National Agricultural Cooperative Marketing Federation and the State Governments through Corporations and Boards are trying to interfere by providing price support to poultry farmers but so far no serious impact is seen. The government role to promote egg and meat marketing societies may be useful. Much needed attention is required towards the export of egg and meat in India, being at strategic position near the Middle East and Gulf countries, where there is a huge potential of export. To compete the international market, high quality, hygienic product at most competitive rates will be required. This scenario appears to be a long goal to achieve. A separate body from Agricultural Product Export Development authority

(APEDA) may be required to give full attention to promotion of eggs and meat and their products.

(iv) Increased awareness of the Nutritive value of eggs and Enhanced Purchasing Power

The increasing awareness of the nutritive value of eggs and thereby need for balance nutrition has led to changes in eating habits with vegetarians accepting eggs as part of their diet.

Simultaneously, there has been an increase in purchasing power, and more money is available for spending on quality food. With the changing food habits and increasing availability of eggs, there has been an increase in demand which is growing at about 10 per cent a year. Despite this, the egg industry experiences periodic slumps.

The key to the problem of slow growth is not per capita consumption, but per capita availability of eggs. Surveys conducted by the NECC in rural areas have shown that the demand for eggs and chicken is unfulfilled because they are not available in sufficient quantities, consequently, their prices are high. NECC is promoting egg consumption through television and other advertising media.

(v) Financing of Poultry Schemes

For the sake of supporting the full-fledged self sufficient poultry industry with complete sophistication in the fields of production, breeding stocks, high quality feeds, pharmaceuticals, medicines, poultry vaccines and equipments, the National Agricultural Bank and Rural Development (NABARD) along with National Commercial and Co-operative banks are financing a large number of poultry schemes all over the country for increasing production of eggs and broiler meat. This indicates the role that is being played by banking institutions in poultry development. The NABARD provides refinance assistance for poultry development for the following purposes:

1. Schemes for poultry breeding including financing of pure line poultry projects to produce grand parent stocks.
2. Financial assistance to hatcheries to produce commercial one day old broiler or layer chicks from poultry breeding stocks.
3. Financing for the setting up of commercial egg production farms of different sizes by small, medium and large farmers.
4. Financing for the setting up to commercial egg production farms of different sizes by small, medium and large commercial broiler farmers.
5. Financial assistance for the manufacture of poultry medicines and vaccines.
6. Financial assistance for egg marketing, broiler processing, preservation and marketing of poultry meat.

Apart from these, for small farmers there are several incentive schemes offered through District Rural Development Agencies (DRDA).

(vi) Education and Training of Poultry Science in India

There is well laid infrastructure for poultry education and training in the country. There are about 56 State Agricultural Universities (SAUs), many of them imparting graduate and post-graduate courses in poultry science. Besides the Central Avian Research

Institute (CARI); IPDA, Atwah, Surat, Gujarat, Institute of Poultry Management of India (IPMI) at Urulikanchan and Project Directorate on Poultry, Rajendranagar, Hyderabad are serving the purpose. The Central Poultry Development Organisations (CPDOs) located at four regions viz. Chandigarh, Bhubaneswar, Mumbai and Hasserghata have been playing a pivotal role in the implementation of the policies of the Government with respect to poultry. More specialised poultry training institutes for middle and lower levels are required.

(vii) Recent Advances in Poultry Nutrition

Nutrition is the science of the interaction of a nutrient with some part of a living organism. It is concerned with providing those elements of the external environment to the internal system of the birds which are essential to maintain the homeostatic conditions in them including maintenance of life, growth, egg production and resistance to diseases.

The salient findings regarding recent advances in poultry nutrition are as follows:

1. Alternate Feed Resources

In the early sixties the priorities in poultry nutrition research were to eliminate from poultry ration feeds that man can use for himself. By the late seventies it is known that maize was not indispensible for poultry as energy source and that rice polishing, deoiled rice bran, tapioca, many kinds of millets, viz., jowar, bajra and ragi may be used as maize substitutes. Less damaged grain can replace 50% of the maize in poultry ration. Similarly the protein need may be met by judicious use of many oil seed meal other than conventional groundnut oil cakes, viz., sunflower oil meal, guar meal, mustard oil cakes, niger oil cake, cotton seed cake, karanja cake etc.

Alternative to fish meal which is scarce and too expensive have also been found to be meat meal, meat-cum-bone-meal, liver residue meal etc.

2. Feed Processing

These findings helped to save maize and similar feeds from being used for poultry and feed costs were also considerably reduced. Haryana Agricultural University workers have attempted greater utilization of guar meal by appropriate ration modification while Punjab Agricultural University scientists have adopted fermentation technique for the same purpose. Using biotechnological approach the feeding value of guar meal, a by-product of guar gum industry has now been enhanced. Research has shown that deoiled sal seed meal could be used upto 5% in chick ration and upto 8% in layer diets as an energy source.

3. In-vitro Evaluation

Another area of considerable activity has been the development of in-vitro methodology for evaluation of feed ingredients and their protein quality. These methods employed the existence of correlation between the energy value of certain chemical identities in feed and the concentration of utilizable energy in the bird.

(*) ME = 432 + 27.91 (% C.P. + % EE × 2.25 + % available CHO)

(**) ME = 51.98 (% C.P. + % EE × 2.25 + % available carbohydrate)

(*) = Simple type of regression

(**) = Multiple type of regression

4. Nutrient Requirement

Scientists of the Poultry Research Division, IVRI; Punjab Agricultural University; Jawaharlal Nehru Krishi Viswavidyalaya, Jabalpur, Andhra Pradesh Agricultural University, Hyderabad are perhaps the leaders in this area. Based on the available information from the sources, specifications for some of the major nutrients in poultry rations have been developed by the BIS from time to time.

5. Limiting and Deleterious Factors

Considerable data are now available regarding some problematic feeding stuffs. In mustard oil cake, it is known that the presence of volatile isothiocynates and vinyl oxazolidienithone may limit the utilization of the cake to a great extent. The role of the various tannin components as well as of erucic acid may however be more important in inhibition of utilization of the cake by poultry. The different tannin fractions in the oil meals of Brassica species namely gallic acid, pyrogallol and pyrocatechol may not play a significant role in inhibiting the availability of the protein in the gut. On the other hand, Erucic acid - a major component of the fatty acid complement of mustard oil caused a significant depression in the body weight gain of chicks fed on the expeller mustard oil cake The toxicity due to erucic acid could be totally eliminated when the fatty acid was extracted from the cake.

Attempt has also been made to increase the level of guar meal (upto 20%) in poultry diet by enzymatic hydrolysis or fungal fermentation of the hemicellulosic gum components in the meal.

Tamil Nadu Veterinary & Animal Science University workers identified and quantified certain fatty acid fractions which inhibited the use of expeller rubber seed meal by poultry. Methods have been adopted to detoxify these factors for enhancing their use in birds.

Andhra Pradesh Agricultural University workers and also the workers of Bidhan Chandra Krishi Viswavidyalaya (BCKV) attempted to utilize the totally inedible Neem seed cake in poultry. The main neem seed toxin, azadirachtin, and others like melianloriol and salannin, all triterpenoid compounds are known to cause severe anti-feeding property either by a direct on palatability or by an indirect effect on the satiety centre in the brain. APAU worker has located a major portion of these toxic principles in the non-saponifiable fraction of the residual neem oil and employed known chemical methods to totally detoxify the deleterious factor.

BCKV nutrition workers took the initiative not only to detoxify Karaja cake but also become successful in isolating some of the toxic principles and thereby made it possible for use of the processed deoiled cake throughout the country as livestock including poultry feed but with an exception of swine.

6. Mycotoxins in Feeds

Central Avian Research Institute and Jawaharlal Nehru Krishi Viswavidyalaya have contributed significantly to our knowledge on Aflatoxin. The tolerance level appear to be 0.5 ppm for broiler chicks beyond which growth depression, low feed intake and reduce feed efficiency were noticeable. The most effective methods are either autoclaving of infested material pretreated with a mixture of calcium hydroxide and formaldehyde or treatment with 5% ammonium solution.

7. Limitations

The essential component for fast and steady growth of poultry industry is production of economical balanced feed. At present, there are about 150 feed mills compounding about 30 million tons of feed of which about 1/3rd is consumed by birds. Except a few feed companies, most of them lack qualified staff, sufficient infrastructure and thus producing poor quality feed. There is no legislation to put the feed composition or proximate analysis on feed bags. As such poor quality and undesirable feed ingredients are commonly used for feed compounding. Added with this the feed testing laboratories are also inadequate where such feed could be got analysed at the time of poor performance. The shortage of good quality feed ingredients is currently the most serious hindrance in the progress of this industry and also in future, shortage of feed is likely to be a serious factor because poultry being the monogastric directly competes with human being for supply of cereal grains and other feed components.

Keeping in view the present rate of growth of poultry industry, feed requirement will increase in future. Nutritionists may have to look for more alternative sources of feed ingredients and this may also be the reason why most of research laboratories are involved in testing various non-conventional feeds like agricultural and industrial waste or by-products as feed.

(viii) Insurance of poultry

The scheme of poultry insurance has been first introduced in this country for the poultry farmers by the General Insurance Corporation (GIC) of India mainly to give financial security to investors of poultry. The policy covers loss against death of birds due to accident (including fire, lightening, flood, cyclone, famine, strike riot, etc.) or disease contracted or occurring during the period of insurance subject to some limitations. The details of these have been discussed in a chapter separately.

WORLD CHICKEN POPULATION

The Food and Agriculture Organisation of the United Nations estimated that in 2002 there were nearly sixteen billion chickens in the world, counting a total population of 15,853,900,000. The figures from the Global Livestock Production and Health Atlas for 2004 are presented in Table 7 while Table 8 shows the egg production parameters of poultry.

Table 7 World Chicken Population

Sl. No.	Country	Populations
1.	China	3,860,000,000
2.	United States	1,970,000,000
3.	Indonesia	1,200,000,000
4.	Brazil	1,100,000,000
5.	Mexico	540,000,000
6.	India	425,000,000
7.	Russia	340,000,000
8.	Japan	286,000,000
9.	Iran	280,000,000
10.	Turkey	250,000,000
11.	Nigeria	740,000,000

It is evident from the Table that China has the highest population of chicken followed by United States, Indonesia and Brazil.

NUTRITIVE VALUE OF EGGS AND POULTRY MEAT

Eggs :

Of all the foods available to man, the egg most nearly approaches a perfect balance of all the nutrients. This is evidenced by the fact that the egg is the total source of nutrition for the developing embryo. Chick requires all the essential nutrients that we need for growth, maintenance, lactation, reproduction, etc. The edible portion of the egg is made up of the yolk and the albumen. Chemical composition of the egg are presented in Table 9 while Table 10 shows the nutritive value of eggs.

Table 8 Egg Production of Poultry

Species	Age of Sexual Maturity	Eggs/Year	Egg Size
	(month)	(no)	(g)
Chicken:			
Light-type	5–6	240	57
Broiler-type		170	
Turkey	7	105	85
Goose	24	15–60	215
Duck (pekin)	7–8	110–175	80
Pheasant	8–10	40–60	32
Quail (bobwhite)	8–10	150–200	9
Pigeon	6	12–15	17
Guinea fowl	10–12	40–60	40

A hen's egg, weighing 57 gms, gives us about 51 gms of food material made up of by 18 gms yolk and 33 gms albumen. The nutrients contain include proteins, fats, vitamins and minerals.

Table 9 Chemical Composition of The Egg

	Whole Egg	White	Yolk	Shell
		(percent of whole egg)		
	100	58	31	11
	←·················· (%) ··················→			
Water ...	65.5	88.0	48.0	–
Protein ...	11.8	11.0	17.5	–
Fat ...	11.0	0.2	32.5	–
Ash ...	11.7	0.8	2.0	96.0
Total ...	100.0	100.0	100.0	96.0

Protein

The yolk and the albumen contain about 17.5 per cent and 10.0 per cent proteins by weight, respectively. The total quantity of proteins available in the edible portion of 57 gram eggs is about 6.5 gms (about 3.5 gms. in the albumen and about 3 gms in the yolk). The protein fraction of eggs is highly digestible and of high quality, having a biological value of 94 on a scale of 100. the highest rating of any food. The reason for this high quality of protein is that egg proteins are complete proteins, that is, they contain all the essential amino acids required to maintain life and promote growth and health.

Fats

These are found in the yolk only as albumen is almost devoid of fat. The yolk contains about 6 gms. of very well-emulsified unsaturated fats, which are easily digestible.

Energy

Eggs are moderate from the standpoint of calorie content, a medium-size egg supplies about 80 calories of energy to our body.

Vitamins

It contains almost all the known vitamins which are stored in the yolk portion. The amount of vitamin A varies from 200 to 1,000 I.U. The component is present in pure form as well as in precursor, form i.e., as carotenoid pigments. The quantity of vitamin D depends upon the amount of direct sunshine the layers get or on the quantity of vitamin D supplement included in their diet. Amount present in eggs increases during spring and summer months. One egg supplies about 15 per cent of the daily needs of an adult person in respect of this vitamin. Vitamin E and K are also found at various concentrations. Among water soluble vitamins, all members of B complex including vitamin B_{12} are present in appreciable amounts.

Table 10 Nutritive Value of Eggs

	Recommended daily allowance for moderately active man	Quantity in 1 egg	Quantity in ½ pint milk (approx. 280 ml)
Energy (calories)	3,000	90	205
Proteins (g)	70	6.6	9.9
Fat (g)	50	5.5	10.3
Carbohydrate (g)	570	–	14.0
Calcium (g)	0.8	0.03	0.37
Phosphorus (g)	0.9	0.12	0.28
Iron (mg)	12	1.6	0.10
Vitamin A (l.U.)	5,000	600	600
Vitamin D (l.U.)	400	50	–
Vitamin B_1 (mg)	1.5	0.095	0.10
Vitamin C (mg)	75	0.0	6
Riboflavin (mg)	2.0	0.19	0.25
Nicotinic acid (mg)	18	0.04	0.08

Average composition of rice and a few animal protein sources are presented in Table 11 while Table 12 shows the composition of protein showing approximate amino acid contents (in % of protein).

Table 11 Average composition in per cent of rice and a few animal protein sources

Component	Rice	Cow milk (whole)	Eggs Hen	Eggs Duck	Chicken meat
Water	13.0	87.3	74.0	71.0	66.0
Protein	7.1	3.5	12.4	13.0	20.2
Fat	1.1	3.5	11.7	14.5	12.2
Carbohydrate	78.0	5.0	0.9	0.5	0
Fibre	0.7	0	–	–	-
Ash	0.8	0.7	1.0	1.0	1.0
Calories per 100g	359.0	65.0	163.0	189.0	200.0

Source : CHATFIELD CHARLOTTE. 1953, 1954. *Food Composition Table*, 'Minerals and Vitamins' *for International Use.* pp 25-28. F. A.O., Rome

Minerals

The egg contains a large number of mineral elements. Phosphorus amounts to about 116 mgm of which 110 mgm is found in the yolk. The element is present as phosphoproteins, phospholipids and inorganic phosphorus. Iron content is about 2 mgm, mostly in the yolk. Calcium in the edible portion is about 2 gms per egg. Other minerals such as Na, K, Mg, S, Cl, Zn, Cu, Mn, etc are also present.

Table 12 Composition of protein showing approximate amino acid contents in per cent of Protein (N X 6.25)

Amino acid (per cent)	Rice	Cow milk (whole)	Hen eggs	Chicken meat
Arginine	7.2	4.2	6.6	7.1
Histidine	1.7	2.6	2.4	2.3
Lysine	3.2	8.7	7.0	8.4
Tyrosine	5.7	6.0	4.5	4.3
Tryptophan	1.3	1.5	1.5	1.2
Phenylalanine	5.0	5.5	6.3	4.6
Cystine	1.3	1.0	2.4	1.3
Methionine	3(?)	3.2	4.0	3.2
Threonine	3.8	4.7	4.3	4.7
Serine	–	4.3	–	4.7
Leucine	8.2	11.0	9.2	–
Isoleucine	5.2	7.5	7.7	–
Valine	6.2	7.0	7.2	–

Source : BLOCK, RICHARD J. and BOLLING DIANA. 1951. *The amino acid composition of Proteins and Foods*, pp. 447-82. Springfield, Illinois, U.S.A

Table 13 Comparison of Nutrient Composition of Cooked Turkey, Chicken and Beef

	Protein	Fat	Moisture	Food Energy Calories
	←·········· (%) ··········→			(per 3½ oz or 100 g)[2]
Turkey (mature, roasted and boned)				
Breast (white meat)	32.9	3.9	62.1	176
Leg (dark meat)	30.0	8.4	60.5	204
Chicken (16 weeks old, roasted and boned)				
Breast (white meat)	32.4	5.0	61.3	182
Leg (dark meat)	29.2	6.5	62.7	185
Beef (cooked and boned) :				
Round steak	28.6	15.4	54.7	261
Rump roast	23 6	27.3	48.1	347
Hamburger	24.2	20.3	54.2	286

1. Source: Nutritive value of American Foods, Ag. Hdbk, No. 456, USDA, 1975
2. Standard portion size.

Poultry Meat

Nutritionally, people eat poultry meat for its high quality protein and its low fat content. Turkey and chicken meat is higher in protein and lower in fat than beef and other red meats (Table 13). Data on dressed, eviscerated and edible meet yields of different types of poultry are presented in Table 14.

EFFECT OF FEEDING RAW AND COOKED EGGS

Eating of Raw Egg

Since the nutrients in the egg are in an easily digestible form, and also because the chick embryo can utilise these nutrients from the raw contents, one may think that it is preferable to consume the egg contents in the raw state rather than after cooking. But this is not so for the following two reasons :

1. Raw egg white (albumen) contain an anti-trypsin factor and also a particular protein, *avidin* which are in combination of vitamin biotin thus render the vitamin unavailable. By continuous feeding of raw eggs, deficiency of biotin takes place which is responsible for the disease "egg white injury" in human. Symptoms include a fine scaly dermatitis, loss of appetite, nausea, pain in muscle, inflammation of the skin and high levels of blood cholesterol. By cooking harmful properties of albumen are destroyed and it also become more digestible.
2. The contents of raw egg may be infected with some organisms capable of causing diseases. This infection will be destroyed by cooking.
3. Cooked eggs also stimulate more secretion of the acid in the stomach required for protein digestion:

Eating of Cooked Eggs

1. Of all the various methods of cooking, half boiling is the best. There is little or no loss of proteins and vitamins.
2. In fried eggs, the loss of proteins depends upon the temperature at which egg contents are fried. If frying is done at a low temperature, only about 0.1 gm protein (out of 6.5 gms) may be lost. At high temperature as much as 0.6 gms of proteins and significant amount of vitamins are lost.
3. In omelettes and poached eggs, the loss of proteins is about 0.2 and 0.5 gms respectively. While in scrambled eggs the loss is about 1.0 gram.

From the point of view of nutrients, half boiled egg is the best followed by full boiled, omlettes, poached, scrambled egg and spiced egg curry (Indian type) in order of nutritive value.

Weight Yield of Poultry at Different Stages of Processing

The average weight yield of chicken, turkeys, ducks and geese at different stages of processing is given below :

Table 14 Dressed, Eviscerated and Edible Meat Yields of Different Types of Poultry

	Live (kg)	Dressed (kg)	Live weight %	Ready to cook (kg)	Live weight %	Edible meat (kg)	Live weight %
Chicken							
Broilers	1.4	1.2	86	0.9	64	0.6	43
Roosters	2.3	2.0	87	1.5	65	1.1	47
Hens	2.5	2.2	88	1.7	68	1.4	56
Turkey							
Young fryers	3.2	2.8	88	2.3	72	1.7	53
Mature birds	8.2	7.3	89	6.3	77	4.6	56
Duck	2.7	2.4	89	1.9	70	1.5	56
Goose	6.4	5.6	88	4.6	72	3.6	56

Source : STEWART, G.F. and ABBOTT, J.C. 1961. *Marketing Eggs and Poultry*, F.A.O. Marketing Guide No. 4, pp. 57-60.

HEALTH PROBLEMS RELATED TO POULTRY PRODUCTS

People are becoming more and more health and diet conscious. Unfortunately, much of the nutritional information that they receive is not authoritative. Worse yet, passions and prejudices sometimes trigger such changes as "poultry products cause allergies and heart disease". Such accusations must be answered by more than simple denial.

Allergies

Occasionally, a highly sensitive child exhibits an allergy symptom to eggs. In most cases, the white of the egg is the portion that creates the reaction, and the yolk is generally tolerated. However, these cases are rare, and most infants and children allergic to eggs can follow a diet that provides for some heat-treated or cooked eggs.

Cholesterol, Animal Fat, and Heart Diseases

Numerous types of heart disease contribute to the death toll of few million persons in the world every year; among them, hypertension, cerebro-vascular disease (stroke), congestive heart failure and atherosclerosis are common. Much attention has been given to the role of animal fats in artherosclerosis, a type of disease wherein a build-up of soft, amorphous lipids and connective tissue develops on the walls of the arteries of the heart. When these deposits become sufficiently large, clots may form and subsequently decrease the diameter of the arterial lumen. In some cases blood flow is greately impaired resulting a heart attack.

Research indicated that individuals with high serum cholesterol levels had a higher rate of artherosclerosis than people with normal levels. Increased serum cholesterol levels can be induced in susceptible individuals when animal fats which are highly saturated and foods high in cholesterol as in eggs are consumed. Thus, the hypothesis that cholesterol is responsible for heart disease become accepted by many as fact. In recent years, research has clearly indicated that this position is entirely too simplistic. For example, studies have shown that certain African tribes whose diets consist almost entirely of animal products do not have elevated serum cholesterol levels.

It is fact that dietary fat is implicated in artherosclerosis, but it must be realised from further research that it is not the sole cause, rather, a number of factors enter into the cause of heart disease, many of which are more important than cholesterol; among them, stress, heredity, hypertension, diabetes mellitus, smoking, lack of exercise, and obesity.

When heart disease is correlated with the consumption of animal products one must also consider the benefits against the hazards. Countries with the highest life expectancies (70 to 72 years) such as, Sweden, Norway, Denmark, Japan, Israel and Switzerland are noted for their high egg production and per capita egg consumption. The nutrients supplied by eggs and meat provide well balanced nutrition, hence, poultry products must not be eliminated from the diet. Rather, a well-planned diet, along with exercise and a minimum of stress provides the best prevention against heart disease.

COMPARATIVE EFFICIENCY OF CONVERSION OF ANIMAL FEED

FEED EFFICIENCY

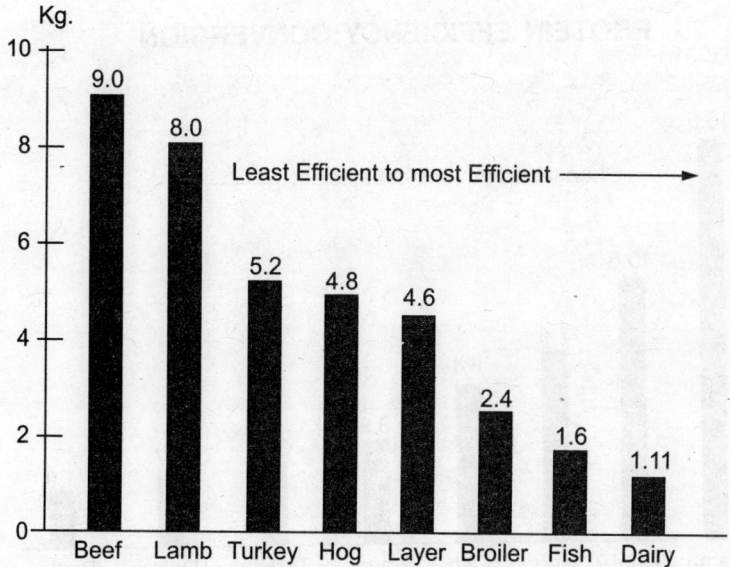

Figure 1 Kilogram of feed required to produce one kg. of product.

This shows that it takes 9.0 kg. of feed to produce 1 kg. of beef, whereas it takes only 1.1 kg. of feed to produce 1 litre of milk.

ENERGY (CALORIE) EFFICIENCY CONVERSION

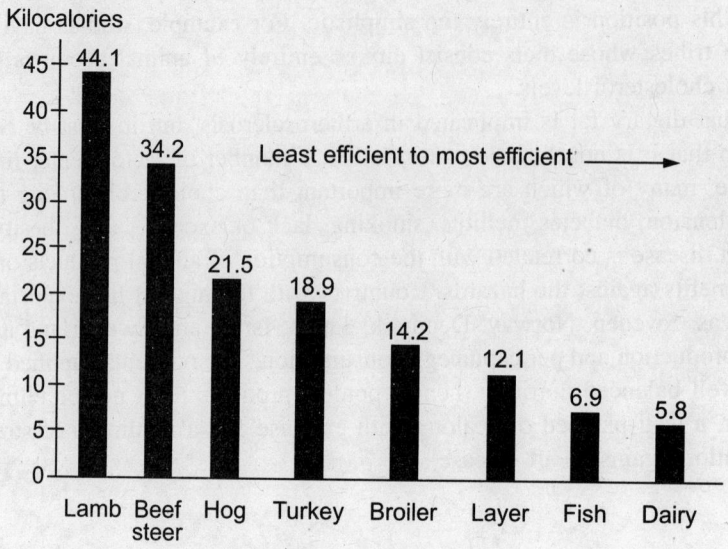

Figure 2 Kilocalories in feed required to produce i kcal of product.

This shows that it takes 44.1 kcal in feed to produce 1 kcal in lamb, whereas only 5.8 kcal in feed will produce 1 kcal in milk.

PROTEIN EFFICIENCY CONVERSION

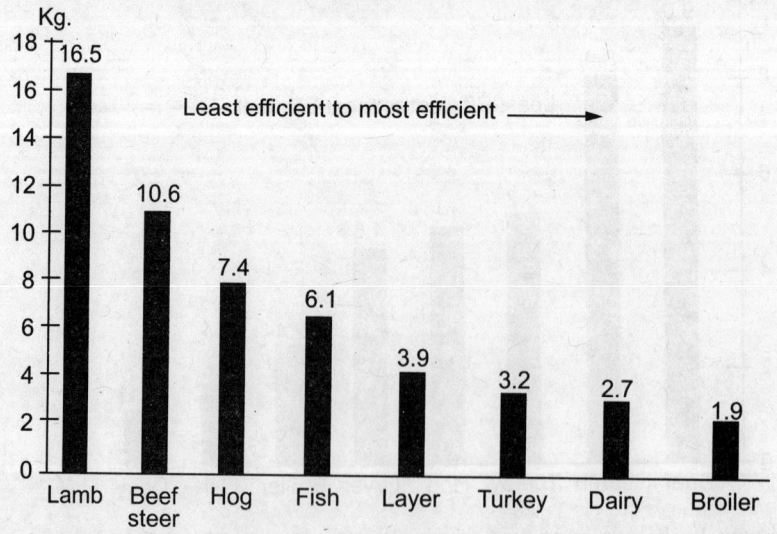

Figure 3 Kologram of feed protein required to produce one kg. of product protein.

This shows that it takes 16.5 kg. of feed protein to produce 1.0 kg. of lamb protein, whereas only 1.9 kg. of feed protein will produce 1.0 kg. of broiler protein.

BREEDS OF CHICKEN

While discussing breeds of chicken in details, a knowledge about the external body parts of a fowl (Figure 4) and details of male combs (Figure 4) are essentials in understanding the description of characteristics of any breed including external anatomy (Figure 5).

There are 8 types of combs; of these only single, rose and pea (Figure 6) are common which distinguishes fowl from other birds.

Regarding colour patterns there are about 13 common colours observed in poultry birds, these are (1) White, (2) Buff (light yellow), (3) Blue, (4) Black, (5) Barred, (6) Red, (7) Spanglad (glittering spot), (8) Mottled (two colours folded together), (9) Laced, (10) Crecentic penciled, (11) Parallel penciled, (12) Stippled (painted in dots or separated touches), (13) Striped (having stripes of different colours).

From the point of economy, original Indian breeds of fowl such as Aseel, Chittagong, Ghagus are now obsolete. Among exotic breeds of fowl which are listed in the *American Standard of Perfection*, only few are commercially important and are described in the following pages.

Classification of Fowls

Fowl may be classified on the basis of utility, economic value or fancy purpose and these include (1) Meat type, (2) Egg type, (3) Dual purpose, (4) Game, (5) Ornamental, (6) Bantam.

Birds of distinct type and colour patterns admitted to the standard are termed as standard breed. They are further classified as (1) Class, (2) Breed, (3) Variety, and (4) Strain.

The term "Class" is used to designate groups of breeds which have been developed in certain regions or geographical areas; thus the class name-Asiatic, Mediterranean, English, Polish, American, French, etc.

The term "breed" denotes an established group of bird having the same general body shape, weight and some common characteristics.

"Varieties" represent a sub-division of a breed, distinguished either by colour pattern, shape, comb type or feather pattern. For example in Leghorns, some of the varieties are Single Comb White Leghorn, Rose Comb Leghorn, Rose Comb Brown Leghorn, Single Comb Buff Leghorn, etc.

The term "strain" is used to denote a given breeder who has done the breeding on the bird and has introduced certain economic characters in the bird.

To sum up we have Classes, Breeds, Varieties and Strains and we might say that a particular bird is a Banerjee Single Comb White Leghorn indicating that Mr. Banerjee is the breeder of the strain, the variety is a single Comb White, the breed is Leghorn and it is in the Mediterranean class.

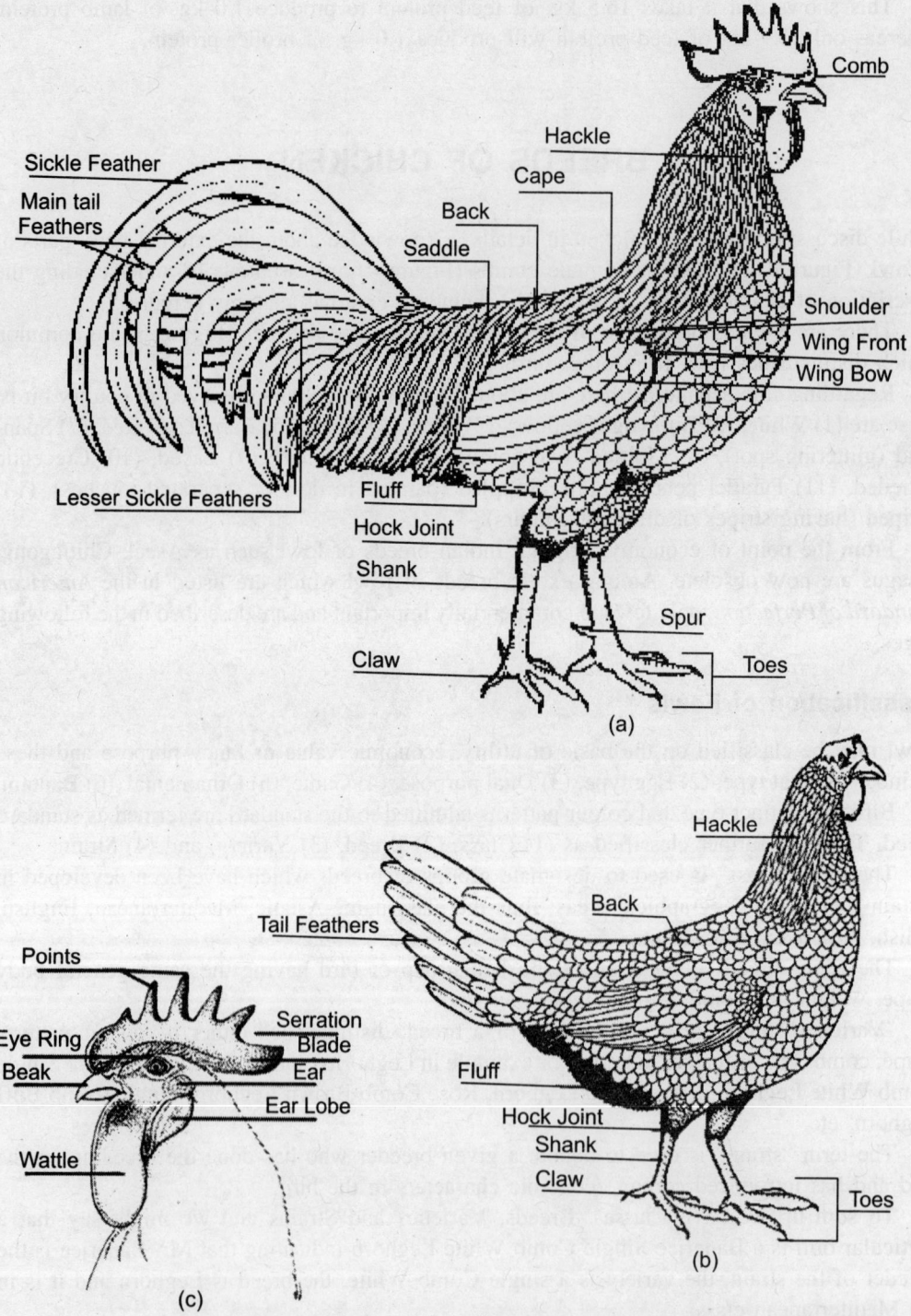

Figure 4 External parts of Fowl. (a) male, (b) female, (c) the head of the chicken.

Table 15 Indications of Sex in Poultry[1]

	Males	Females
Head	Usually larger with larger and longer attachments, such as comb and wattles; courser than that of females in appearance	Smaller, rather fine and delicate in appearance compared with males. Hen turkeys have hair on center line of head.
Plumage	Feathers usually long and 'pointed' at the ends. Tail feathers in chickens long and curved. Parti-colored varieties, have more brilliant colors than the females. Most male ducks have a curl in the tail feathers	Feathers inclined to be shorter and more blunt than those of the male. Tail feathers short and straight in comparison with the male. Modest colors in parti-colored varieties
Body	Larger and generally more angular than the female. Depth from keel lo back greater on same weight birds. Bones, including shanks, longer, larger, and coarser	Finer boned, body more rounded
Skin	Slightly coarser, particularly in old birds. Feather follicles larger. Less fat under skin between heavy feather tracts and over back	Smoother, generally a better distribution of fat between feather tracts. Feather tracts narrower but carrying more fat
Keel	Longer with fleshing tending lo taper at the base	Shorter with more rounded appearance over the breast
Legs	Drumstick and thigh relatively long with flesh tending to show less full until mature	Drumstick and thigh relatively shorter with drumstick more inclined to roundness, increasingly so with age

[1] 'Poultry Grading Manual' Ag Hdbk No. 31 USDA 1971, pp 4 and 5

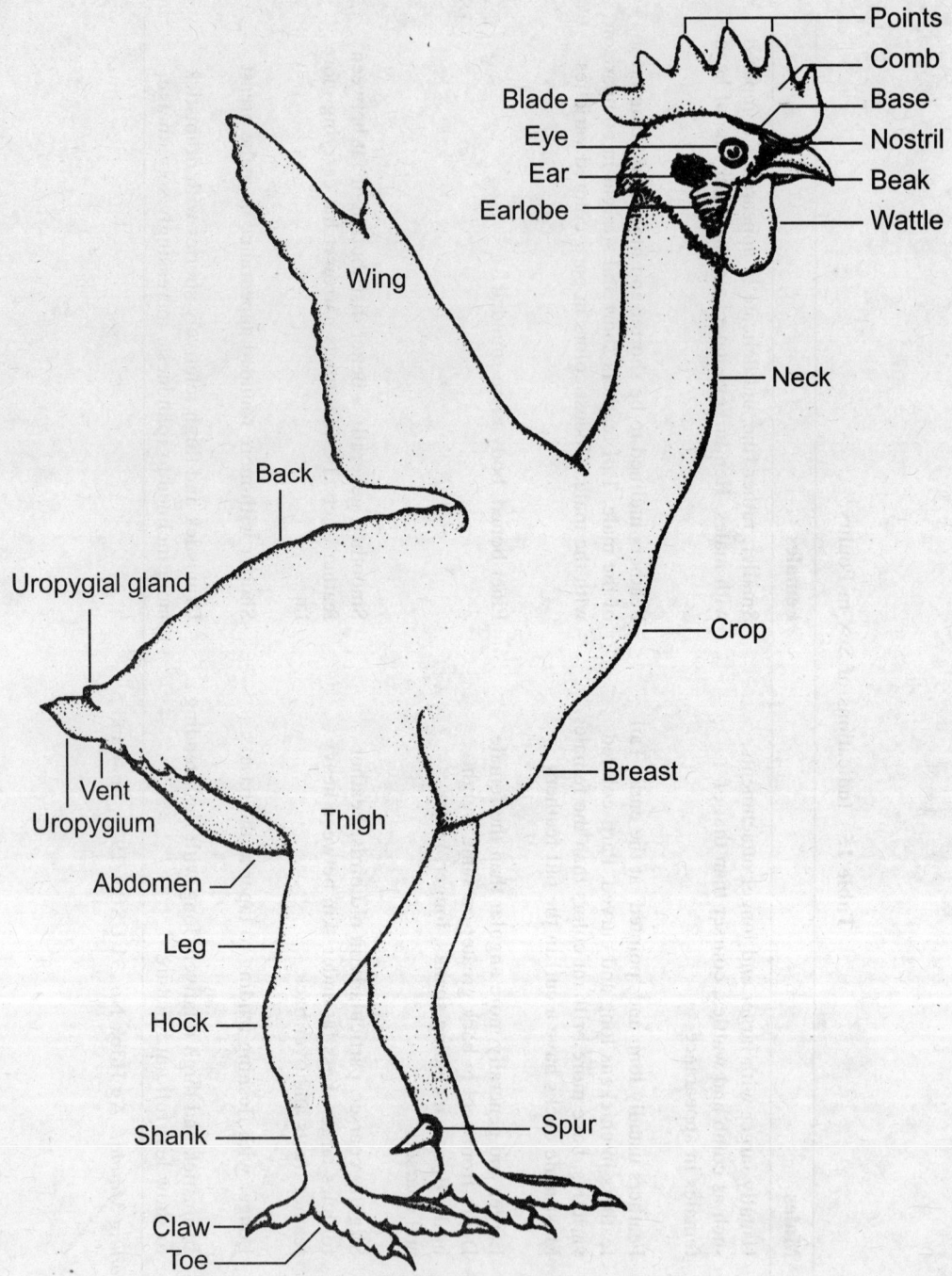

Figure 5 External anatomy of fowl.

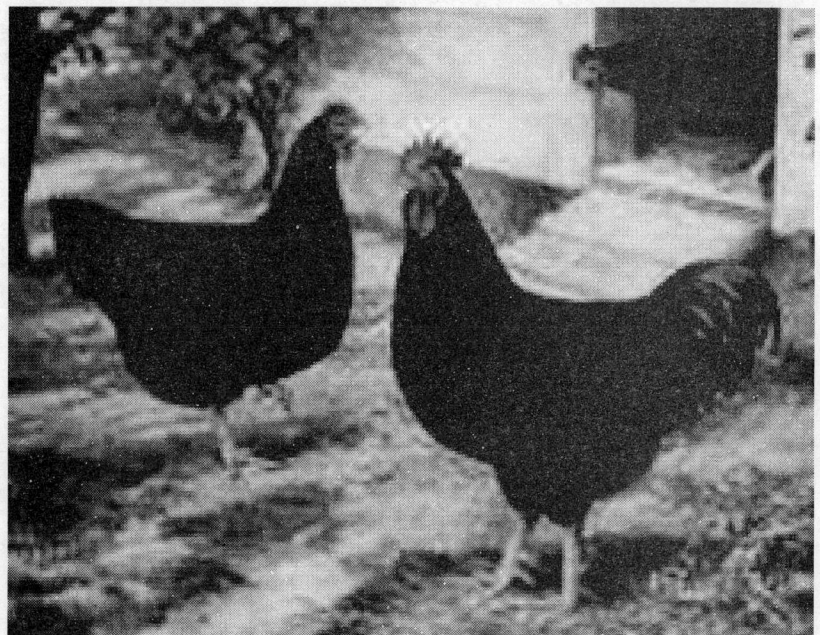

Plate 1. S.C. Rhode Island Red.

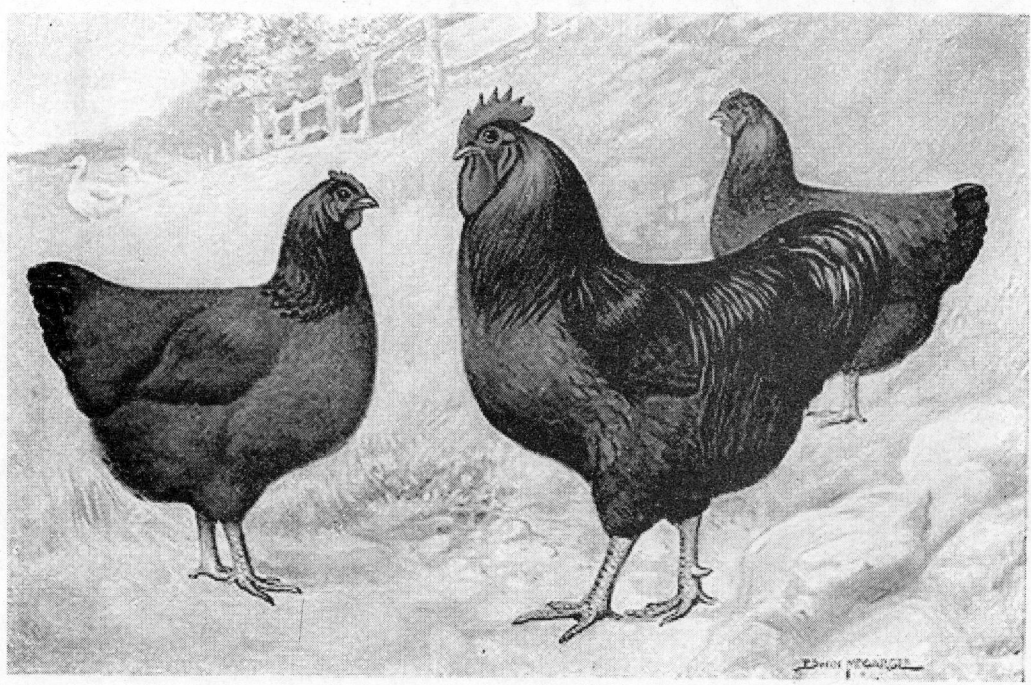

Plate 2. New Hampshires.

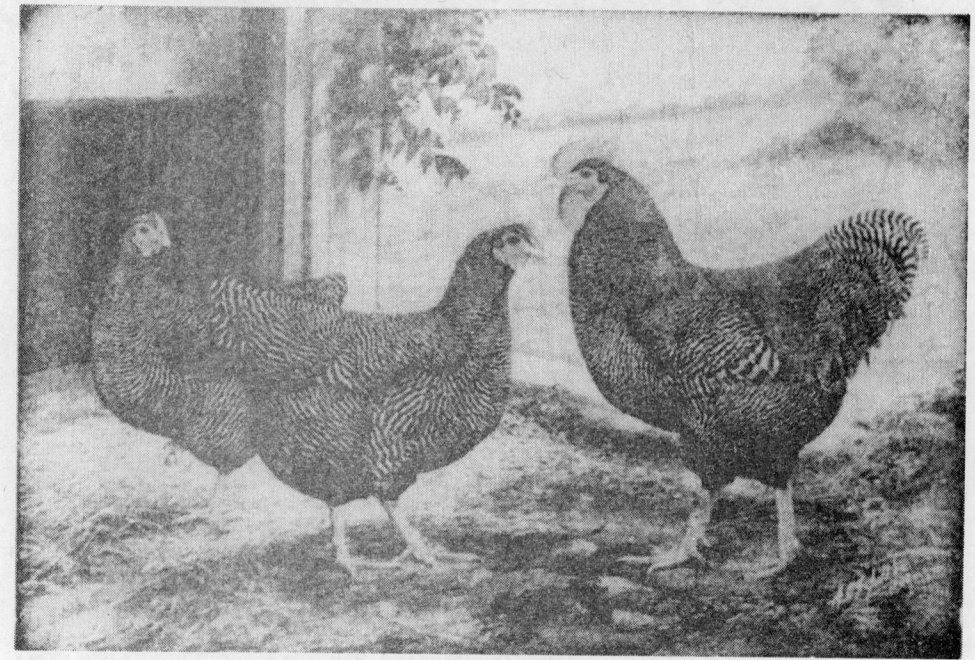

Plate 3. Barred Plymouth Rocks.

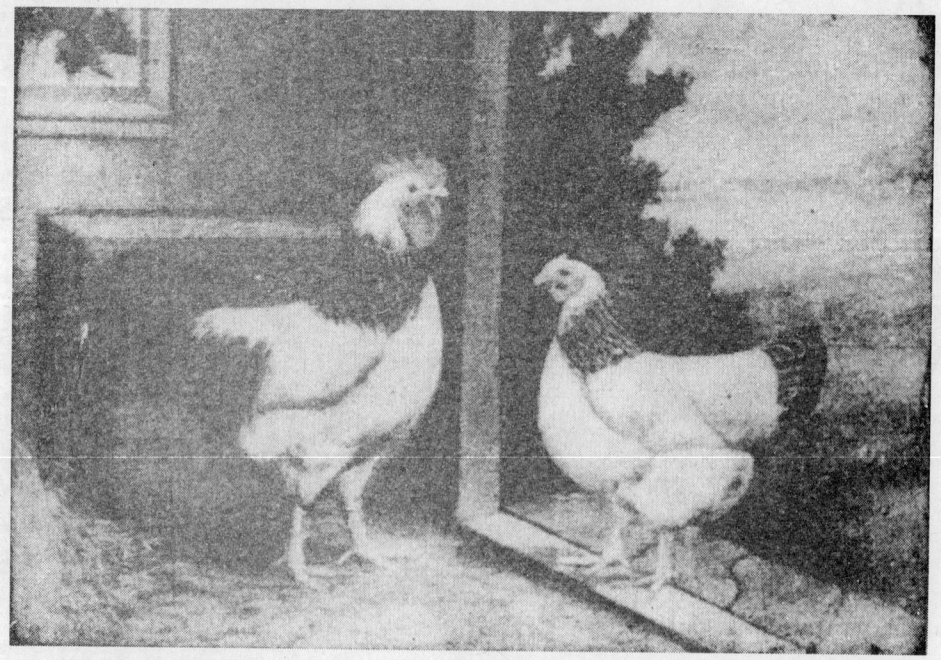

Plate 4. Light Sussex.

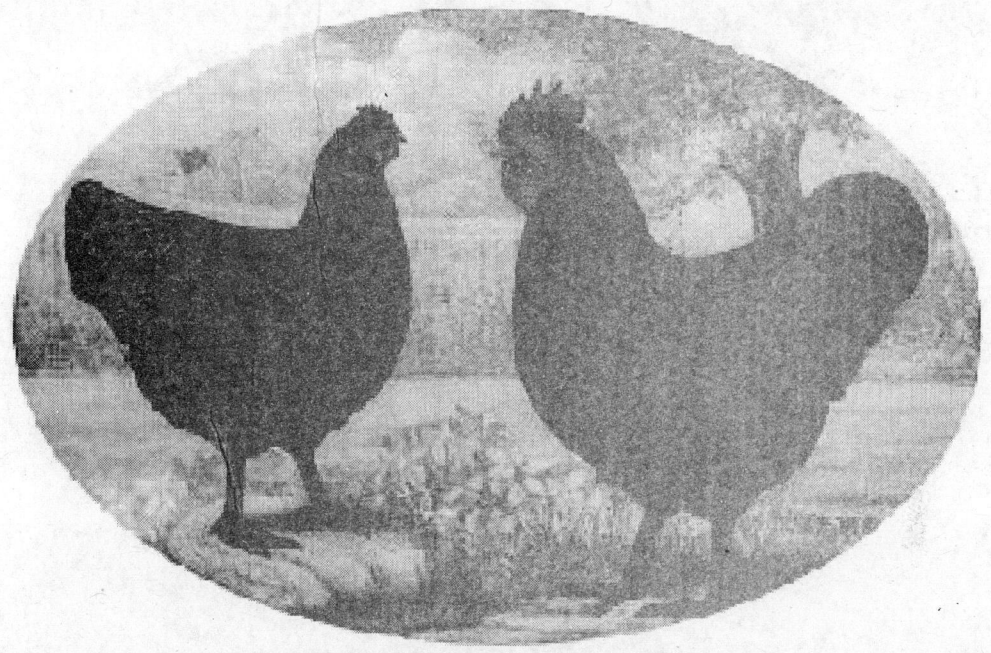

Plate 5.   Australorps.

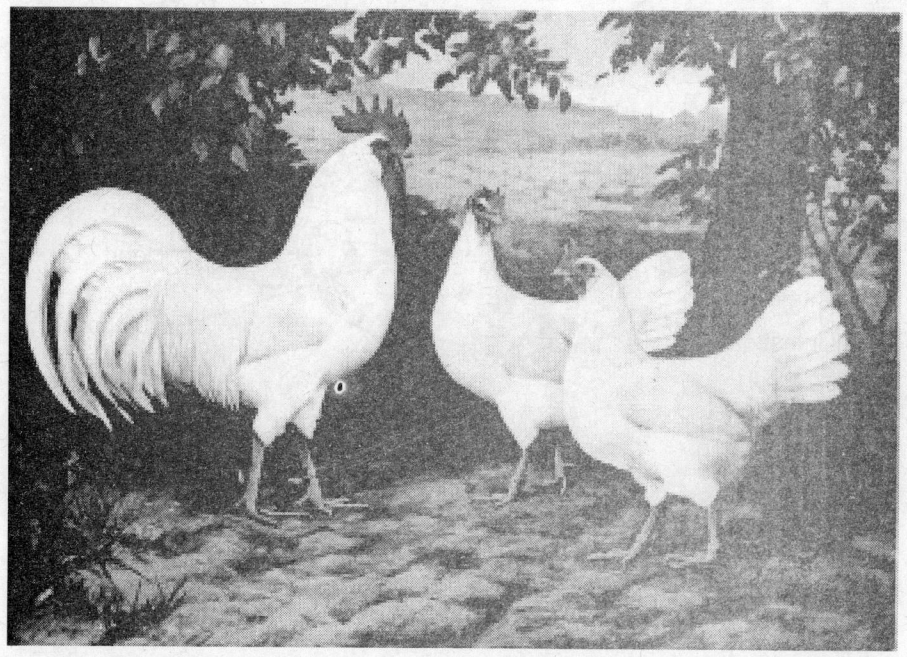

Plate 6.   S.C. White Leghorns.

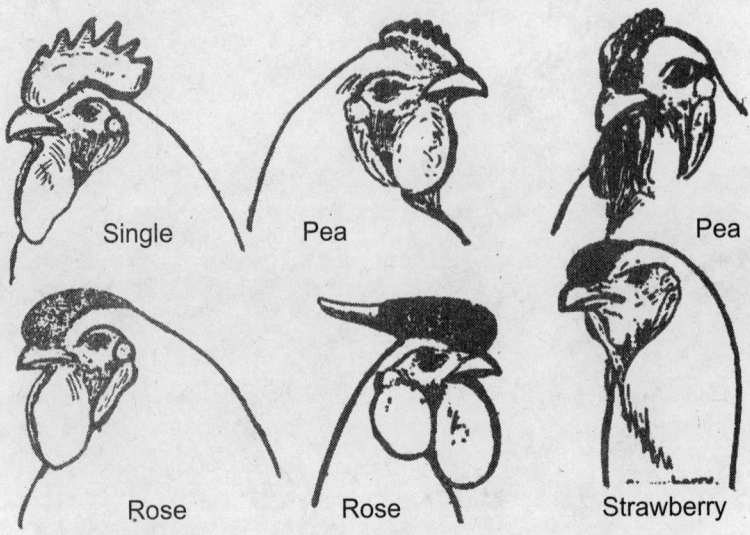

Single   Pea   Pea

Rose   Rose   Strawberry

Figure 6   Types of Standard male combs

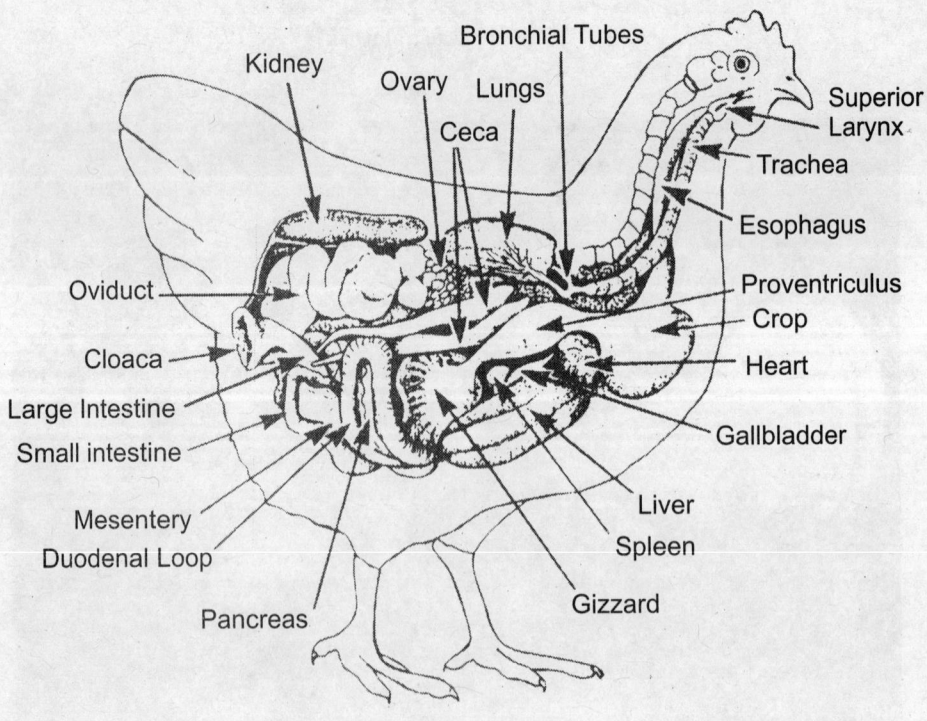

Figure 7   Schematic of a chicken

AMERICAN CLASS

Rhode Island Red

Rhode Island Red originated from Rhode Island in New England after crossing with the red Malay Game, Leghorn and Asiatic native stock.

The bird has a somewhat long, rectangular body, which is also broad and deep. The back is flat and the breast is carried well forward–characteristics which make it a good meat producing bird. The plumage of the Rhode Island Red is rich dark or brownish red in colour, evenly distributed over the entire surface, and is well glossed. The wing when spread shows black both in primaries and secondaries. The tail coverts, sickle feathers, and main tail feathers are also black. In the lower neck feathers of the female, there is also slight black marking at the base. The usual colour of the breed is, brownish red, but buff, white and brown are not uncommon.

There are two varieties of this breed: (1) Single Comb, and (2) Rose Comb. The characteristics of the varieties are identical aside from the type of comb. In both cases the skin and shanks are yellow and the ear lobes red. The Single Comb is the more popular of the two.

The standard weight in kg is: Cock–3.8; Hen–3.0; Cockerel–3.4 and Pullet–2.5. Colour of egg shells, brown to dark brown.

Plymouth Rock

The Plymouth Rock is one of the most popular breeds in America, largely because it is a bird of good size, with excellent fleshing properties and good egg laying abilities. Birds of this breed have long bodies and have good depth of body. They have single combs. Mature birds weigh from 3.5 to 4.5 kg. There are seven varieties of Plymouth Rocks, each distinguished by its plumage. They are: (1) Barred, (2) White, (3) Buff, (4) Silver-pencilled, (5) Blue, (6) Partridge, and (7) Columbian.

In general, the plumage is greyish white, each feather crossed by almost black bars which should be even in width, straight and should extend down to the skin. Each feather should end with a narrow, dark tip which, with the alternate dark and light bars, give a bluish cast or shade to the surface colour.

Solid black or partly black feathers may occur in some birds of practically all strains in this variety. Black spots on the shanks are also common, particularly in females. All these strains indicate purity of breeds.

Barred Plymouth Rock. In this variety, the male birds have black and white bars of equal width, whereas in female the white bars should be as wide as the black bars.

White Plymouth Rock. White Plymouth Rocks have been used extensively in broiler production. The plumage is white throughout and usually free from black ticking, brassiness and creaminess. The variety was developed from a sport of the Barred variety.

Table 16 Some Breeds and Varieties of Poultry and their Characteristics

Breed and Variety	Plumage	Standard Weight Pounds		Type of Comb	Color of Ear Lobe	Color of Skin	Color of Shank	Shanks Feathered?	Color of Egg
		Cock	Hen						
American									
White Plymouth Rock	White	9½	7½	Single	Red	Yellow	Yellow	No	Brown
White Wyandotte	White	8½	6½	Rose	Red	Yellow	Yellow	No	Brown
Rhode Island Red	Red	8½	6½	Single and rose	Red	Yellow	Yellow	No	Brown
New Hampshire	Red	8½	6½	Single	Red	Yellow	Yellow	No	Brown
Asiatic									
Brahma (Light)	Columbian Pattern	12	9½	Pea	Red	Yellow	Yellow	Yea	Brown
Cochin (buff)	Buff	11	8½	Single	Red	Yellow	Yellow	Yes	Brown
English									
Australorp	Black	8½	6½	Single	Red	White	Dark slate	No	Brown
White Cornish	White	10½	8	Pea	Red	Yellow	Yellow	No	Brown
Mediterranean									
White Leghorn	White	6	4½	Single and rose	White	Yellow	Yellow	No	White

New Hampshire

The shape of the body of the bird is less rectangular than that of the Rhode Island Red. The plumage is chestnut red, but is not so well established as in the Rhode Island Red. It has a single comb. In females, the lower neck feathers are distinctly tipped with black. The main tail feathers are black, edge with medium chestnut red. In both sexes, the under colour is light salmon.

The breed is a good-producer of large brown shelled eggs. The standard weight in kg Cock 3.8; Hen 2.7; Cockerel 3.4; Pullet 2.5.

ASIATIC CLASS

Brahma

The breed was developed in India and exported to America and England about one hundred years ago. The original birds were light in colour. Brahmas are massive in appearance, well feathered and well proportioned. They have pea combs. Mature birds weigh from 4 to 5 kg. Three varieties of Brahmas have been produced: (1) Light, (2) Dark, and (3) Buff.

Light Brahma. The light Brahma is most popular because of its colour and its size. Mature birds weigh about 500 gm more than birds of the other two varieties.

The colour pattern of the light Brahma is similar to that of the Columbian Plymouth Rock and the Columbian White, the hackle feathers are black with white edging, and the main tail feathers are black, with the exception of top feathers of the female, which are laced with white. The shanks, toes and beak are yellow.

Dark Brahma, In the male, the hackle is greenish black with an edging of white. Plumage in front of the neck is black. The wing bow is white and the primary wing feathers and tail feathers are black.

In the female, the head and the upper neck are silver grey, the wing bows are steel-grey with black pencilling and the primary wing feathers are black with a narrow edge of steel-grey. The back is steel-grey, with the same black pencilling as on the breast, body and fluff. The tail is black except for the top two feathers, which are grey underneath. The shanks, toes and beak are yellow.

Cochin

It is also known as Shanghai fowl. It originated in Shanghai (China). Characterized by massive appearance, thickly feathered shanks, single comb and a cushion-like structure at the base of the tail. The popular varieties are buff, patridge, white and black. Standard weight (kg): Cock, 4.9; hen, 3.8; cockerel, 3.6; pullet, 3.1.

Langshan

It is a graceful bird with a well-proportioned body. It originated from Langshan region of China. The principal breed characteristics are shorter but deeper body than Brahma or Cohin, large tail feathers, tail carried high, long legs and single comb. Black and White are the two main varieties. Black Langshan is known for its dark brown beak, bluish-black shanks and pinkish-white toe. White Langshan has the plumage colour as that of White Plymouth Rock except slaty white to pinkish-blue back, slaty blue shanks and toes with pink between scales.

ENGLISH CLASS

Sussex

The breed developed in England about 200 years ago primarily as table birds. It has a long body, shoulders are broad with a good depth from front to rear and the bird in general has excellent fleshing qualities. Males of this breed have a single comb and coloured beaks, shanks and toes. The standard weights in kg are Cock 4.0; Hen 3.1; Cockerel 3.4; Pullet 2.7. The varieties are described below:

Light Sussex. The plumage is quite similar to that of the Columbian Plymouth Rock and Columbian Wyandote. This variety appears to lay well during summer months in India.

Red Sussex. The plumage is deep rich red in both sexes. The only exception to the Red are found principally in the primaries where the lower webs are black with a narrow edging of red, and in the secondaries, where the upper webs are black like that of the tail colour. The under colour of all sections in both sexes is red with a slight bar of slate.

Australorp

The breed was developed in Australia where for many years it has been bred principally for egg production rather than meat. It is also very fleshy which makes it a good dual purpose breed.

The back is somewhat long, and the body slopes gradually towards the tail. It has a good depth of body, and more closely feathered than the Orpington. The comb is single, the body is black, plumage is lustrous greenish black in all the sections, the under colouring is dull black.

The "Austro White" a hybrid cross between the Australorp male and the White Leghorn female, has proved to be an excellent layer with good vigour and is maintained in large flocks in commercial egg farms of India. The standard weight of Australorp in kg is: Cock 3.8; Hen 3.0; Cockerel 3.4; Pullet 2.5.

Orpington

Orpingtons were developed in Kent in England. They are long, deep and broad and well rounded, with a full breast and a broad back. They are little more loosely feathered than breeds of American class. Orpingtons have single combs. Mature birds weigh from 4.5 kg.

There are four varieties: (1) Buff; (2) Black; (3) White; (4) Blue. Only the Buff Orpington has made much popularity in America.

Buff orpington.   It was evolved from Buff Cochin, Dark Dorkings, and Golden spangled Hamburgs. The plumage is the same as in other Buff breeds, such as the Buff Plymouth Rock. The shanks and toes are white.

MEDITERRANEAN CLASS

Leghorn

Out of tue important breeds classified as Mediterranean breeds, the Leghorn is by far the most popular. It is the word's number one egg producer. The breed originated in Itlay and so far there are 12 varieties. Only three varieties, however, have become popular. They are:

(1) Single Comb White; (2) Single Comb Buff; and (3) Single Comb Light Brown.

The breed is small, active, and reputed for the harmony of its various parts. In appearance, the Leghorn is the neatest of all birds. It is small and very compact in form, carries the tail rather low and has a small head with well set comb and wattles. It has a relatively long back, prominent breast, and comparatively long shanks.

The shape of comb is quite important to Leghorn fanciers. The single comb of the male should be of medium size and should stand erect, with five uniform, deeply serrated points. The front point of the female should stand erect, but the remainder of the comb should gradually slope to one side.

The White, Buff and Brown varieties are subdivided further on the basis of the character of the comb, i.e., whether it is rose or single comb. All the varieties have yellow beaks, skin, shanks (legs) and toes.

In India about 50 years ago White Leghorn fowls were introduced by Christian missionaries and fanciers in U.P., Travancore-Cochin and few other States; the indigenous non-descript fowls in the villages were graded up with the White Leghorns. Today, White Leghorns are one of the most popular breeds throughout the plains of India.

Leghorns are known for their stylish carriage. Mature birds weigh from 2.0 to 2.7 kg.

Minorca

Minorcas, originally called Red-Faced Black Spanish, are the largest and heaviest of Mediterranean breeds of poultry. Long strong bodies, large combs, long wattles, large white ear lobes, large and full tail moderately elevated, with firm muscular legs set squarely under the powerful looking body, are the distinct characteristics of this breed. The beak, shanks and toes are black.

An excellent producer of large white eggs. Colour of skin white; the egg shell is chalk white in colour. This breed was at one time even more popular than the Leghorn because of the superior size of its white eggs, but is now dropping out of favour probably because of the decline in production. The standard weight in kg. : Cock 4.1; Cockerel 3.4; Hen 3.0; Pullet 2.8.

THE SKELETAL SYSTEM

The skeleton serves as a framework for the body and the attachment of muscles, protects vital organs, holds the bone marrow and contains air spaces which aid in respiration and flight although domestic fowls are no longer prone to the skill of flying. The bone marrow produces the red blood cells and part of the white cells.

The *head* is small in comparison with other parts of the body. The relative position of nostrils and the opening in the upper and lower parts of the mouth should be noted. The nasal cavities open into the roof of the mouth from a point just back of the upper mandible. The *neck* is long and very flexible. The cervical vertebrate fit upon each other in such a way that there is a great freedom of movement of the head and neck for eating, care of plumage, defence, and other purposes. The *backbone* shows much fusion of vertebrate. The *hind limbs* are adapted for walking and perching. The tibia or "drumstick" is the largest bone of the limb. Most breeds of chicken have four toes, three extending forward and one backward. The ribs are attached above to the spinal column and below to the sternum. They are braced to each other by additional bones to give a finer framework. The *sternum* or breastbone is very large and projects back beyond the ribs, forming a part of the abdominal floor. The *pactoral girdle*, corresponding to the shoulder girdle in mammals, consists of the scapulae or shoulder blades, the coracoids, and the clavicle or "Wishbone". The *pelvic girdle* makes reproduction or egg laying less difficult. It consists of the ilia, ischia, and pubis or "lay bones" in the hen. The pubis has a tendency to straighten out when a bird is in production. There is a tendency of the rear of the keel to drop down when a bird is in production and to be drawn up towards the pubis when the bird is out of production. Figure 8 reprents the skeleton of a fowl.

BLOOD VASCULAR SYSTEM

In birds, the blood vascular system operates at a much higher pulse rate and blood pressure level. Considering that some birds live to be more than 100 years old with such an arrangement, there should be little question of its efficiency or effectiveness. Figure 9 represents the heart of a chicken.

Table 17   Heart Rates in Birds

Type of Bird	Heart Rate Beats/Minute
Canary	1,000
Quail	500–600
Chicken	350–475
TurKey	200–275
Pigeon	220
Goose	200

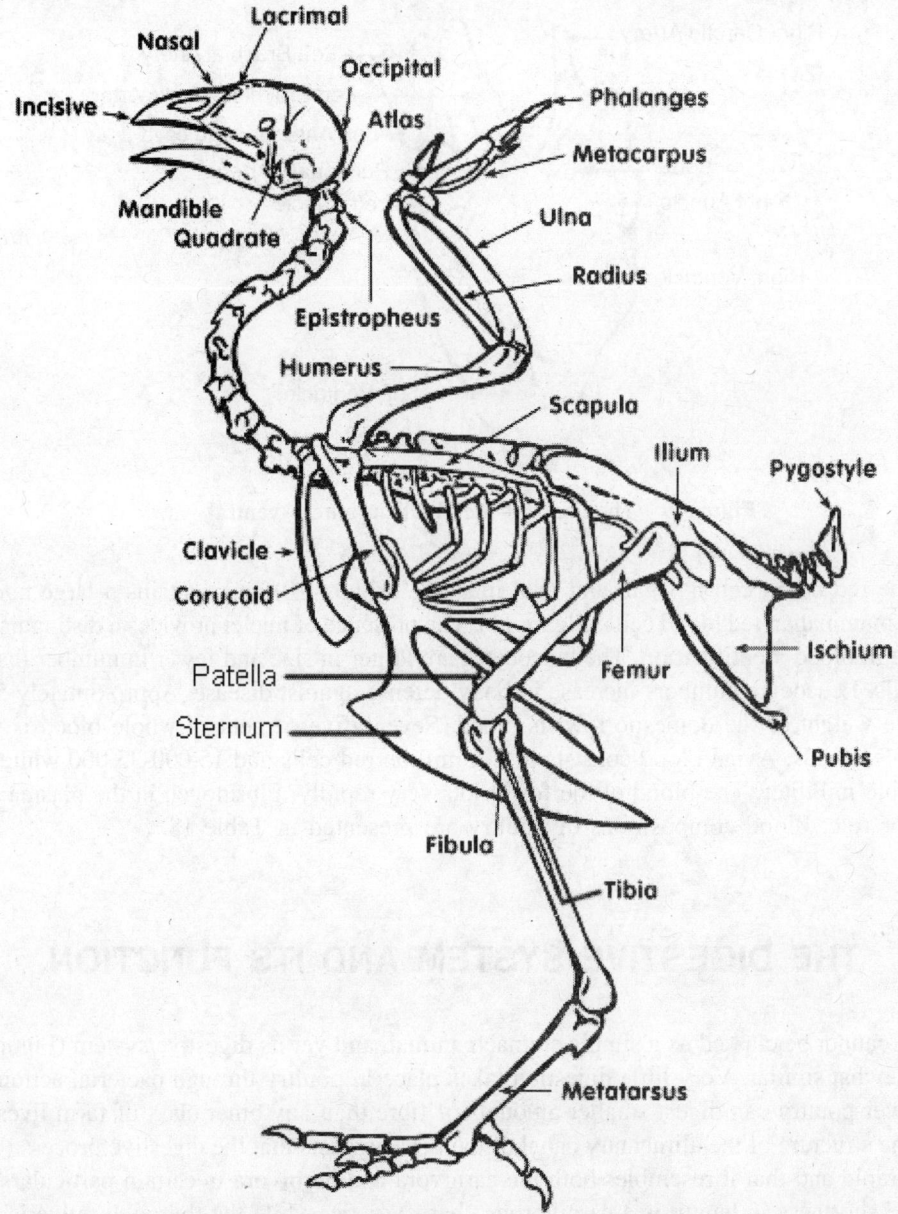

Figure 8 The skeleton of a fowl

The main difference in the vascular system lies in the heart. The right atrium of the chicken is larger than the left but the mass of the left ventricle is nearly three times that of the right. The right A-V valve is simply a muscular flap, but the left A-V valves are membranous as in mammals. The aortic and pulmonary valves are similar to those in mammals. Heart rates in birds are presented in Table-17.

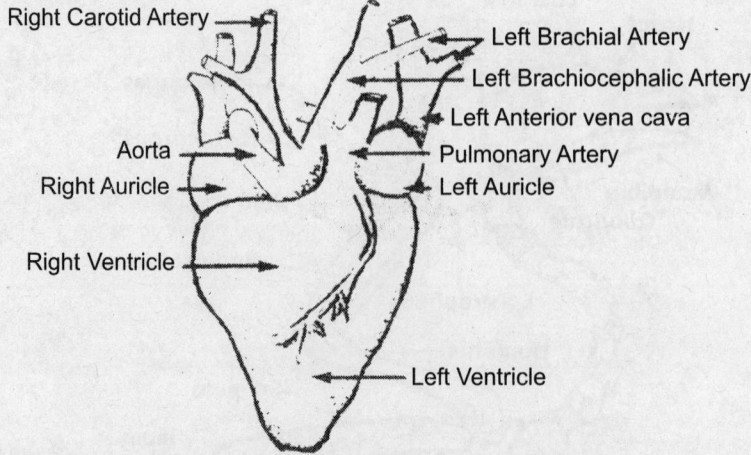

Figure 9 The heart of the chicken; antero-ventral view

The red blood cell is small and oval in shape (Figure 10) and contains a large nucleus, unlike mammalian red blood cells (Figure 11). The presence of nuclei provides a distinguishable feature in blood identification. The leucocytes are larger in size and fewer in number than the red cells. Leucocyte numbers increase in body defense against disease. Approximately 5% of the live weight of the domestic fowl is blood. Seventyfive percent of whole blood is water and 25%, solids. Avian blood consists of 2-4 million red cells and 15,000-35,000 white cells per cubic milliliter. The blood of the fowl clots very rapidly. Fibrinogen in the plasma plays a major role. Blood compositions of poultry are presented in Table 18.

THE DIGESTIVE SYSTEM AND ITS FUNCTION

A bird cannot be classed as a simple stomach animal, and yet its digestive system (Figure 12) is somewhat similar. Very little digestion takes place in poultry through bacterial action, and moreover poultry can digest smaller amounts of fibre than any other class of farm livestock.

The structure of the alimentary canal of the bird suggests that the digestive process (Table 19) is rapid and that it resembles both the carnivora and herbivora in certain particulars. The relative shortness in length is a carnivorous characteristic, while the thorough pulverising of the feed in the gizzard corresponds to mastication in the herbivora.

Following is a brief description of the digestive organs in poultry and its function.

Mouth Parts

The distinctive character of the mouth of the bird is the absence of lips and teeth. These parts are replaced by a horny mandible on each jaw, forming the beak.

Table 18 Blood compositions of Poultry

Type of Poultry	Total Leukocytes thousands per mm^3	Lymphocytes	Heterophils	Eosinophils	Basophils	Monocytes	Thrombocytes thousands per mm^3
Chicken	20.0	59 0	27.2	2.0	1.7	10.2	25.4
Chick	29.4	66.0	20.9	1.9	3.1	8.1	26.5
Duck	23.4	61.7	24.3	2.1	1.5	10.8	23.4

(partly from Kolb. *Lehrbuch der Physiologie der Haustiere*)

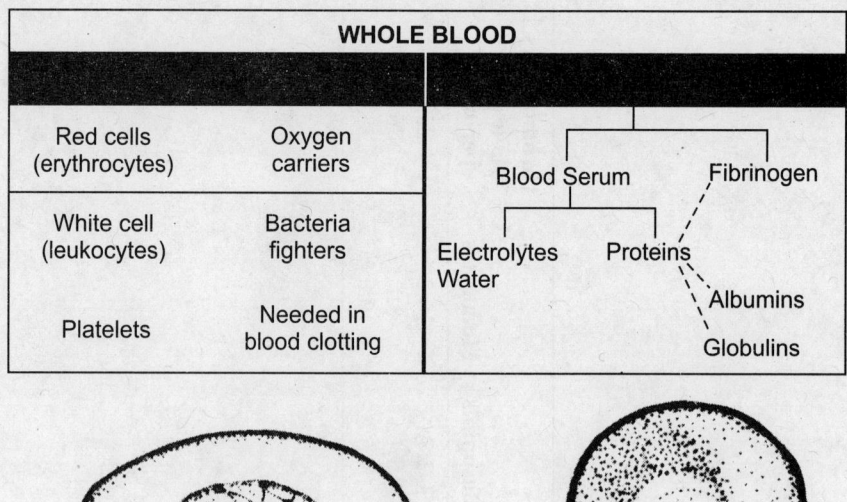

WHOLE BLOOD	
Red cells (erythrocytes) — Oxygen carriers	Blood Serum / Fibrinogen
White cell (leukocytes) — Bacteria fighters	Electrolytes Water — Proteins
Platelets — Needed in blood clotting	Albumins / Globulins

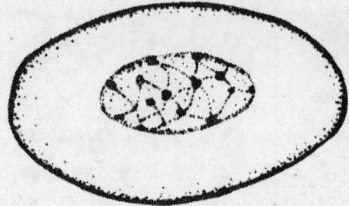

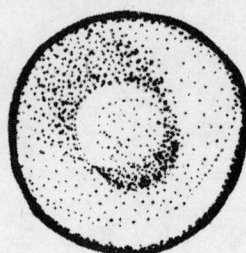

Figure 10 Avian   **Figure 11** Mammalian

Red blood cells

The tongue is shaped like the barbed head of an arrow with the point directed forward. The barb-like projections at the back of the tongue serve the purpose of foreing the grain toward the entrance to the gullet when the tongue is moved from front to back. The amount of saliva is very small.

Esophagus

The esophagus or gullet is distinguished by its enormous expansibility. Food passes from the mouth through the esophagus to the crop and onwards.

Crop

The crop is an enlargement of the esophagus, and is used for storing and softening the food. Food is gradually sent to the stomach as needed by contraction of the walls of the crop.

Proventriculus

Two or three inches beyond the crop, an enlarged muscular portion of the esophagus will be seen, about ½ to ¾ inch in diameter and from 1¼ to 2 inches long. This is the proventriculus, a small organ which receives the feed from the crop. On the inner surface, are the openings of various glands, which secrete gastric juice and some acids. These liquids are mixed with the food and assist in further softening it. This glandular stomach does not appreciably detain the food.

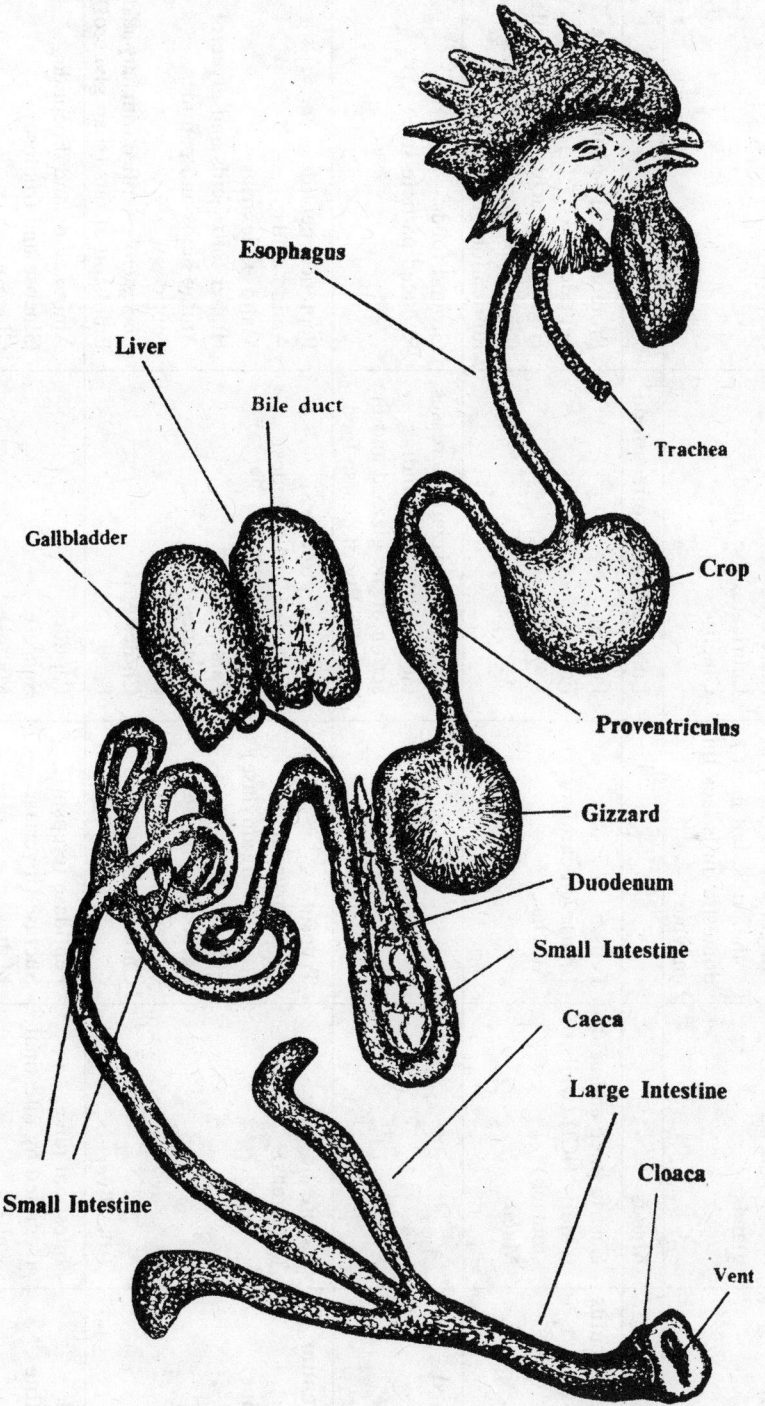

Figure 12 The digestive system in a chicken.

Table 19 Digestive Processes in Poultry

Region	Secretion (secreted by)	Enzyme	Enzyme Acts on. or Function	End Product of Digestion
Mouth	Saliva (salivary glands)	Amylase is secreted in some birds, but most domestic birds lack this enzyme	Starch, dextrins Lubricates the food Glucose	Dextrins
Crop	Mucus		Lubricates and softens food	
Proventriculus	Gastric juice and acids (chiefly HCl) (walls of stomach) Mucus	Pepsin Lipase (in carnivores) Amylase	Protein Fat	Proteoses, poly-peptides, peptides Higher fatty acids and glycerol Coating of stomach lining of lubrication of food
Gizzard			Grit in the gizzard increases the motility and grinding action of the gizzard and the digestibility of coarse feed	Ground foods Reduced particle size
Duodenum (small intestine)	Pancreatic juice (pancreas) Bile (liver)	Trypsin Chymotrypsin Amylopsin (amylase) Steapsin (lipase) Carbozypeptidase Collagenase Cholesterol esterase	Proteins, proteoses, peptones, and peptides Starch, dextrins Fats Peptides Collagen Cholesterol Fats	Peptones, peptides Amino acids Maltose, dextrins Higher fatty acids and glycerol Amino acids and peptides Peptides Cholesterol esterified with fatty acids Emulsion of fats (soap glycerol)
Small Intestine	Intestinal juice (secreted by intestinal wall)	Peptidase (erepsin) Sucrase (invertase) Maltase Lactase Polynucleotidase	Peptides Sucrose Maltose Lactose Nucleic acid	Amino acids and dipeptides Glucose and fructose Glucose Glucose and galactose Mononucleotides
Caeca	A limited amount of microbial activity		Cellulose, polysacharides, starches, sugars	Volatile fatty acids, Microbial protein, B-vitamins, Vitamin K

Gizzard

The gizzard is heavily muscled, reddish-green colour, and located just back of the proventriculus. Probably some gastric digestion takes place in the gizzard, but this organ functions chiefly in crushing and grinding feed. It is the largest single organ of the body. The gizzard is composed of two pairs of thick, powerful muscles covered internally with a thick, horny epithelium.

In fact, the gizzard functions as a filter, in such a way that fine materials enter the duodenum in about one minute after ingestion by a fowl, while coarse materials are retained much longer to be ground by the contractions of the gizzard.

Duodenum

Placed in the section of the small intestine which forms a fold immediately after the digestive canal leaves the gizzard, this loop, or fold of the intestine is the duodenum, which supports the pancreas.

Gastric digestion, together with some pancreatic digestion, takes place in the duodenum.

Pancreas

Lying between the folds of the duodenum, this organ is relatively longer in birds than in mammals. It secretes a fluid known as the pancreatic juice, that contains proteolytic, amylolytic and lipolytic enzymes which vigorously hydrolyse proteoses, peptones, starches and fats. The pancreatic juice empties into the duodenum.

Liver

This is a large, several lobed, dark red organ. It is more or less flat, even more so at the extremities. It is the largest gland in the body. The liver secretes the bile.

Two ducts convey the bile from the liver to the terminal part of the duodenum. The one from the right lobe of the liver is enlarged to form the gall bladder in which the bile is temporarily stored. The one from the left lobe has no such enlargement. They enter the duodenum together. The gall bladder can be easily identified by its dark green colour. Bile aids in the digestion of fat.

Spleen

This round reddish body is found near the liver. It is usually from ¼ to ½ inch in diameter. Its function is little known. Some authorities believe that the white corpuscles of the blood accumulated in the spleen are rebuilt or cast from the body.

Small Intestine

It makes up the digestive tract from the gizzard to the caeca. It is about 2½ feet long in mature bird. The inner surface is lined with mature villi, which may be seen washing under water.

Besides its digestive function, the small intestine also acts as an organ of absorption of the feed ingredients in simpler form.

Caeca

At the junction of the small and large intestines are two blind sacs, 5-7 inches in length. These open into the intestine as one end, but have no outlet at the other. They appear to serve as temporary storage organs for faecal materials, and some absorption may take place in them. They also aid in the digestion of fibre.

Large Intestine

It lies between the junction of the caeca and extends for a short distance up to the exterior opening of the cloaca. Short villi project into the lumen of the tract for further absorption of the digested materials (in mammals villi are absent in the large intestine).

Cloaca

The faecal materials from the rectum and urine from the kidneys pass into this organ. The materials are mixed and excreted through the vent.

Urinary System

From each kidney, the urine, in the form of a white pasty material, passes through the ureter to the cloaca, where it is subsequently voided with the faecal matter from the cloaca.

HORMONES

Hormones are substances produced by specialized tissues called the endocrines or the ductless glands and liberated into the blood stream to be carried to a remote tissue or viscera called the target organ on which they exert characteristic physiological effects. Like vitamins and enzymes the hormones are effective in minute amounts. Though the name hormone indicates that its action is to stimulate ('hormaein' in Greek means 'to excite'), not all of them are excitatory. They differ from enzymes in that they are not all of them protein in nature and as a rule do not act on the endocrine gland which has produced them. In fact, the hormones in many cases, act by influencing the enzymes. Functions of hormones are presented in Table 20 while Figure 13 shows the endocrine glands of the chicken.

MALE REPRODUCTIVE SYSTEM

The male reproductive system produces male reproductive cells (spermatozoa), meant for introducing them into the oviduct of the female for fertilisation of the egg and secondly for producing a hormone which influences sex characters.

The male reproductive system consists of the testes, vas deferens, and papillae or rudimentary copulatory organs (Figure 14).

Table 20 Hormones of the fowl

Gland	Hormone	Type of Hormono	Functions of Hormone
Hypophysis (pituitary gland);			
1. Adenohypophysis (anterior lobe)	Gonadotropic hormones		
	1 Follicle stimulating hormone (FSH)	Protein	Stimulates growth of ovarian follicles in females Maturation of sperm in males
	2 Lutenizmg hormone(LH)	Protein	Triggers ovulation in females. Acts on Leydig cells of testes to produce androgen
	3 Prolactin	Protein	Causes broodiness in chickens. Initiates crop-sac secretion in pigeons.
	Growth hormone (GH) or Somatotropin (STH)	Protein	Growth promotion. Protein synthesis
	Adrenocorticotropin (ACTH)	Protein	Stimulation of the adrenal cortex and release of the adrenal corticoids
	Thyrotropin (TSH)	Protein	Stimulation of the thyroid glands to (1) re-lease thyroxine, and (2) absorb iodine
	Melanotropin (MSH)	Protein	Function is not known in birds
	Oxytocin (storage)	Protein	Stimulates uterine tissue
2. Neurohypophysis (posterior lobe)	Vasotocin (storage)	Protein	Antidiuretic hormone. May initiate the contraction of the uterus that begins oviposition
Hypothalamus	Oxytocin	Protein	See Neurohypophysis
	Vasotocin	Protein	See Neurohypophysis.
	Releasing factors for		Stimulates the adenohypophysis to release its hormones
	1. LH		
	2. FSH		
	3. TSH		
	4. ACTH		
Thyroid glands	Thyroxine and Triiodotyrosine	Protein	Affects metabolic rate. Affects feather growth and color
Ultimobranchial glands	Calcitonin	Protein	Calcium metabolism. May play a role in the regulation of serum phosphorus
Parathyroid glands	Parathyroid hormone (PTH)	Protein	Calcium mobilization and also phosphorus metabolism.

Table 20 (Contd.)

Adrenals:		
1. Cortex		
Aldosterone	Steroid	Electrolyte and water metabolism. Carbohydrate, fat, and protein metabolism
Corticosteroids	Steroid	
Catecholamines		
2. Medulla		
1. Adrenaline (epinephrine)	Protein derivative	Initiates sympathetic neural responses
2. Noradrenaline (norepinephnne)	Protein derivative	Neural transmitter
Pancreas		
Glucagon	Protein	Carbohydrate, fat, and protein metabolism
Insulin	Protein	Carbohydrate, fat, and protein metabolism
Testes (male)		
Testosterone	Steroid	Secondary sex characteristics. Sexual behavior, Spermatogenesis
Ovary (female)		
Estrogens: estradiol, estriol, estrone	Steroid	Secondary sex characteristics. Affects growth and fat deposition. May be involved with the growth and development of the follicle involved in albumen synthesis
Progesterone	Steroid	Involved in albumen synthesis. Antagonistic to ovulation
Pineal gland		
Melatonin	Protein	Functions unclear in poultry

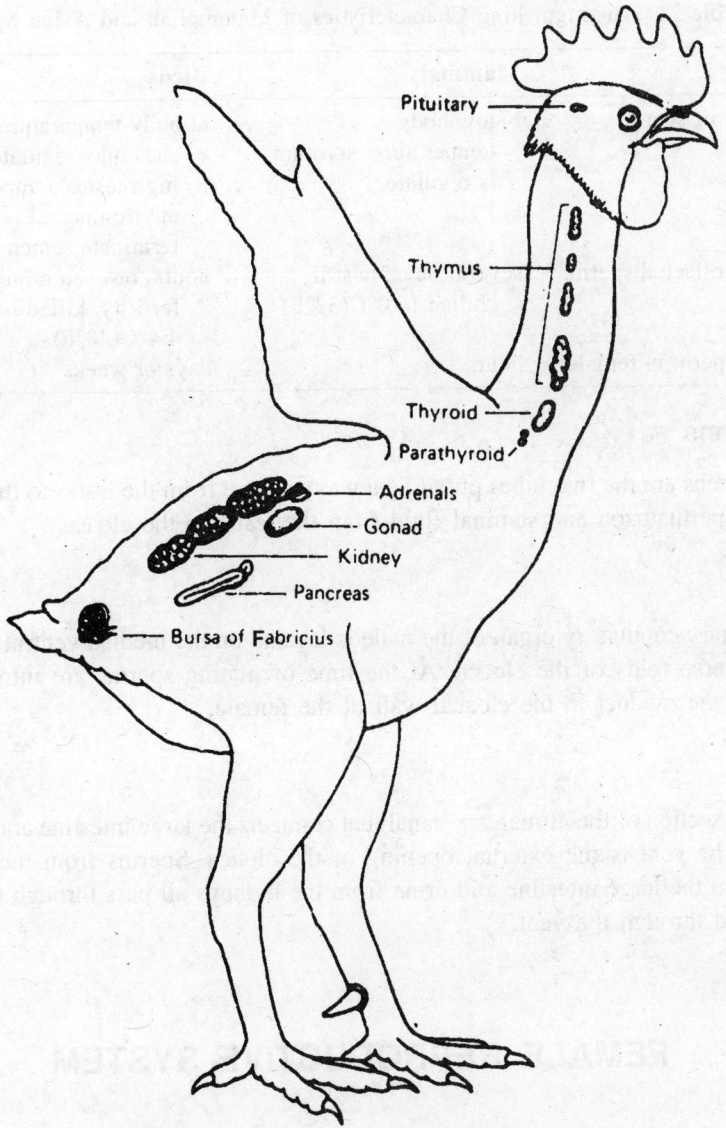

Pituitary

Thymus

Thyroid

Parathyroid

Adrenals

Gonad

Kidney

Pancreas

Bursa of Fabricius

Figure 13 Endocrine glands of the chicken.

Testes

The testes are two small ovoid organs situated at the anterior end of the kidneys in the dorsal body wall. The left testis is usually larger than the right one. Each testis consists of a larger number of slender tubes, called seminiferous tubules, from the linings of which the reproductive cells are given off. The spermatozoa are then carried out of the testes by the seminal fluid, which is also produced in the testes. Millions of these are produced and expelled in the seminal fluid. Distinguishing characteristics of mammalian and avian sperms are presented in Table 21.

Table 21 Distinguishing Characteristics of Mammalian and Avian Sperms

	Mammals	Birds
Development of sperm:	below body temperature; scrotum is regulator	at body temperature, except air sacs may regulate otherwise high testes' temperature. High environmental temperature may terminate semen production
Viability of collected sperm:	several days; best if chilled to 0°C(32°F)	hours, or even minutes for high fertility, killed below 4.4°C(40°F)
Viability of sperm in female:	hours	days or weeks

Vas Deferens

The vas deferens are the two tubes pursuing a wavy course from the testes to the cloaca. They convey the spermatozoa and seminal fluid from the testis to the cloaca.

Papillae

The rudimentary copulatory organ of the male is located on the median ventral portion of one of the transverse folds of the cloaca. At the time of mating sperms are introduced by the papillae into the oviduct in the cloacal wall of the female.

Cloaca

The enlarged section of the alimentary canal that connects the large intestine and vent is called the cloaca. The vent is the external opening of the cloaca. Sperms from the testes, faecal materials from the large intestine and urine from tne kidneys all pass through the cloaca and are eliminated through the vent.

FEMALE REPRODUCTIVE SYSTEM

The female reproductive system differs greatly from that of mammals. The reproductive cell, also known as a gamete, ovum or egg, is an article of food. It is large and enclosed with a food supply for embryo development.

The reproductive system of the female consists of primary and accessory sexual organs, the ovary and the oviduct with its five parts: infundibulum, magnum, isthmus, uterus, and vagina (Figure 15).

Ovary

At hatching time the female chick has two ovaries and two oviducts. Normally, only the left one develops, the right persisting if at all, only as a functionless rudiment. A few cases have

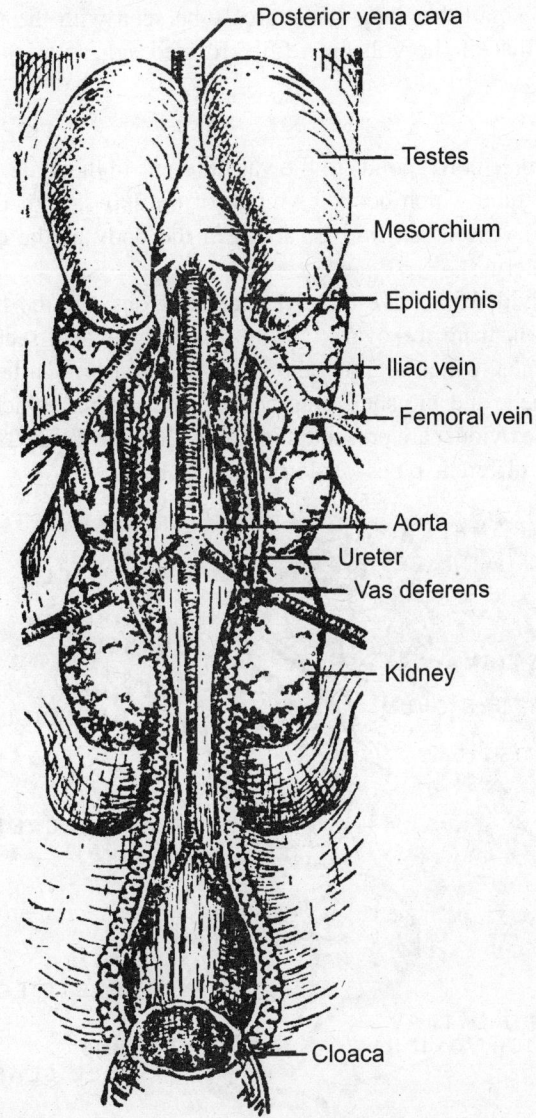

Posterior vena cava

Testes

Mesorchium

Epididymis

Iliac vein

Femoral vein

Aorta

Ureter

Vas deferens

Kidney

Cloaca

Figure 14 Male urinary and reproductive organs

been reported, however, in which both right and left ovary and oviduct were present and functioning in a mature pullet. This is very rare.

The functioning ovary appears as a cluster of many spheres, each of which is independently attached by a very slender stalk. Each sphere is a more or less developed ovum or yolk enclosed in a thin membrane or follicle. The yolk vary in colour from pale straw colour to deep reddish-yellow or orange. Each yolk contains a germinal disc, from which the embryo develops. In a hen in laying condition, as many as 900 to over 3,600 ova have been counted.

Many of them are so small that they can scarcely be seen with the naked eye, while others vary in size even to that of the yolk in a fully formed egg.

Oviduct

The oviduct in the female corresponds to the vas deferens in the male. The oviduct in a laying hen is a large, coiled tube which occupies much of the left side of the abdominal cavity. It is covered with blood vessels and moves about in the body as the eggs are developed and moved towards the uterus.

The oviduct is divided into five rather defined regions: (1) the funnel or infundibulum, which receives the yolk from the ovary; (2) the magnum, which secretes the thick albumen or white; (3) the isthmus, which secretes the shell membranes; (4) the uterus, which secretes the thin white, the shell, and the shell pigment; (5) the vagina, which holds the egg until it is laid. Functions of the oviduct are presented in Table 23 while Table 22 shows the comparative reproductive traits in different types of domesticated birds.

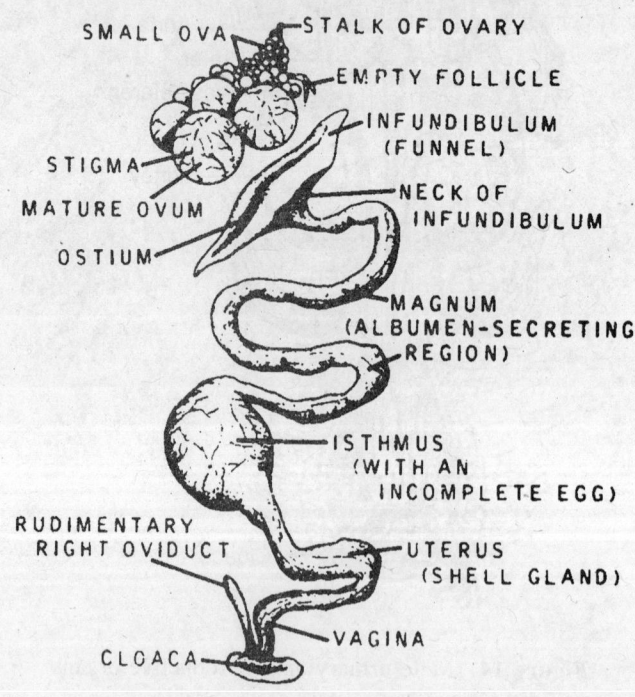

Figure 15 Female reproductive organs

FORMATION AND STRUCTURE OF THE EGGS

The knowledge of the formation (Figure 16) and structure of the egg (Figure 17) is essential for an understanding of fertility, embryo development, egg quality, any disease of the female reproductive organs.

Table 22 Comparative reproductive traits in domestic poultry, the pheasant, the coturnix quail

Species	Incubation period (days)	Age at sexual maturity (months)	No. eggs per year	Egg weight (gm)	Fertility %	Hatchability of fertile eggs %
Chicken (*Gallus gallus*)	21	5–6	230	58	90	80
Turkey (*Meleagris gallopavo*)	28	7–8	80	85	75	65
Duck (*Anas platyrhyncos*)	27–28	6–7	120–180	60	95	70
Goose (*Anser anser*)						
Small type	30	9–10	60	135	70	80
Large type	33	10–12	50	215	65	75
Pheasant (*Phasianus colchicus*)	24–26	10–12	40	30	95	85
Guinea fowl (*Numida meleagris*)	27–28	10–12	40–70	40	90	95
Quail (*Coturnix japonka*)	15–16	1.6–2	210	10	75	65

Yolk Formation

The ovarian tisssue appears as a cluster of tiny ova or yolks. During the early stages of yolk formation, the oocytes grow very slowly by the gradual accumulation of light yolk. Food materials is carried to the developing ovum by the blood circulation in the follicle. When the ovary starts to function, a few of the ova starts to increase in size. The ovum is enclosed in a thin membrane, the *Vitelline membrane*. The yolk and its vitelline membrane are in turn enclosed in a highly vascular coat of connective tissue, the *follicle*. As the ovum or yolk increases in size it is suspended in its follicle and held to the ovary by a slender stalk, the follicle *stalk*.

Each yolk grows very slowly for about 10 days before it is ready to leave the ovary. When a diameter of about 6 mm is reached, a few ova suddenly begin to grow at an enormously increased rate. They add 4 mm to their diameter every twenty-four hours, until full size of about 40 mm in diameter is reached. An ovum within 7 to 9 days of laying contains less than 1 per cent of its final complement of yolk, yet within these few days it is sufficient to supply the missing 99 parts instead of slow growth for last 3 days.

It is during the period of rapid growth that the concentric layers of light and dark yolk are formed. The thickness of each layer of light and dark layers, representing the growth in a 24-hour period, is from 1.5 to 2 mm. The visible white and yellow bands result from periodic deposition of different amounts of carotinoid pigment.

The size of the yolk influences the size of the finished egg. Large yolks stimulate the albumen and shell glands to greater secretion.

Ovulation

When the yolk has reached maturity, the follicle ruptures along a definite line, the stigma, where there are normally no blood vessels. In most instances the ovum probably is discharged into the body cavity and is later engulfed by the funnel of the oviduct through repeated advances and recessions of the edge of the infundibulum over the surface of the ovum. Once completely enclosed, it appears to be forced along by wave-like contractions of the muscles of the oviduct. If the yolk fails to get back into the oviduct the bird is known as internal layer. The yolks may rupture and the liquid be reabsorbed into the circulation, leaving an abnormal deposit of yellow solids, or the yolks may dry up, leaving masses of caked egg yolk material in the body cavity.

Fertilisation

Fertilisation usually takes place shortly after ovulation in funnel of the oviduct, provided that the hen has been mated, and the sperm cells have had time to move to the funnel of the oviduct. Sperms will remain in the oviduct for 2-3 weeks after mating, but the newest sperm is the one most likely to fertilise the egg. It is possible to fertilise eggs within 24 hours after mating.

Since the sperm must penetrate the vitelline membrane, which surrounds the yolk, in order to reach the germinal disc, it is of interest to note that the vitelline membrane on the freshly ovulated yolk has been found to be only 4 microns thick. But after the short time in the

Table 23 Functions Of The Oviduct

Part	Approximate Time Egg Spends in Section	Functions
Infundibulum (Funnel)	15 min	Picks up yolk from the body cavity after it is released from the follicle If live sperm are present fertilization occurs in this section
Magnum (albumen secreting region)	3 hrs	Thick white (albumen) is deposited around the yolk. This layer later forms the chalaziferous layer, the chalaza. and inner thin and thick white
Isthmus	1¼ hrs	Inner and outer shell membranes are added with some water and mineral salts. These membranes give some protection to the egg contents from outside contamination
Shell Gland (uterus)	21 hrs	During the first part ot the egg's stay in the shell gland, water and minerals pass through the shell membranes into the white inflating the egg and giving rise to the outer layer of thin white. Soon after the egg is inflated the shell gland starts to add calcium over the shell membranes continuing this process until just prior to laying. If the shell is going to be colored pigment is added in this section
Vagina	Entire time from ovulation to laying is slightly more than 24 hours	The egg passes mto this section just prior to laying. Its function is not known. Some believe it adds a protein sealer to the shell to seal the pores which then functions as a protective layer

oviduct, the membrane becomes swollen and thickens, as a result of the contact with the secretions of the oviduct. The complete vitelline membrane of the yolk of laid egg is about 48 microns thick.

Embryo Development

The fertilised ovum starts cell division and embryo development soon after fertilisation. It continues during the period approximately by 24 hours when the egg remains in the oviduct. The germ spot or blastoderm increases in size and there is some change in the consistency of the white and yolk. Unless the fertile egg is held below 82°F after it is laid, there will be further germ development. It is, therefore, desirable to produce infertile eggs at all times except when they are not needed for hatching.

Secretion of Thick White

Immediately upon being grasped by the mouth of the oviduct, the ovum or yolk is forced through the oviduct by ciliary action or by peristaltic movements of the walls of the oviduct

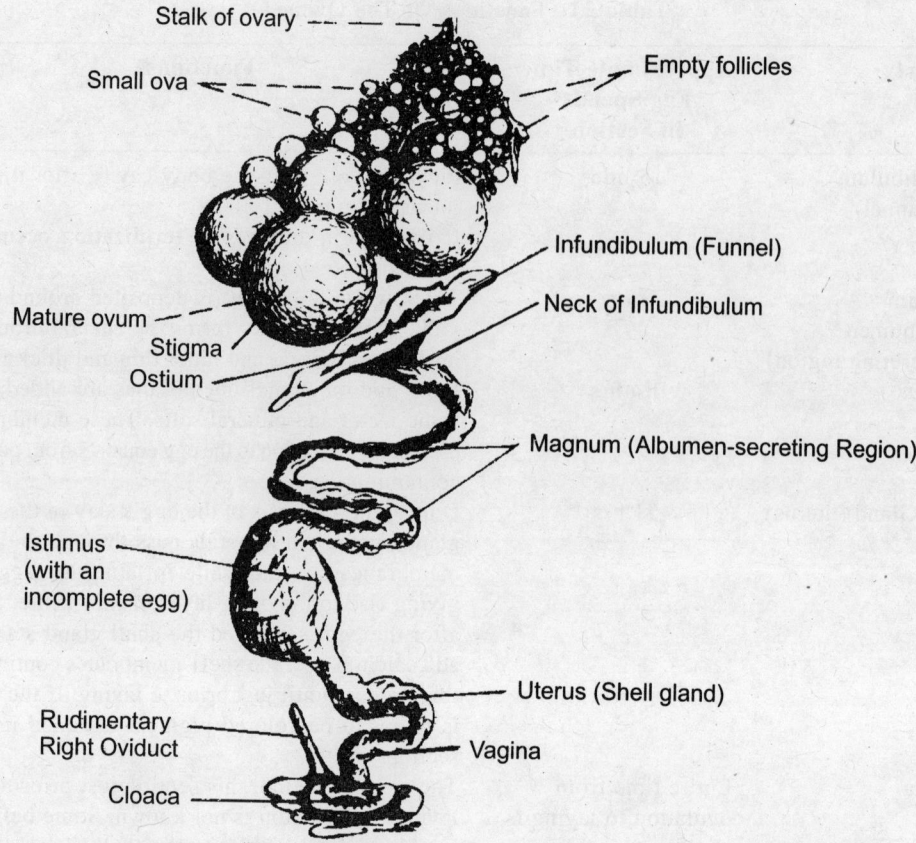

Stalk of ovary

Small ova

Empty follicles

Infundibulum (Funnel)

Neck of Infundibulum

Mature ovum

Stigma

Ostium

Magnum (Albumen-secreting Region)

Isthmus
(with an
incomplete egg)

Uterus (Shell gland)

Rudimentary
Right Oviduct

Vagina

Cloaca

Figure 16 Formation of egg in the reproductive organs of the hen

to the magnum region. It requires about 3 hours to pass through this region. The inner surface of the magnum section of the oviduct is lined with goblet cells that secrete albumen. At this region the yolk acquires the mass of firm white albumen, which make's up about one-half of the total white, by volume. Hens that lay eggs containing a relatively high percentage of thick white have more goblet cells. The thick white percentage tends to decrease from about April to July in most flocks.

Formation of the Shell Membranes

The yolk, surrounded with its thick white, passes from the magnum through a short section of the oviduct known as the isthmus. Here the two shell membranes are added and the shape of the egg is determined. An isthmus of large diameter tends to result in thick round eggs, while one of small diameter tends to result in long slender eggs.

It is an interesting fact that these membranes are so formed as to enclose the yolk and thick white rather loosely. They do not plump out until the egg receives its final quota of white in the uterus.

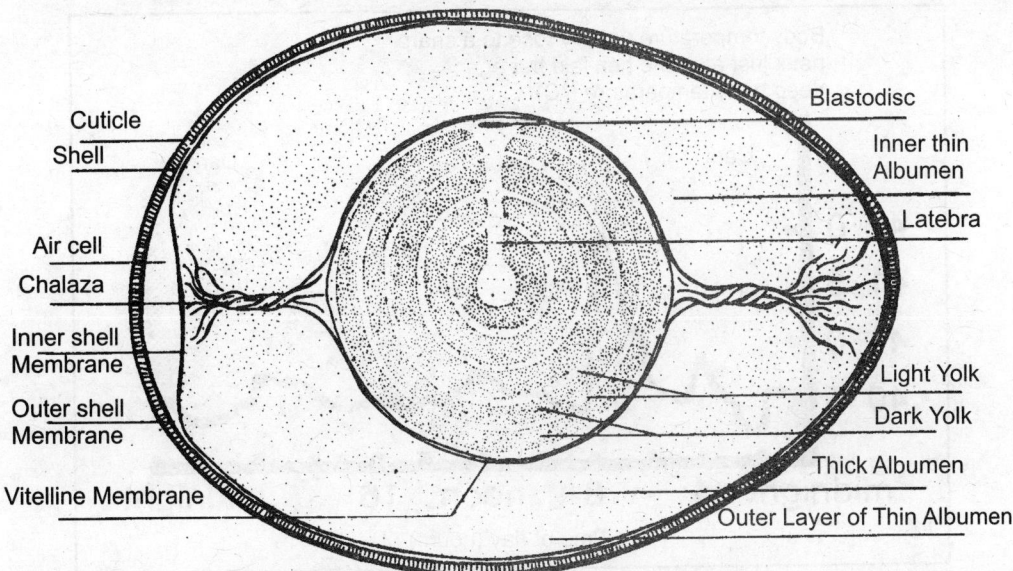

Figure 17 Structural features of the chicken egg

Addition of Thin White and Shell

The developing egg passes from the isthmus into the uterus, where it remains for about 24 hours. The inner layer, between the inner and outer layers of thick white, becomes apparent while the egg is in the uterus as a result of the albumen rotating around the yolk. The thin white, composed of water and a mineral solution consists largely of sodium, calcium and potassium. The inner and outer layers of thin white each comprise about 20-25 per cent of the total white.

In addition to the formation of the inner and outer layers of thin white,, the uterine glands also secrete material for the shell, consisting largely of calcium carbonate. It is carried to the uterus by the blood circulation. It is interesting to note that the calcium of blood is nearly double at the laying stage. High temperature always tends to reduce shell thickness.

Chemical Compositions and Nutritive Value of Eggs

Chemial Compositions of the egg are presented in Table 24 while Table 25 shows the nutritive value of eggs.

Table 24 Chemical Composition of the Egg

	Percent	Water	Protein	Fat	Ash
		(%)	1%)	(%)	(%)
Whole egg	100	65.5	11.8	11.0	11.7
White	58	88.0	11.0	0.2	0.8
Yolk	31	48.0	17.5	32.5	2.0
Shell	11	—	—	—	96.0

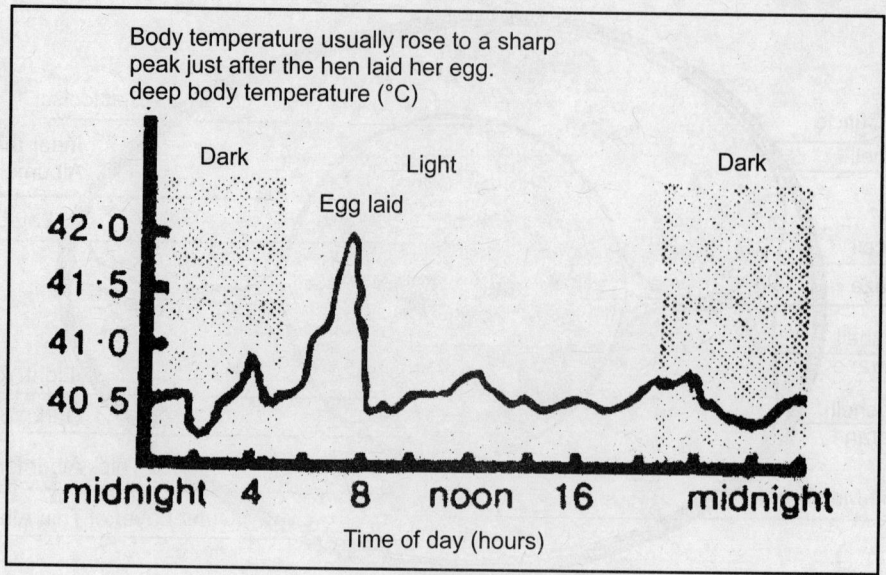

Figure 18   How a laying hen's temperature changes

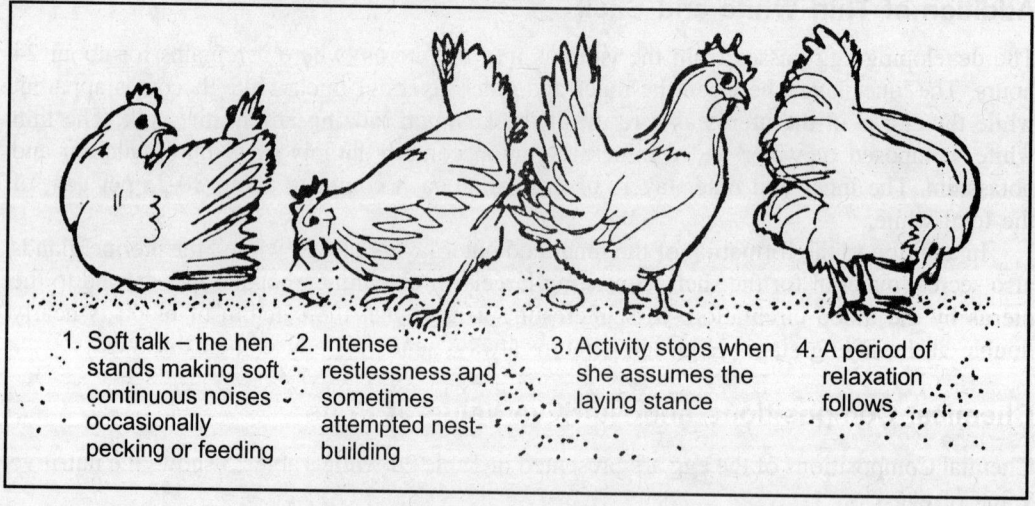

1. Soft talk – the hen stands making soft continuous noises occasionally pecking or feeding

2. Intense restlessness and sometimes attempted nest-building

3. Activity stops when she assumes the laying stance

4. A period of relaxation follows

Figure 19   Typical laying behaviour in a battery hen.

EGG PRODUCING CARRIER OF A LAYING HEN

A laying hen will produce eggs for a number of years, but it is only economical to keep the layers up to the age of their.18 months. Egg production commences at about 22 weeks of age (five and half months), rises sharply, reaching a peak at about 32-35 weeks of age, and then gradually declines at the rate of half a week. It is thus an usual routine practice to replace the layers at the age of their 18 months.

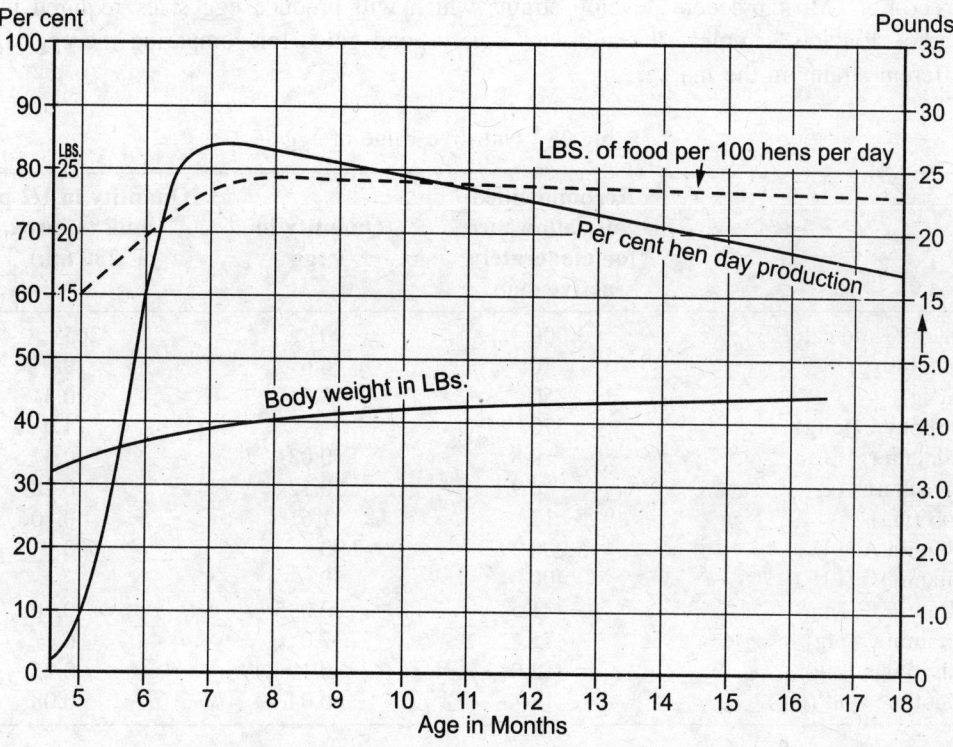

Note the changes in egg production, body weight and feed consumption of Single Comb White Leghorn hens during their production period.

Figure 20 Egg producing carrier of a laying hen

The production cycle may be conveniently divided into three stages (popularly called phases).

Phase I is the period from 22 weeks (age of first laying) of age to 42 weeks of age and during this period the layer is expected to (1) increase in egg production from zero to a peak of approximately 85% production; (2) increase in body weight to attain mature body weights; (3) produce eggs of gradually increasing size from about 36 gms per egg at 22 weeks of age to approximately 58 gms per egg at 42 weeks of age.

Phase II is the period from 43 weeks to 62 weeks of age. Egg production declines upto 65 per cent.

Phase III is the period from 63 weeks upto 72 weeks. The egg production is loss than 65 per cent.

A typical production, body weight and feed consumption curve for a laying flock is snown in Figure 20.

TEN FACTORS AFFECTING EGG SIZE

Breeding. Most breeders develop strains which will produce egg sizes required by the market. Random sample test results are a very good guide for comparing the egg size of different strains in the market.

Table 25 Nutritive value of eggs

	Recommended daily allowance for moderately active man	Quantity in 1 egg	Quantity in 1/2 pint milk (approx. 280 ml.)
Energy (kilo calories)	3,000	90	205
Proteins (g)	70	6.6	9.6
Fat (g)	50	5.5	10.3
Carbohydrate (g)	570	–	14.0
Calcium (g)	0.8	0.03	0.37
Phosphorus (g)	0.9	0.12	0.28
Iron (mg)	12	1.6	0.10
Vitamin A (I.U.)	5,000	600	600
Vitamin D (I.U)	400	50	–
Vitamin B_1 (mg)	1.5	0.095	0.10
Vitamin C (mg)	75	2.0	6
Riboflavin (mg)	2.0	0.19	0.25
Nicotinic acid (mg)	18	0.04	0.08

Feeds. Most rations in the market arc well balanced. However, if an unbalanced stale, or badly mixed feed is given, smaller eggs may result.

Feed restriction. All birds should be able to get food when they want it. Any restriction on feed, whether due to lack of enough feeder space, forgetting to feed the birds or from using stale feed, will lower feed consumption and reduce egg size.

Lack of water. Water that is too hot. too cold or dirty will be unpalatable to the birds– they will not drink enough, food consumption will fall and egg size will suffer. Keep the water fresh and clean and look out for any faulty drinkers supply.

Protein level. Rations containing less than 15 per cent protein are liable to give smaller egg size. Although this is not likely to be a problem with commercially compounded rations, home mixers should keep a careful check on the point.

Laying-house temperature. Experiments have shown that egg size can be less at least by 1 oz. per dozen at temperatures over 70°F than at 55°. It is important, therefore, to keep house as cool as possible during hot weather.

Disease. Most disease will upset the birds, giving decreased feed consumption. This can only lead to lower production and egg size. Good hygiene and management will reduce this risk.

Age of maturity. Birds which mature early, such as those reared during increasing day-length, will lay smaller eggs than birds reared on a constant day length or a decreasing daylength.

Age of birds. Birds at 20 to 26 weeks of age will lay smaller eggs than at 40 to 50 weeks. Maximum egg size can be expected when the birds reach about one year old. Egg size tends to get smaller just before birds stop laying.

Egg cooling and storage. It is important to cool eggs as quickly as possible after they are laid and to store them at a temperature of 50 to 55°F, otherwise they will lose weight by evaporation. This may result in poorer grading results, and so a poorer economic return.

ABNORMAL EGGS

Double-yolked eggs. Such types are due probably from two ova ripening at the same time, or one ovum being pushed back into the oviduct at the same time when another ovulation takes place. The type is more common in pullets than older birds. Probably newly functioning ovary and oviduct takes time to work normally.

Meat spots. Sometimes found either on the yolk or in the white of egg. Spots are generally degenerated blood clots resulting from haemorrhages in the ovary or oviduct.

Blood spots. May be found as a result of haemorrhages of small blood vessel in the ovary or oviduct. The follicle probably does not rupture along the stigma, where there are normally no blood vessels, or else the rupture occurs before ovulation. If the spots are found in the white of the egg, it indicates a haemorrhage in the wall of the oviduct.

Soft shelled eggs. The conditions generally result from the failure of the shell glands to secrete normal composition (may be due to calcium deficiency) or from the peristaltic constrictions becoming so violent as to hurry the egg through the uterus.

Small yolkless eggs. This type of egg is due to the stimulus produced by some foreign substance, such as a blood clot or piece of membrane, gaining entrance into the oviduct and passing along in the same manner as the yolk. The passage of the particle will stimulate the albumen, shell membrane and shell glands to secrete their particular products.

An egg within an egg. After an egg has been formed it may be forced back up to the tunnel region by reverse peristaltic action. As it again passes the oviduct, albumen, shell membranes and shell are added.

Foreign-matter in eggs. Feather, and other foreign-matter, sometimes find their way into the oviduct and become included in the albumen; they pass through the egg formation stages and thus become embodied in the egg.

Pale yolks. These may be caused by constitutional anaemia, but are more likely due to lack of carotene and other colouring substances. Pale yolks usually occur during the winter months, and by increasing the amount of maize or maize meal in the ration, this defect may be rectified.

Rotten new-laid eggs. These are laid by an over-fat hen, a bird with oviduct disease, or one with vent gleet, which has affected the oviduct. The egg, when completely formed, has been unable to pass out of the oviduct on account of one of these reasons and has, therefore, remained bad.

SELECTION AND IMPROVEMENT

Selection, as used in connection with breeding, refers to the choosing of parents for the next generation. Its skilled performance is the foundation of constructive breeding practice. Success in poultry production is just as dependent upon the use of good breeding stock as it is in crop production. A farmer who plants seed with poor yielding ability gets, a poor yield, likewise a poultry breeder who selects poor males and hens for the breeding flock to start poultry farm will definitely run at a loss, no matter, whether good feed, management and disease control practices are adopted.

Therefore, before selecting birds for starting a poultry farm a hasty or hurried decision should be avoided or selection should not be made for sentimental reasons or because of someone having purchased a particular pair of birds from a definite farm running profitably.

Careful selection of birds pays a poultryman in different ways and to get a really good foundation stock, a few basic points noted below may be followed.

1. Number of necessary removals during the laying year is reduced.
2. Culls are eliminated.
3. Average egg production is higher.
4. Profit is greater.
5. Segregation of best birds for breeding purposes is made possible.
6. Appearance of improved flock from the standardisation view-point.
7. Late maturing individuals can be excluded.
8. Production of subsequent generation of higher quality individuals is aided.
9. The spread of disease is retarded through the elimination of diseased individuals.

Selection of individual males and females for breeding may be based on:

1. The past in which the pedigree of the individual examined for several preceding generations.
2. The present in which the appearance or performance of the individual and its sibs (sisters and brothers) is used in making final judgement.
3. The future in which the breeding worth of the individuals is judged by the appearance or performance of its descendants, usually only its sons and daughters.

Two or more of these bases may sometimes be used in combination, especially the second and third. The constructive breeder attempts by selecting individuals which are pure for certain desirable genes and through intelligent mating, to assemble in new individuals still more desirable combination of genes.

Pedigree Selection

A good individual with a good ancestry is preferable to an equally good individual with a poor ancestry, but it should be emphasised that a good ancestry only improves the chances for better breeding performance and is no guarantee for such performance.

Since genes and chromosomes occur in pairs and are halved for any individual in each generation, it is immediately apparent that a particular remote ancestor can have very little influence on the genetic make-up of an individual which is considered in selection.

Pedigree selection is of value in a broad sense in that one would certainly choose a breeding cockerel whose dam had laid 250 eggs in preference to one whose record was only 150. But one should also remember that two cockerels from the 250 eggs hen may give widely differing performance as measured by the egg production of their daughters. Furthermore, a difference between 250 eggs and 150 eggs in a dam's record may be important in selection, whereas a difference between 275 and 250, or even between 300 and 250 would seem negligible.

Appearance and Performance

Vigour.   Good health or vigour is the first prerequisite qualification in a bird to be used for breeding purposes. This is evident by its behaviour and body characteristics.

Birds with good vigour are active and take an interest in things going on around them. They walk, run, fly, scratch, sing, cackle or crow, and show sex interest.

They have a broad, long, deep body, with a good capacity for handling feed and producing eggs.

The head gives a good indication of the health of the bird. Rice said,—"The bird carries its health certificate on top of its head". This refers to the comb. A large bright red comb indicates good vigour, while a small, pale or dark comb indicates low vitality or disease condition.

Breed type.   Birds to be maintained as breeders should be representative of the breed and variety to which they belong. A variety is a sub-division of a breed used to distinguish groups of the same breed as fowls differing in colour of plumage, shape of comb, and other characteristics.

Head.   The appearance of the head is variable because of differences in size, shape and expression. Hens with coarse, phlegmatic, masculine, or "beefy" heads are not likely to lay many eggs. Those with clear-cut rugged, alert heads that are at the same time fine in quality, arc likely to be among the best layers in the flock.

Eye.   A good individual should have bright, prominent, well-placed eyes. They should not be depressed nor show evidence of physical debility. The so-called "pearly" eye and the retraced pupil are commonly associated with fowl paralysis.

Beak.   The beak should be relatively short, strong, well-curved and in proportion to the head of the bird. The mandibles should meet properly and not overlap each other nor be deformed in any other manner. Such deformities are likely to interfere with the food consumption of the bird and consequently with the production.

Face. The face of the individual should be clean-cut and lean, yet should not present a pinched-in appearance. If (in facing the front of the bird's head) the face of the fowl is narrow and the eyes appear to be closed, it is undesirable and is usually an indication of low vitality.

The comb and wattles should be of reasonable size, well placed and fine in texture. A smooth, velvety feel indicates good texture.

Condition of comb, vent and abdomen. With some simple practice it has become a minor matter to distinguish a layer from a non-layer. This can be done by closely examining the following parts of the bird.

(a) *Comb:* The comb is a secondary sexual character. It tells us what is going on in the ovary. If the comb is dry, hard and scaly, the hen may still be laying but she will soon stop.

If the hen has been out of laying but the ovaries are expanded and she is coming back into production, the comb indicates the fact. It begins to swell; the blood rushes to the tips of the points, and they become hot, soft, waxy, brighter in colour and fall.

The comb is reddest and hottest just before laying commences. As soon as laying starts, the comb gradually cools and becomes somewhat lighter in colour.

(b) *Pubic bones:* When a bird is laying, the pubic bones–the two small bones extending along the sides of the body towards the vent are spread apart to such an extent that 2 or 3 fingers can be placed between them. During non-laying period the pubic bones become thin and pliable. In a poor-layer, the pubic bones are close together and can barely accommodate one finger space between them.

(c) *Vent:* When a hen is laying heavily the vent is greatly stretched during the exclusion of egg. It is, therefore, much larger than when she is not laying. During laying period it is oval in shape, pliable and moist.

(d) *Abdomen:* When the bird is laying heavily the abdomen is much larger than at other times. The intestines and oviduct are expanded in the laying hen because they are distended and stretched by larger quantities of food and by egg. It has also been found that the heart, gizzard, crop, etc., are much larger than in a poor layer. The skin covering the abdomen is soft and pliable. Usually 3 or 4 fingers are accommodated between the end of the keel and the ends of the pubic bones. The abdomen is constricted, the skin becomes thick and the space between the end of the pubic bones and of the keel shortens in case of non- layers

Body conformation. To lay a large number of eggs a bird should have a good body with the following characteristics:

1. A flat, broad back that carries well but towards the pubic bones.
2. A wide heart girth.
3. Good depth of body that increases towards the abdomen in a bird in laying condition
4. Good span between the pubic bones and keel bones.
5. Thin, straight pubic bones set well apart.
6. Good quality of skin.

7. Body wedge-shaped from back to keel bone.
8. Legs set well apart.
9. Good fleshing in all parts of the body.
10. Reasonably long keel bone.
11. A widespread of lateral processes.

Proportionate Measurements

Body measurements should be considered from the standpoint of their relationship to the size of the individual. A bird of the Asiatic or American class, for instance, may actually have large body measurements than one of the Mediterranean class, but in proportion to the size of the individuals, the former may have a much smaller proportionate capacity and consequently be a poorer producer. Each breed should be judged on the basis of the characteristic breed size. A bird should be well proportioned and have skeletal development consistent with its size.

Quality. Quality is devoted by the character of the bird, as evidenced by the examination of the shanks, keel and pubic bones. The bone formation should be sufficiently rugged for the size of the individual but should not tend towards coarseness. The shanks should appear wedge-shaped. Rounded shanks are not good. The pubic bones should be pliable, pointed and thin when bird is in production. The keel should be sufficiently long to support the abdomen and should be refined in nature.

The skin should be loose, pliable and of velvety quality.

Plumage is sometimes used as an index in selection. This is particularly possible when the hen is nearing the end of her laying year, at this time the feathers of a high producer are usually brittle, rough, broken and soiled, whereas normally in such birds, due to the pliability of the skin the feathering is generally loose.

Pigmentation

This also gives some information regarding a bird's past production, in case of hens having yellow skin and shanks. During the period of production, the yellow xanthophyl pigment in the feed eaten is used for colouring the yolks and the body gradually loses its reserve supply of yellow pigment. The order of disappearance of pigment from the body and the approximate period of egg production required to bleach the body structures are follows:

Vent	1–2 weeks
Eye rings and Ear lobes	2–4 weeks
Beak	6–8 weeks
Shanks	12–20 weeks

The pigment first leaves those structures having the best blood circulation. When a bird stops production, the pigment return in the same order it left and approximately twice as fast.

Moulting

Moulting is the act or process of shedding and renewing feathers. The shedding and renewal of feathers normally occurs once a year, though it may occur in certain individuals twice in a year and more rarely, only once in a period of two years. Hens usually moult in the following order: (1) head, (2) neck, (3) body (including breast, back and abdomen), wing and tail. Not only this, but there is a high degree of regularity about the order of moult within the several sections. The wing primaries, for example, begin to drop before the secondaries. The first primary to be shed is the inside one, next to the axial feather, and the remainder are shed in succession until the last one to be dropped is the outermost primary near the tip of the wing.

Birds inherit the tendency to shed their plumage annually. An early moulter, under normal conditions, is a poor layer. A late moulter, under normal conditions, is a good layer. The nature of moulting both at the starting time and its duration should be considered while judging a bird's laying ability.

Hens seldom lay and shed feathers at the same time. A high producing bird may, for a short time, moult and lay simultaneously; but usually she sheds more rapidly, and is declining in production when moulting begins. When her wing feathers commence to drop, it is a sign that she is nearly or quite through laying. The fact that a hen sheds rapidly though early, stamps her as being better than the common early moulter that sheds slowly. Presumably, a hen does not stop laying because she moults, but rather moults or stops laying because her physical condition is such that she cannot support egg prpduction and continue nourishment of the feathers.

In general it may be said that there are three kinds of moulters in the birds hatched during the usual spring season: early, medium and late.

1. *Early moulter.* The bird ceasing to lay in June, July or early August, shows that she has a short laying period, that she probably started late and lacks the vitality, laying capacity, or inherited tendency to discontinue.
   The early moulter sheds and grows feathers so gradually that a person may not observe the process unless the bird is handled. She seldom completes her moult in less than 3 or 4 months. She then rests for a short time and frequently does not get back into production for some time. In brief, she takes a longer vacation and should be culled.

2. *Medium moulter.* Birds moulting late August or September are termed medium moulters. If artificial illumination is to be used, birds moulting in September may be segregated, allowed to recuperate under favourable conditions for renewing their plumage and recovering their body weight, and placed under lights in October. If after about 4 weeks of non-laying the birds are to be kept for another year they may be culled.

3. *Late moulter.* A hen moulting in October or later is termed a late moulter. The feathers are dropped rapidly, and in a short time the plumage appears rough. There may be a few old feathers clinging to the bird, and her body will soon be covered with pin feathers. Hens are rarely seen during July or August in this ragged condition. While moulting, the late moulter is quite timid and dislikes to be handled. This is due to active circulation and sensitive nerve development in the feather follicles while new plumage is being grown. At this time the slightest touch hurts the bird.

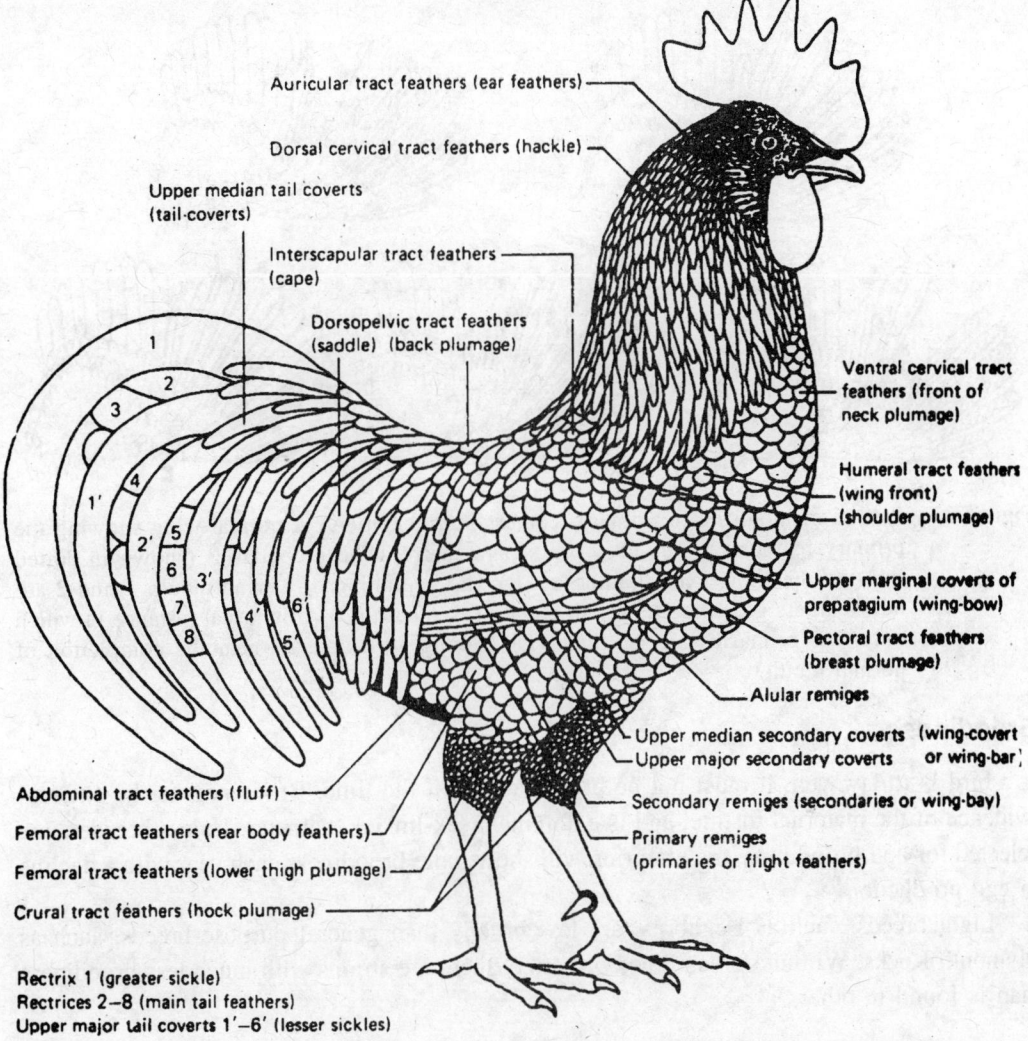

Figure 21 Feather coat of the male single comb white Leghorn chicken – right lateral view.

The feathers grow in rapidly, as soon as the moult is over and most of the birds are back in production as early moulters. Such a moult indicates that the bird has high vitality and therefore usually is a superior producer. Pattern of moulting in primary feathers in chicken is presented in Figure 22 while Figure 21 shows the feather coat of a male single comb White Leghorn chicken.

Temperament

A good layer is more active, more alert, and yet at the same time more easily handled than a poor layer. She is among the first off the perch in the morning among the last on it at night. When not on the nest she is busy and business-like, scratching or ranging in an eager search for food. The appetite of a great layer is seldom satisfied.

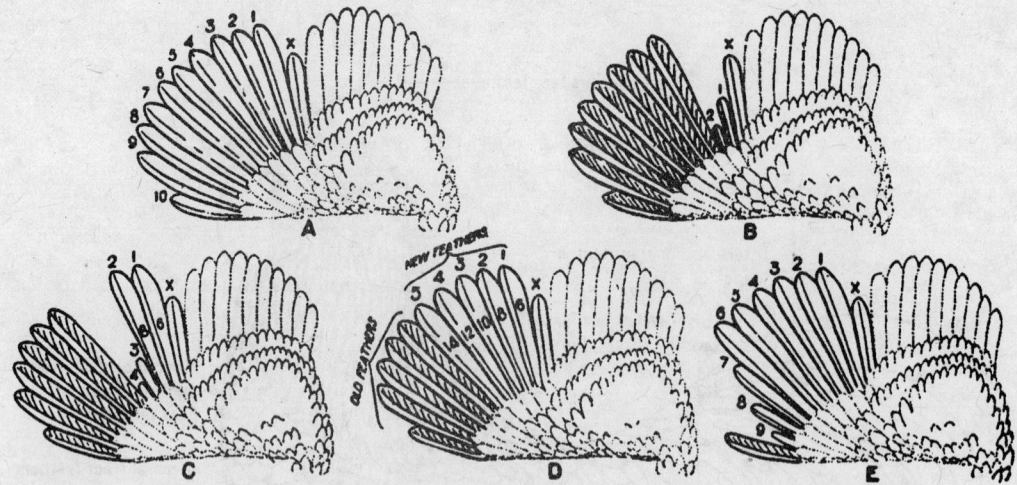

Figure 22 Pattern of moulting in primary feathers in chicken (A) A normal wing showing the primary feathers, 1–10. They are separated from the secondaries (shown in dotted line) by the short axial feather, x. (B) The beginning of a wing moult. 1 and 2 are new feathers growing in. (C) An eight week moult. (D) An unusual instance in which only five primaries are moulted. (E) A wing as it appears near the completion of normal moult.

Broodiness

If a bird is to lay well, it must not be broody much of the time. Broodiness is the external evidence of the maternal instinct and is a dominant sex-linked character. Unless breeders are selected for non-broodiness, the offspring will show more broodiness each year with a decline in egg production.

Light breeds, such as Leghorns, are less broody than general purpose breeds, such as Plymouth Rocks. Within a given breed or variety there are strains with much less broodiness than is found in others.

Precosity or Sexual Maturity

By sexual maturity is meant the number of days between the date a pullet is hatched and the date she lays her first egg. Early sexual maturity is determined by at least two dominant genes; one is autosomal and the other is sex linked, although probably other genes are involved.

Pullets hatched during February. March and April are of two types regarding sexual maturity. Those hatched early, i.e., in February and the beginning of March are definitely better than those hatched in the latter part of this period. It has been suggested that this difference is associated with the relative length of dayiight.

Females for breeding purposes shouid be selected on the basis of their earliness of sexual maturity as that of their dams and their sisters.

Persistency

Implies that a bird continues to lay well toward the close of her first laying year. Length of laying during a year is influenced not only at the beginning of the first egg laid, but also at the end of the period the last egg is laid. The tendency to continue laying eggs up to a longer time say up to the next winter is known as persistency and it has much the same effect at the end of the year as early maturity does at the beginning.

Lack of persistency is easily determined, as a rule, by the beginning of an early moult. Some hens moult as early as June and others as late as, December, so that it is easily possible to have a difference of one hundred and eighty days of a laying year on account of this one factor.

The common practice of culling laying flocks in late summer is based on the fact that persistency is highly correlated with total annual egg production. Culling out the early moulters automatically removes many of the low producers from the flock.

Trapnest Records

From all considerations trapnesting is the only means of obtaining a definite check on the productivity of an individual. It also provides the opportunity to study egg size, colour, texture and shape and production intensity and persistency. Naturally, it gives a material index for use in the selection of birds. Many poultrymen have a tendency to pay considerable attention to "trapnesting records" and not enough to physical make-up. A wise procedure is to first select the birds according to handling qualities and then resort to the trapnest for conformation of the selection. Neither method of selection is as efficient as the combination of both.

Progeny Test

Family and progeny records are essential in breeding for improvement in characters of low heritability such as egg production, hatchability and viability. The final and most valuable test for a breeder is the kind of progeny that it produces. It is not, how many eggs a hen lays that counts, but the number her daughters will lay. If a bird is to be valued as a breeder, it must be able to transmit desirable characters to its offspring. The progeny test is also used for the purpose of distinguishing between individuals which are homozygous and those which are heterozygous for some simple character such as rose comb and white skin colour.

It is highly important to select sires of superior breeding value because the average sire has about ten times as many chicks as the average dam.

The breeding programme should be bared on the selection of outstanding families.

CULLING FOR BETTER PROFITS

Birds which do not perform well are culled to optimize profits. Culling is practised on the basis of outward appearance or available records. Culling on the basis of stunted growth and physical deformity do not pose any problem. Culling for poor production or non-production requires handling of the flock thereby causing a drop in production, so it should be practised in the night.

Culling on the basis of moulting

Moulting which refers to the shedding of feathers provides some indication about the laying capacity of a bird. Good layers not only moult late but also complete the moulting period quickly and sometimes continue to lay even during moulting. Poor layers on the other hand moult early, take a long time to complete the process and do not lay any eggs during the moulting period. It is possible to determine the beginning of moulting by counting the stiff primary feathers in the wing. The first one to be dropped is the inner one next to the axial feather which separates the primaries from the secondaries. It takes about 6-weeks for the first new primary feather and 2 weeks for each additional full-grown feather. A wing having 4 new primaries during moulting season indicates that the bird has been in moulting for 12 weeks.

Culling from outward appearance

The appearance of a bird though not an index of its laying ability, gives an idea about its health and vigour. The main characteristics for distinguishing a layer from a non-layer are given below:

Table 26 Guide for selection and culling layers

	Character	Good layer: keep	Poor layer: cull
I.	**Vigour**	Strong	Weak, unthrifty
II.	**Breed type**	Wedge shape body	Shallow and tendency towards rocker keel
III.	**Head**	Neat, refined	Beefy, crow head
	1. Comb and Wattles	Full, red, waxy, warm and velvety	Very long, thin and sharp pointed
	2. Eyes	Full bright, alert	Dull, sleepy
	3. Beak	Stocky, well curved	Very long, thin and sharp pointed
	4. Ear lobes	Full waxy and velvety	Shrunked and coarse
IV.	**Neck**	Stocky, rather short	Long and thin
V.	**Body**	Capacious	Limited capacity
	1. Back	Broad and straight	Narrow and crooked
	2. Sides	Deep, straight	Shallow, barrel-shaped
	3. Keel bone	Long and properly curved	Short and crooked
	4. Pelvic bones	Wide apart, thin	Close together, thick
	5. Skin	Thin, soft, oily	Thick, dry, rough
	6. Abdomen	Large, soft, free from fat	Small, hard, with thick fat
	7. Vent	Full, larger and moist	Small, dry
	8. Feathers	Warm and soiled	Clean and perfect
VI.	**Legs**	Wide apart, well-set	Close together, knock-kneed
	1. Shanks	Thin and soft in back	Full, hard and round in the back
	2. Toe nails	Stocky, well curved	Long, thin
VII.	**Temperament**	Alert, active, friendiy	Shy, nervous, quacky
VIII.	**Moult**	Late and rapid	Early and slow

Figure 23 shows the selection of a good layer based on the measurement of pelvic bone.

Culling on the basis of pigmentation

Yellow pigmentation of the skin surface especially vent, eye rings, ear lobes, beak, shanks, etc. of a hen provide an indication about its laying ability. Yellow pigmentation of the skin, especially in yellow skinned breeds like White Leghorn and Rhode Island Red, is because of carotenoid pigment known as xanthophylls from the ration containing yellow maize. Birds in lay lose their pigments and the exposed parts present a bleached appearance. Vent loses the pigment earliest as compared to other parts. A white or pink vent in yellow-skinned variety is an indication that the bird is laying. The inner edges of the eye-lids lose their yellow pigment more slowly than the vent. The ear lobes in the Mediterranean breeds lose their pigment even more slowly. The beak is next to lose colour, starting at the base and gradually extending to the tip. Normally the beak loses its colour 4 to 6 weeks after heavy laying. The shanks are the last to lose their colour. The appearance of bleached shanks indicates that a bird has been laying at a good rate for the last 3 to 4 months. When a bird stops laying the yellow pigment reappears in the same order as it disappeared and comes back twice as fast. The approximate period for which a bird has been in production may be judged from the disappearance of yellow pigment from different parts of body in the following order: vent, 1 to 2 weeks; eye rings and ear lobes, 2 to 4 weeks; beak, 6 to 8 weeks; and shanks, 12 to 20 weeks.

HATCHING THE EGGS

The process of hatching, by which, in the span of 21 days, a microscopic germ is changed into a downy chick, capable of walking, eating and expressing its needs by its voice and actions seems nearly magical. With such rapid development and change within the egg, great care must be exercised to provide correct conditions if a good percentage of strong chicks is to be hatched. No detail should be overlooked in giving the eggs every chance to hatch, and each chick a chance to live, since upon their ability to do this may rest the success or failure of the poultry enterprise. Let this problem be discussed starting from the selection of hatching eggs.

Selection and Care of Hatching Eggs

1. **Egg size.** The size of the eggs used for hatching is important because there is a high correlation between the size of eggs used and the size of the chicks hatched. Neither small sized egg nor very big sized egg should be selected. It is always desirable to select eggs approximately 58 gm each. Eggs in which the proportion of white to yolk is about 2:1 usually hatch better than eggs having wider or narrow ratios. The yolk portion is rich in carotene, hence a growth promoting substance is always desirable. Abnormal shaped egg should always be discarded.

2. **Shell colour.** In case of varieties of chickens that lay white shelled eggs, all eggs used for incubation should be free from tints, except for the first few tinted eggs laid at sexual maturity.

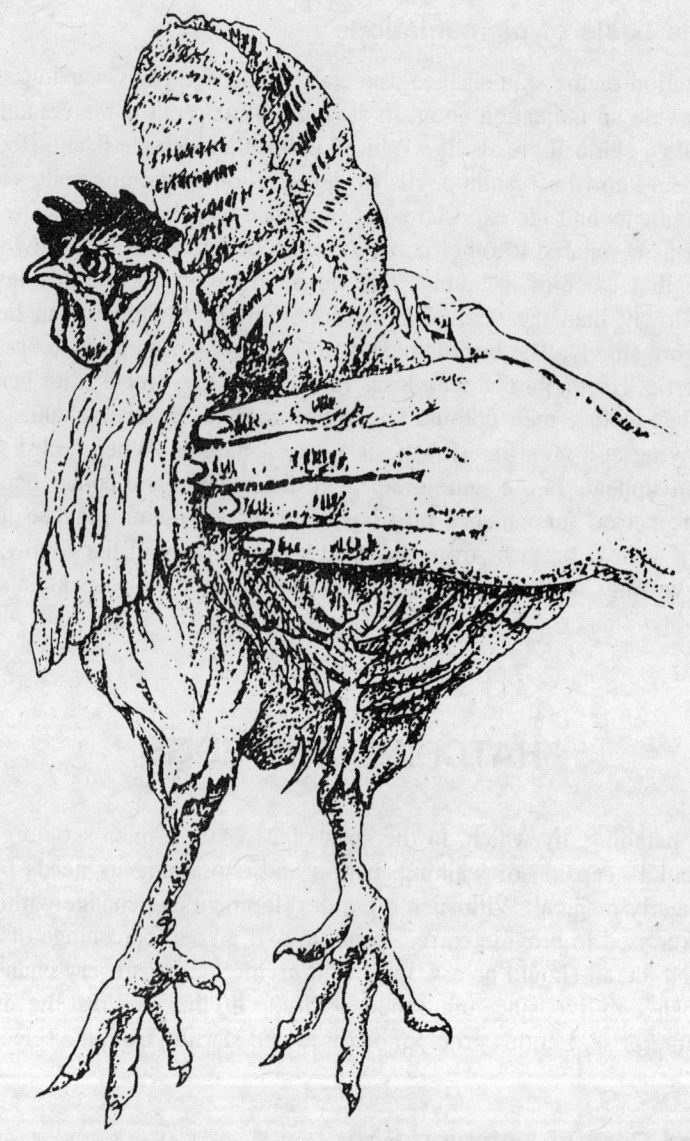

Figure 23 Selection of good layer, which permits four fingers to be placed between the pelvic bone and the end of the breast bone in a hen in full lay.

For brown coloured eggs, medium and dark brown eggs hatch better than light brown eggs.

3. **Shell texture.**   When shell texture is poor due to deficiency of calcium or vitamin D the result, of course, is associated with low hatchability, otherwise the mottled appearance of the egg shell as observed by candling does not appear to be related to hatching results.

4. **Cracked shells.**   All eggs should be tested for cracked shells, and this can be done quite readily by tapping two eggs together. If there is a resonant sound, both eggs are sound in shell; but if there is dull sound, one of the eggs is cracked and should not be used for incubation.

5. **Tremulous air cells.**   Care should be taken in shipping or delivering eggs to a hatchery to avoid excessive shaking which sometimes results in a condition known as "tremulous air cells", a condition that tends to lower hatchability.

6. **Soiled egg.**   Soiled eggs should not be washed in water before setting, as washing with water opens up the pores and this interferes with the hatching results. If the dirt is not excessive, it should be removed with a knife. Highly soiled eggs should not be set.

7. **Age of egg.**   In hot weather, eggs should not be kept for more than 3 days but in winter they may be kept for 7 to 10 days.

8. **Turning.**   Turning eggs is not necessary if they are not held longer than one week during the storage period.

Always collect the hatching eggs from the best birds where good, strong and healthy males are used for mating.

The Best Time to Start Hatching

The best time to raise chickens altogether depends upon the climate in which the chickens are to be raised.

July, August and September are the most favourable months for raising chickens in Punjab, U.P. and Madhya Pradesh because of (1) low rainfall, (2) suitable room temperature. Before July the heat is very great and after September the winter is too much. Both the conditions are unfavourable for chickens.

In places like Simla, Nainital, Mussoorie, Darjeeling, Assam and where ever the cold is severe during the cold season and moisty air during the rain, March, April, May and June are the favourable months for raising chickens.

In West Bengal and all other places of India where there are no westerly hot winds, chickens can be raised most successfully from October to end of March.

Natural Hatching

Natural hatching or hatching of eggs by hen is a primitive but most effective method to get a high percentage of success. It is particularly claimed that the hen is more to be trusted and consequently some breeders trust special sittings of egg which are to produce future stock cockerels.

Selection of the hatching hen.   Pullets are not recommended for this purpose. The ordinary *deshi* hen is ideal for hatching chickens as she is a close sitter, and owing to her light weight, there is little possibility of eggs being broken.

The hen should be thoroughly broody. A broody hen can be recognised by her constant determination to sit in her nest. The hen must be in perfect health, and have all her feathers on her. Hens in moult should always be rejected.

The hen should be thoroughly dusted with a good insecticide, such as gammaxane or sodium fluoride. A further dusting ten days later will ensure its complete freedom from lice and ticks.

Sometimes hens will lay several eggs during natural hatching. Every egg placed under a hen should be marked distinctly so that if any eggs are laid in the nest may be detected and removed.

Best time to set hen. The best time to set a hen is at night, as at this time she is more likely to settle down to her job. Besides, when eggs are put under the hen at night, the chickens are more likely to appear on the night of the 21st day, and will have the whole night to rest and gain strength.

The nest. The nest on which the hen is placed must be made in a quiet corner because she will not be disturbed. An earthen pot, about 15 inches in diameter and 8 inches in depth be filled three-quarters with earth or ashes. Over the earth a fine, soft hay, straw or leaves are placed, and the latter pressed down to make a hollow. A quantity of flours of sulphur or an insecticide powder is sprinkled over the nest, and after the eggs have been placed on the hollow, the hen is gently seated on them and left undisturbed.

Apart from an earthen pot any other vessels of wood or tin, etc., of any specification can be made use of on the same principles. Great care should be taken to provide a nest just large enough for the hen to properly sit in. The nest must not be too large, or else the eggs will roll away from under the hen and become chilled and spoiled.

A sitting hen must not be kept in a damp, dirty, draughty or badly ventilated place.

Care of sitting hens. Before putting the hen on the eggs she must be placed under a basket and fed and watered; a plentiful supply of good grain must be given. It is a good plan to set a hen on half a dozen dummy eggs, and allow her to sit and settle down for 2 or 3 days. By this way the hen will acquire all the qualities of broodiness and then the dummy eggs should be removed and the good eggs are placed under her.

The sitting birds should receive clean water twice daily and adequate amount of whole grains and limestone grit. Sloppy foods of all description should be avoided as they tend to produce loose droppings and consequent soiling of the eggs.

Hens ought to come off their eggs at least once every day. The temporary change from the cramped position is good for the hen and the exposure to the fresh air gently benefits the eggs. If the hen does not come off her nest, she may have to be lifted off the eggs.

It becomes important to see that she gets her food and a little exercise at the same time of the day. She should be allowed to go back to her nest after about 20 minutes.

Care of the hatching eggs. Some breeders insist that the eggs should be laid on their sides which aids the foster mother to turn the eggs regularly every day. Eggs should be placed about 1¼" apart.

After the eggs have been placed under the hen, all that needs to be done is to inspect them every day to see that they are all right.

When the weather is very hot and dry it may be necessary to sprinkle warm water of 102°F over the eggs in order to give moisture. In West Bengal it is generally not necessary due to normal humidity.

It is a sound practice to sprinkle flours of sulphur over the nests and eggs just a day or two before the chickens appear.

Rats often are a nuisance as they steel eggs from under the hens. The only remedy is to keep the hen with her eggs in a box with a good strong bottom and ½" mesh wire-netting sides.

Infertile and addled eggs are generally examined from the nest after the 7th or 10th day of sitting. For this purpose there are different methods of testing, of which candling of eggs (Figure 24) is the most common. If the egg is perfectly transparent, like a new-laid egg, it is infertile; but if a small dark body is seen floating about the centre of the egg, it contains a chicken. After 21 days, if the egg has a partly-formed chicken in it, or is rotten, then it is addled. If the chicken is fully formed and is dead in the shell, it is spoiled. If the germ has formed in the egg and not hatched, it is fertile, but has been addled or spoiled by some cause, for which the eggs may be to blame.

The other method of testing fertile good eggs is as follows:

On the 19th or 20th day of hatching fill a large bowl with hot water (exactly at 102°F), place the testing eggs in the water. After a minute the fertile eggs containing live chickens will wriggle in the water; this is caused by the chickens endeavouring to make escape from the shells. The infertile and addled eggs will float about, but will not wriggle.

The eggs must be allowed to remain only one minute in the water, and then taken out. properly dried and put back under the hen.

Number of eggs under a hen. The size of the hen and the state of the weather must decide the number of eggs to be placed under her. It is better to place a few. Small country hens should have only 6 eggs in the warm weather and 4 in the cold weather. Under no condition should the number of hatching eggs exceed 7 or 8 under a country hen.

Artificial Incubation

Improvement in the design and construction of incubators, have made artificial incubation so reliable that machines have largely, and on most farms completely, replaced broody hens. Incubators can be roughly classified as: (a) hot water radiation from pipes in the egg chamber; (b) hot air infusion, or warm air pouring directly into the egg chamber; (c) forced-draft, where the air is driven by fans or agitated by paddles. Out of these hot air flat type and hot air mammoths are very common and are discussed below:

Hot Air Flat Type Incubators

The flat type incubator is usually of small capacity, ranging from 50-500 eggs. Full instructions about their use are supplied with the machines, and these instructions are to be followed very strictly. In general fresh air enters get warmed by the hot air tubes at the side of the machine, and as it cools, sinks towards the floor and escapes by the vent or openings at lower levels. Figure 25 illustrates a typical flat type of incubator, heated by oil lamp attached to the side of the incubator. The eggs rest on wire bottomed trays fitted some 6-8 inches below the

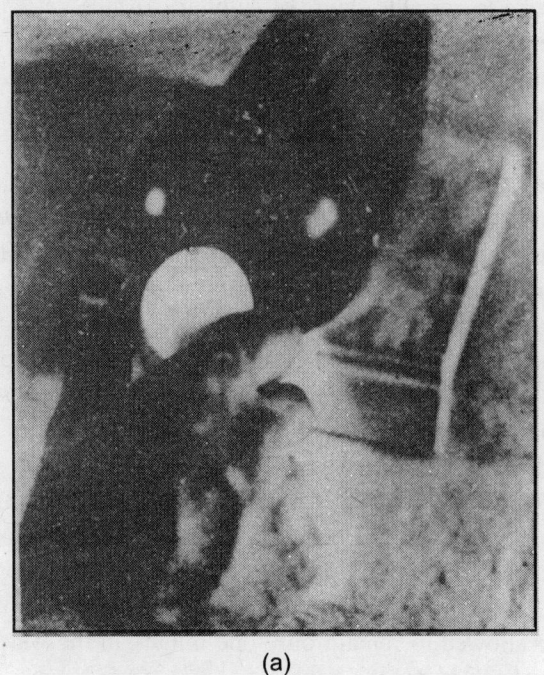

(a)

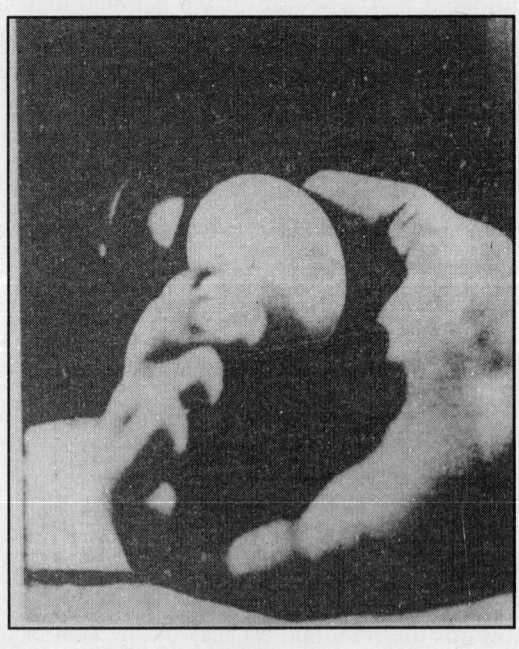

(b)

Figure 24 Hand candling of eggs: (a) Egg placed at candling light with palm of hand down. (b) Hand turned with a snap of the wrist to cause egg contents to move within the shell.

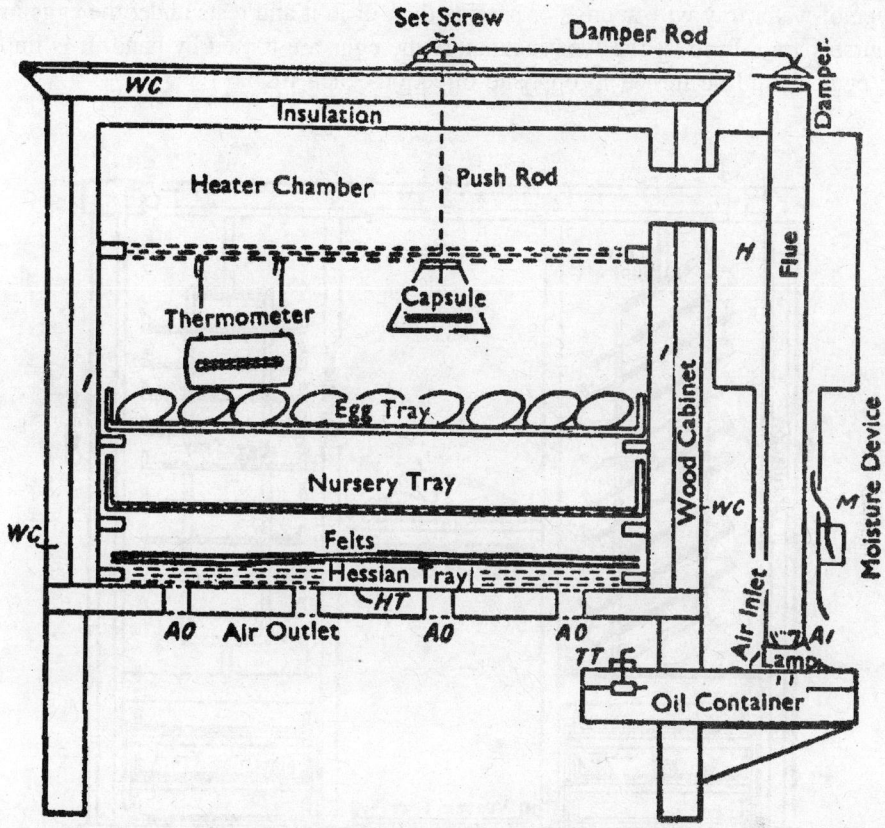

Figure 25 Hot Air Incubator. WC = Wood carbinet; H = hot air; AO = air outlet.

hessian of the heating chambers. Under this tray is another tray, this having a floor of hessian, and is known as the nursery tray. Most of the machines of this type have a glass window fitted to the front of the hatching egg tray. The tray itself is especially made short, so that when pushed fully back there is a space of two inches between its front edge and the front of the machine, the idea being that the dried chicks, being attracted by the light, come forward to the window and fall through to the cooler and less crowded nursery tray below. The heat regulating principle in these incubators is simple. When the temperature of the incubator rises above the level to which it is previously adjusted, the capsule (made up of two thin metal sheets welded together containing small amount of ether) expands and forces the push rod upwards, and this in turn lifts the damper off the exhaust flue, but as soon as the inside temperature falls below the required point, the damper closes down and all the heat goes into the incubator. In this incubator only one thermometer is necessary. To provide the necessary moisture, one type of machine has a trough fitted with a wick which enters the double wall of the lamp flue, and in evaporation charges the heating and rising air with extra moisture. Some have two small troughs which slide into fitments attached to the two inner side walls of the egg compartment and are filled with warmed water about hatching time. Others fit a small type of water tray with sponge or hessian over or in it and rests under the eggs in place of the nursery tray. In most flat type incubators the eggs are turned by hand. It is important that the eggs should be turned in opposite directions each time.

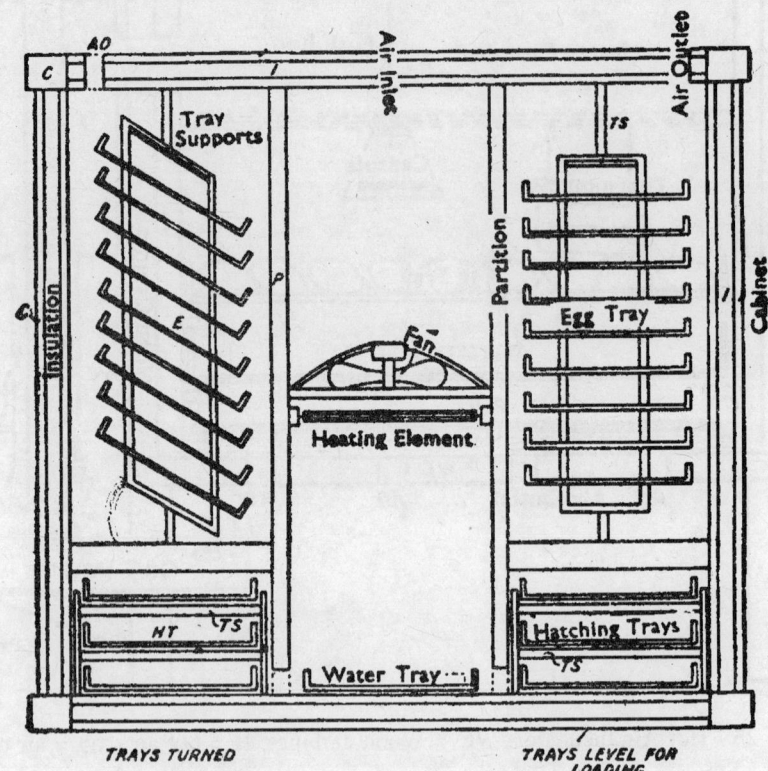

LEFT SECTION WITH TRAYS TIPPED IN TURNED POSITION RIGHT SECTION WITH TRAYS LEVEL FOR LOADING

AO = air outlet; HT = hatching tray; E = egg tray; C = cabinet.

Figure 26   Cabinet incubator

Hot Air Mammoths

The chief difference between these machines aud the flat type are; (1) the eggs are placed in the upright position with the broad end upper-most; (2) the eggs are turned by tilting the trays through 40-45° each side of the horizontal, and (3) the ventilation and internal -air circulation are mechanically controlled by some arrangement of fans. In this case the heat is controlled by a thermostat, which either cuts in or out with the heater unit, and is set at a quarter degree each way. Should the machine rise a quarter degree above the setting, then the heat is turned off and when it drops to a quarter degree the setting, then it cuts in again, thus the incubator

Table 27 Artificial Incubation Requirements for Birds Eggs

Forced-air Incubator Requirements	Chicken	Turkey	Duck	Muscovy Duck	Goose	Guinea Fowl	Pheasant	Peafowl	Coturnix Quail
Incubation period (days)	21	28	28	35-37	28-34	28	23-28	28-30	17
Temperature (degrees C/F, dry bulb)	37.6 99.75	37.4 99.25	37.5 99.5	37.5 99.5	37.4 99.25	37.6 99.75	37.6 99.75	37.4 99.25	37.4 99.25
Humidity (degrees C/F, wet bulb)	29.4-30.6 85-87	28.3-29.4 83-85	28.9-30 84-86	28.9-30 84-86	30.0-31.1 86-88	28.3-29.4 83-85	30.0-31.1 86-88	28.3-29.4 83-85	28.9-30 84-86
Do not turn eggs after	19th day	25th day	25th day	31st day	25th day	25th day	21st day	25th day	15th day
Temperature during last 3 days of incubation (degrees C/F, dry bulb)	37.2 99.0	36.9 98.5	37.1 98.75	37.1 98.75	36.9 98.5	37.2 99.0	37.2 99.0	36.9 98.5	37.2 99.0
Humidity during last 3 days of incubation (degrees C/F, wet bulb)	32.2-34.4 90-94	32.2-34.4 90-94	32.2-34.4 90-94	32.2-34.4 90-94	32.2-34.4 90-94	32.2-34.4 90-94	33.3-35.0 92-95	32.2-34.4 90-94	32.2-34.4 90-94

[1]For still-air incubators add 1–2°C. (2–3°F) to the recommended operating temperatures.

steadily runs to a half degree. The methods of turning the eggs vary with the make of machines some by a wheel attachment at the side and some by a lever, but they all result in the egg tray, which during the period of incubation is tilted at an angle.

MANAGEMENT OF INCUBATORS DURING INCUBATION

1. **Levelling of the incubator.** Levelling may be accomplished by the use of a spirit-level and if the level is not even, the damper rod will not function normally thus will affect the temperature regulation of the incubator.

2. **Sanitation and fumigation.** (1) Sweep the compartment and brush out all fluff and debris. Also clean out the incubator room and when all clearing up has been completed, spray the floor with disinfectant. (2) Scrub the egg trays, carrier-rack and the water trays with disinfectant. Reassemble them and leave them outside the machine for a short time to air. (3) Replace the rack and trays in the compartment. (4) For routine fumigation add about 50 cc of 40% formaldehyde to 25-30 grams of potassium permanganate crystals into an enamel basin near the fan to ensure even distribution. The above quantities are required for 100 cubic feet of incubator capacity.

3. **Regulating incubator.** A trial run of the incubator at the beginning of each hatching season, regardless of the incubator new or old is a must. The thermometer should be checked comparing with a standard thermometer. The wick of the lamp should be new, of sufficient length to last during the incubation period. The thermostat should be regulated according to the manufacturer's instructions, and the machine operated at a temperature of 103°F are at least 24 hours to make sure that the machine is alright.

4. **Placing eggs.** Arrange the eggs in egg tray in rows either on their sides in the case of flat type incubators or upright, with the broad end up in cabinet-type machines.

5. **Regulating temperature.** For flat type incubators the temperature will depend upon the design of the incubator and the height of the thermometer bulb above the eggs. Most satisfactory results are secured with a temperature of 101°F during the first week followed by 102°F during the second week and 103°F during the 3rd week of incubation.

6. **Sufficient ventilation.** When the amount of CO_2 in the air exceeds 2 per cent, the hatchability of eggs decreased rapidly. On the 21st day of incubation about 140 to 150 times as much air is required as on the first day. This emphasises the need for good ventilation and particularly the necessity of keeping the ventilation outlets well opened during the later stages of incubation.

7. **Turning of eggs.** Best hatching results are obtained when the broad end of the eggs is kept uppermost. Eggs should be turned daily, starting with the third day of incubation. The number of turning during the early stages of incubation should be 4 to 6 times daily. After about a week the number of turnings may be regulated at 8 hours equal

interval. Cease turning after 18th day. The object of turning the egg is to prevent the embryo sticking to the shell membrane.

8. **Testing eggs.** Incubated eggs should be tested (candled) on the 7th and 14th day as explained under 'natural hatching'. The infertile eggs may be sorted, hard boiled and later ground up as part of chicken ration.

9. **Care during hatching.** Care of the hatching eggs (sprinkling flours of sulphur, egg testing, etc.) from the day of setting upto 18th day may be taken as same with that as described under natural hatching. On the 19th day the nursery tray should be placed. A good hatch is that when the chicks are out of their shells before the end of 21st day. As activity increased with the pipping of the shells, the temperature is likely to run very high, and the moisture too low. It is of no use to assist a chick to come out of its shell as usually in such cases the chick becomes weak or crippled. The chicks which have hatched should remain in the incubator without any feed for at least 18 to 24 hours. After drying off and fluffed out, the temperature should be gradually reduced to 93° to 95°F for "hardening off" the chicks before transferring them to the brooder.

Artificial incubation requirements for bird's eggs have been presented in Table 27 while Table 28 represents the important events in embryonic development. Successive changes in the position of chick embryo and its embryonic membranes are presented in Figure 27.

Causes of Poor Hatches and "Dead in the Shell"

Poor hatches may be the result of unhealthy stock, incorrect mating, or breeders fed on a deficient ration. Inefficient operation is a major cause of poor hatches, and points to watch are as follows:

1. **Preparation.** Before eggs are set, the machine should be run for a few days to check for temperature variations and general performance. Have on hand spare capsules, the thermometers, mercury tubes, micro switch and an element. Organise these matters in the off season.

2. **Age of eggs.** It has been observed that preserved eggs at 55°F to 60°F give better results only for one week, after this the percentage of hatchability will decrease if eggs are stored beyond 7 days to the extent of 10% for each subsequent day.

3. **Turning of eggs.** The eggs should not be roughly shaken, particularly in the delicate early stages. Turning should be 2 to 3 times during 24 hours up to about 17th day. On 18th day onwards there should not be any turning.

4. **Time of turning.** Turning should take place at night and morning, at the same time each day.

5. **Infertile eggs.** Causes of infertile eggs are as follows:
   (a) Insufficient or too many hens per male bird
   (b) Underfed males
   (c) Lice-infested males
   (d) Eggs held too long
   (e) Over fat hens

    (f) Cross-mating of a light and heavy breed

    (g) Cold conditions early in the season

    (h) Very inbred lines

6. **Moisture Control.** A thick wick in the wet-bulb thermometer will give a lower temperature than required, and a thin wick that becomes hard will give too high a reading. Inefficient wicks can be a major cause of poor hatches.

7. **Control of ventilators.** Ventilators should be neither closed right up to hold humidity nor opened too much to reduce it. Instead the control should be carried out by reducing or increasing the surface area of water in the trays. Insufficient ventilation can cause many "dead in the shell".

8. **Air circulation speed.** Too slow a circulation will result in hot and cold places in the machine, and too high a speed will mean excessive drying out of the eggs. Check the recommendations for the type of machine. If pulleys are replaced on the incubator see that they are of the correct size.

9. **Malformed or crippled chickens.** Excessive low or high temperatures are the principal cause of these, and another cause is incorrect turning of eggs wrong way up in the trays.

10. **Thermometers.** Thermometers should be tested before each hatch. A rough check is to take one's own temperature in the mouth if the reading is 98.4° F the thermometer will be a good one. A thermometer reading with a 2° inaccuracy, particularly if it is 2° under the correct temperature, could cause almost a complete failure in electric forced draught machines.

11. **Dead in shell.** If death in shell comes in early stage (3 to 5 days), insufficient turning, incorrect fumigation, or incorrect temperature could be the cause. If death in shell has occurred between 12 and 14 days, suspect excess moisture in the early stages, general condition of the breeding stock, or incorrect feeding such as insufficient riboflavin in the feed. If death in shell has occurred in the last stage (18-21 days), temperature, humidity or ventilation have not been right. Other causes could be rough handling in transfer or chilling through a delay in the process of transfer or due to failure of electric supply.

12. **Weak and small chickens.** Weak chickens can result from over heating, small chickens from small eggs or insufficient moisture. Chickens breathing heavily may be affected by disease or by too much moisture. Musty chickens often result from low temperatures or insufficient ventilation.

BROODING AND REARING

Systems of Brooding

Brooding units are designed to house chicks from one-day old until they no longer need supplementary heat (0-8 weeks). *Growing pens* are used from the end of the brooding period

Table 28 Important events in embryonic development

Stage or Period	What Takes Place
Before egg laying	Fertilization, division, and growth of living cells, segregation of cells into groups of special function
Between laying and Incubation	No growth: stage of inactive embryonic life
During Incubation:	
First day:	
16 hours	First sign of resemblance to a chick embryo
18 hours	Appearance of alimentary tract
20 hours	Appearance of vertebral column
21 hours	Beginning of formation of nervous system
22 hours	Beginning of formation of head
23 hours	Appearance of blood islands—vitelline circulation
24 hours	Beginning of formation of eye
Second day:	
25 hours	Beginning of formation of heart
35 hours	Beginning of formation of ear
42 hours	Heart begins to beat
Third day:	
50 hours	Beginning of formation of amnion
60 hours	Beginning of formation of nasal structure
62 hours	Beginning of formation of legs
64 hours	Beginning of formation of wings
70 hours	Beginning of formation of allantois
Fourth day	Beginning of formation of tongue
Fifth day	Beginning of formation of reproductive organs and differentiation of sex
Sixth day	Beginning of formation of beak and egg-tooth
Eighth day	Beginning of formation of feathers
Tenth day	Beginning of hardening of beak
Thirteenth day	Appearance of scales and claws
Fourteenth day	Embryo turns its head toward the blunt end of egg
Sixteenth day	Scales, claws, and beak becoming firm and horny
Seventeenth day	Beak turns toward air cell
Nineteenth day	Yolk sac begins to enter body cavity
Twentieth day	Yolk sac completely drawn into body cavity; embryo occupies practically all the space within the egg except the air cell
Twenty-first day	Hatching of chick

until the broilers are sold or the pullets moved into permanent laying houses (upto 20 weeks).

Laying pens or cages are used for pullets and hens from the time they start to lay until they are culled and sold at the end of the laying period (upto 78-80 weeks).

There are two general systems of brooding: (1) natural method, and (2) artificial method.

In deciding on the method of brooding to use, it must be remembered that if artificial methods of incubation have been practised, then artificial methods of brooding should follow.

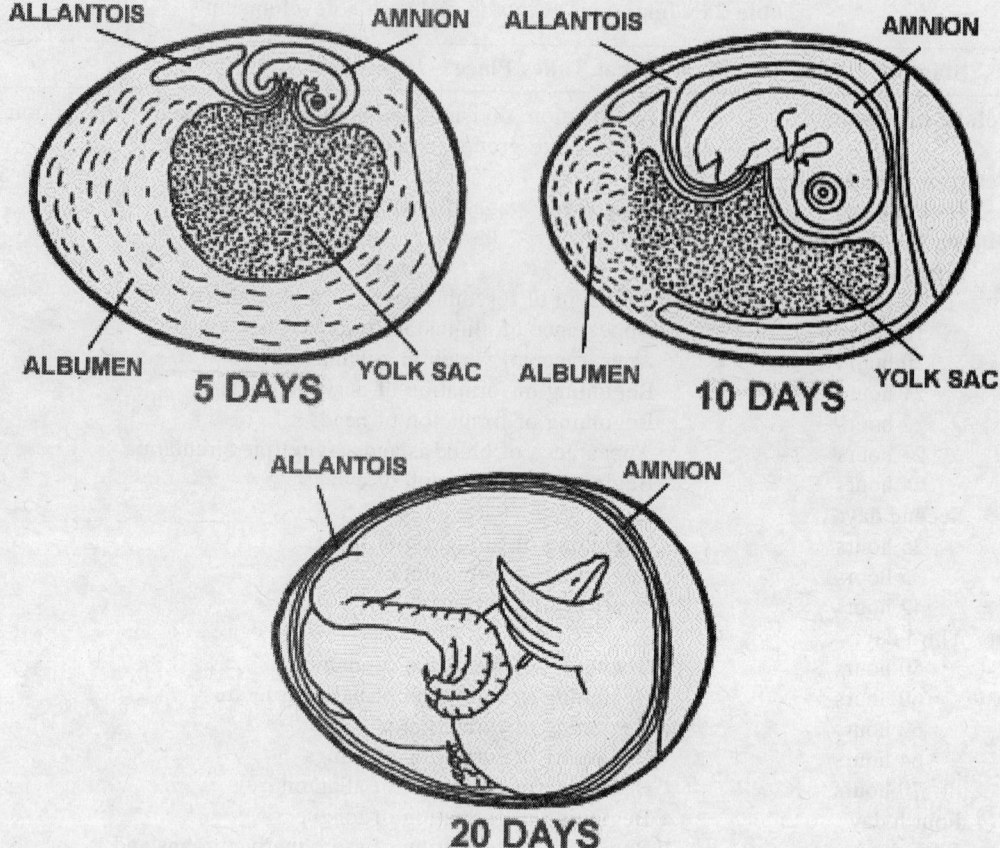

Figure 27 Successive changes in the position of the chicks embryo and its embryonic membranes.

Natural Brooding

Natural brooding once the only method used in brooding chicks, has been quite largely replaced by artificial method. The natural method is used on farms where only few chickens are raised each year. *Deshi* hens as a class are ideal mothers as they possess a strongly developed maternal instinct, moreover, because of their small structure they seldom injure the young chicks by trampling on them. Expending upon her size, a hen will brood 15-20 chickens. The broody hen will provide all the warmth required by the chicks. Before placing the chicks with the hen she should be examined for her good health and free from lice, etc.

Rearing coop. A rearing coop is made up of packing box material which is about 2 feet square, sloping down from front to back, say about 2 feet height in front and 18 inches at the back. The essential requirements of such a coop are dryness, durability, ventilation, cheapness, roominess and safety. Wire enclosed runways are a desirable attachment for brooding coops.

Food for chicks and mother. For the first week, it is advisable to give small quantities of feed frequently, perhaps every two hours; this should consist of a chick mash, mixed with water or milk to a crumbly consistency, and this at first may be given on a board, in or close to the coop.

The hen must not be neglected and she should have a suitable wet or dry balanced growers mash. Care must be taken to see that the feed for the hen is so arranged that the chicks do not get access to it. Clean water must always be available for hen and chicks.

Other managerial practices. The cage should be cleaned and sprayed regularly to hold mites and similar pests under control. Wire netting of suitable mesh should cover the top of the run and the floor of the coop to prevent damage from rats, cats, owls and other predatory animals. During the first week vaccination against Marek's and Ranikhet disease should be provided. Debeaking during the first week is desirable. At the age of 6-8 weeks vaccination should be done to prevent fowl pox and Ranikhet diseases.

Movement of coop and rua. Frequent moving of the coop along with its run to a fresh site will prevent out-break of disease and parasitic infestation. It is also desirable to let the chicks and broody hen in the sun for a short time once or twice a day.

Artificial Brooding

Artificial brooding is the handling of newly born chicks without the aid of hen. It is accomplished by means of a temperature controlled brooder (rearer or foster mother). Artificial brooding has several advantages over the natural method, namely: (1) chicks may be reared at any time of the seasons ; (2) thousands of chicks may be brooded by a single person; (3) sanitary condition may be controlled; (4) temperature may be regulated; and (5) feeding may be undertaken according to plan.

Requirements of floor space, brooder temperature and water space have been presented in Table 29 while Figure 28 and 29 show the distribution of the chicks within the brooder and typical brooder equipment set up respectively.

Table 29 Floor space, temperature and water space for chicks in Artificial Brooder

Age	Floor space	Brooder temperature	Water space
First week	100 to 120 sq. cms. per chick	95°F	Start on shallow pans to avoid crowding, use 4 waterers per brooder.
2-4 weeks	250 to 300 sq. cms. per chick	90°F ... 2nd wk. 85°F ... 3rd wk. 80°F ... 4th wk.	Provide 4-6 waterers of 3 litre capacity per brooder. Fill waterer at least twice daily.
5-8 weeks	700-800 sq. cms. per chick	80°F	Use water trough with adjustable stands. Keep waterers at chicks' shoulder level, 2 cm. space per chick.

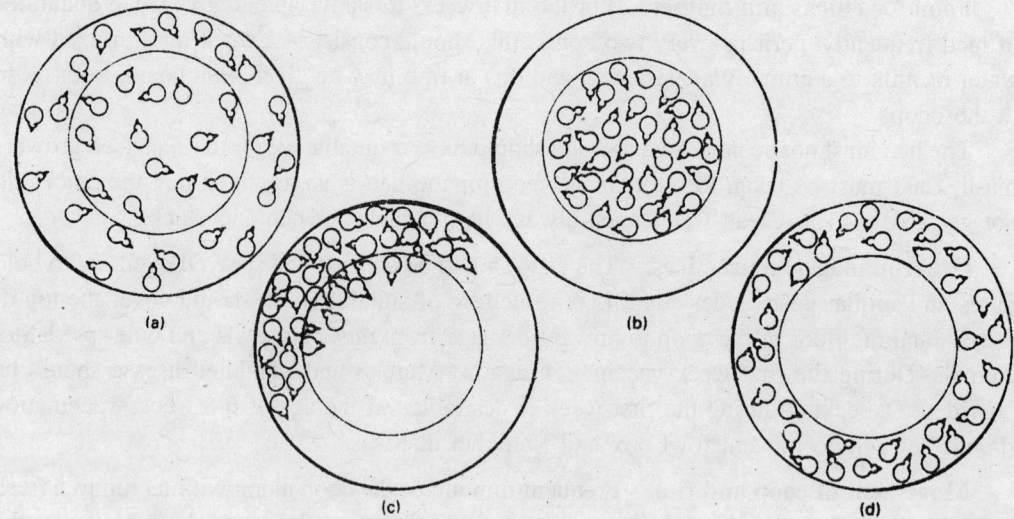

Figure 28 Distribution of the chicks within the brooder indicates their comfort : (a) satisfactory (b) too cold (c) draft; (d) too warm.

There are many types, styles and sizes of brooder units on the market that employ a variety of fuels. The equipment usually is rated by the manufacturer according to the number of chicks that may be started under each unit. The essentials of a good brooder are: a dependable mechanism for controlling temperature and regular supply of fresh air, dryness, adequate light, space, easy disinfection, protection against chick enemies, safety from fire, and economy in construction. For heating such brooders, use of coal, kerosine oil, gas, electricity are used depending upon the availability of such materials and the capacity of the poultrymen. From the point of temperature regulation, electricity is the best. Basket brooders and brooders from packing cases are very popular where small number of chicks are raised. For large number of chicks, battery brooders of multiple tiers having adjustable feeding and water trough with thermostatically heat regulating mechanism are very common now-a-days.

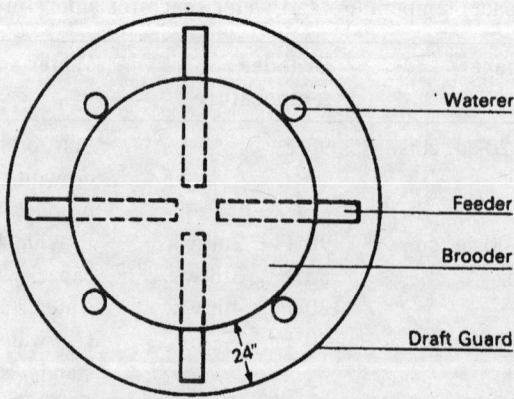

Figure 29 Typical brooder equipment setup

MANAGEMENT OF CHICKS IN THE BROODER

1. Adjust the temperature as per requirement of the chicks. In case of oil heating, see that there is no defect in the stove or lamp. Chicks should not get access in heated parts of the lamp at any cost.
2. Avoid a damp poultry house; in case of dampness, however, a deep litter can solve the problem.
3. Discourage litter eating by the chicks, scatter mash over egg case flats when the chicks are first taken out of their boxes. Keep chick hoppers filled. Provide balanced standard mash.
4. Keep provision for the entrance of fresh air.
5. Chicks may be taught to roost when they are from 4-6 weeks old. Early roosting will help to reduce over crowding and prevent litter borne infections.
6. Provide clean, fresh water in front of the birds at least twice daily.
7. Chicks, after 3 weeks old may be provided chopped green grasses.
8. Clean the brooders including feed hoppers daily.
9. Follow a regular vaccination programme.
10. Avoid overcrowding as this will lead slow growth and mortality.
11. Keep the brooder in such a place that cold wind and rain does not get in.
12. Daily inspect the condition of birds and their faces for any sort of abnormality. Keep in touch with any veterinarian for the help at the time of need.
13. It is always advisable to check the fittings, temperature control, feed and water trough arrangement before shifting the chicks in the brooder.

HOUSING AND EQUIPMENT

Need for Poultry Housing

The chicken as a wild jungle fowl, sought safety and rest on the high limbs of a tree or in the thick underbush. The jungle served for protection against the hot sunlight. Nature's object, with poultry is to cause the hen to reproduce herself and to maintain the race to which she belongs on the basis of survival of the fittest. On such natural conditions of wild state they lay very few eggs, and these only in the spring of the year.

But under modern conditions, the hen is required to lay many eggs throughout the year, and this object can best be achieved if a comfortable shed is provided for them. So, in conclusion, we can say that poultry is housed for comfort, protection, efficient production and convenience of the poultry man.

Essential of Good Housing

Comfort. The best egg production is secured from birds that are comfortable and happy. To be comfortable a house must provide adequate accommodation; be reasonably cool in summer, free from drafts and sufficiently warm during the winter; provide adequate supply of fresh air and sunshine; and remain always dry. Given these the hen responds excellently.

Protection. Includes safeguards against theft and attack from natural enemies of the birds such as the fox, dog, cat, kite, crow, snake, etc. The birds also should be protected against external parasites like ticks, lice and mites.

Convenience. The house should be located at a convenient place, and the equipment so arranged as to allow cleaning and other necessary operations as required.

Location of Poultry House

In planning a poultry house, the location should be taken into consideration. In selecting site for poultry houses, the following factors should be considered.

1. **Relation to other building.** The poultry house should not be close to the home as to create unsanitary conditions. On the other hand, it should not be too far away either because this will require more time in going to and for in caring for the birds. In general at least three trips should be made daily to the poultry house in feeding, watering, gathering the eggs, etc.

2. **Exposure.** The poultry house should face south or east in moist localities. A southern exposure permits more sunlight in the house than any of the other possible exposures. An eastern exposure is almost as good as a southern one. Birds prefer morning sunlight to that of the afternoon. The birds are more active in the morning and will spend more time in the sunlight.

3. **Soil and drainage.** If possible the poultry house should be placed on a sloping hillside rather than a hilltop or in the bottom of a valley. A sloping hillside provides good drainage and affords some protection.

   The type of soil is important if the birds are to be given a range. A fertile well drained soil is desired. This will be a sandy loam rather than a heavy clay soil. A fertile soil will grow good vegetation which is one of the main reasons for providing range.

   If the poultry house is located on flat poorly drained soil, the yards should be tiled, othere wise, the birds should be kept in total confinement.

4. **Shade and protection.** Shade and protection of the poultry house are just as desirable as for the home. Trees serve as a windbreak in the winter and for shade in the summer. They should be tall, with no low limbs. Low shrubbery is no good as in their presence the soil becomes contaminated under the shrubbery, remains damp, and sunlight cannot reach it to destroy the disease germs. One thing should be remembered that plenty of sun shine should be available at the site.

Housing Requirements

Floor space. The smaller the house the more square feet are required for each hen. Bigger pens have more actual usable floor space per bird than smaller pens. The recommendations as suggested might be useful regarding floor, feeders and watering space (Tables 30, 31 and 32 respectively).

For economic production of laying hens it is always better to keep them in small units of 15 to 25 birds This number can go up to a maximum limit of 250 birds. In commercial poultry farms, units of 125 or so are advisable. Where there is a long house, partitioning at every 20 feet should be made to eliminate drafts, etc.

Ventilation.   Ventilation in the poultry house is necessary to provide the birds with fresh air and to carry off moisture. Since the fowl is a small animal with a rapid metabolism, its air requirements per unit of body is high in comparison with that of other animals. A hen weighing 2 kg and on full feed, produces about 52 litres of CO_2 every 24 hours. Since CO_2 content of expired air is about 3.5 per cent, total air breathed amounts to 0.5 litre per kg live weight per minute,

A house that is a tall enough for the attendant to move around comfortably will supply far more air space than will be required by the birds that can be accommodated in the given floor space.

Temperature.   Hens need a moderate temperature of 50°F to 70°F. Birds need a warmer temperature at night, when they are inactive, than during the day. The use of insulation with straw pack or other materials not only keeps the house warmer during the winter months but cooler during the summer months. Cross ventilation also aids in keeping the house comfort-'ble during hot weather.

Dryness.   Absolute dry conditions inside a poultry house is always an ideal condition. Dampness causes discomfort to the birds and also gives rise to diseases like colds, pneumonia, etc. Dampness in poultry house is caused by: (1) moisture rising through the floor; (2) leaky roofs or walls; (3) rain or snow entering through the windows; (4) leaky water containers; (5) exhalation of birds.

Table 30   Floor space requirement per bird

S. No.	Age (weeks)	Floor space per bird (cm^2)	
		Light breeds	**Heavy breeds**
1	0 to 8	700 minimum	700 minimum
2	9 to 12	950 minimum	950 minimum
3	13 to 20	1900 minimum	2350 minimum
4	21 and above	2300 to 2800	2800 to 3700

Table 31   Feeder space requirement per bird

S. No.	Age (weeks)	Feeder space per bird (linear cm.) Minimum
1	0 to 2	2.5
2	3 to 6	4.0
3	7 to 12	7.5
4	13 and above	10.0

Table 32 Watering space requirement per 100 birds

S. No.	Age (weeks)	Watering- space, minimum	
		Running length of channel type of trough (cms).	Capacity of fountain type of trough (litres).
1	0-2	25	9.0
2	3-12	100	18.0
3	13 and above	250	22.5

Light

Records show that light always stimulates egg production in all birds and chicken is no exception. They usually seek or build nests, mate and lay eggs as day length increases after winter, but during winter when day length is at minimum, they cease egg production, molt and regrow feathers. Man has taken the advantage of this phenomenon and with electric lights, given the layers a condition of perpetual spring, the result is year round egg production.

Initially, it was thought that due to light, birds remain more active and consume more feed and hence more egg or meat production. Today, the action of light is further considered physiological; light enters the eye of the bird and sends a message to the brain through optical nerves. The brain takes the information and coordinates it with its memory of the light that it has received in the past. It then stimulates the pituitary gland which releases certain hormones necessary for ovulation. The process is not spontenious but requires couple of hours for completion of the job upto egg laying.

Principle of Lighting

(i) The basic principle underlying the process of lighting is that increasing day length advances sexual maturity and decreasing day length delays it.

(ii) When birds mature earlier than usual (precocious maturity), due to an inappropriate rearing light pattern, will tend to result in a depressed rate of lay and also reduced egg size because of low point-of-lay body weight.

(iii) Best target for maturity is probably the average age of maturity for particular strain. Late maturity will result in depressed rate of lay, but larger eggs.

(iv) Light affects both the growing birds upto 3 to 4 weeks of age and layers. The rays of light not only act by way of the eye, but also penetrates the skull and appears to exert a direct effect on pituitary for release of gonadotrophic hormones. Growers between 4-20 weeks do not require extra light.

(v) Under natural sunlight, hormonal secretions are activated once the total length of the light day reaches 11 to 12 hours, as in spring (February to March). During winter (December to January), the length of the light day is not normally long enough to make for maximum egg production.

Light requirements

About 10 lux (one ft. candle) is normally considered enough for production. This can be obtained by mounting 40 watts bulbs at a height of 7 feet, with a distance of 10 feet. Although further increases in intensity result in slight further increase in production, pecking problems arise and electricity costs go up.

Chickens do not respond to all wave lengths of light. Orange and red lights are most effective. Normal white incandescent bulbs will also serve the purpose.

Blue light minimises the activity of the birds and thus are used in broiler farm during the night when broilers are ready for market and removed by individual catching process.

Lighting schedule for egg production

(a) 0-3 weeks : Brooding light-24 hrs./day to provide additional heat.

(b) 4-20 weeks : Growth period; No additional light is necessary.

(c) After 20 weeks : Give 1 hour light in addition to the day light, i.e. 6 p.m. to 7 p.m. during 20th week. Then increase the lighting period at the rate of 30 minutes for every week till it reaches a total of 17 (sun light + artificial light) hours of light per 24 hours.

Sanitations. The worst enemies of the birds, i.e., lice, ticks, fleas and mites are abundant in poultry houses. They not only transmit diseases but also retard growth and laying capacity. The design of the house should be such which admits easy cleaning and spraying. There should be minimum cracks and crevices. Angle irons for the frame and cement asbestos or metal sheets for the roof and walls are ideal construction materials, as they permit effective disinfection of the house. When wood is to be used, every piece should be treated with coaltar, creosote, or similar strong insecticides before being fitted.

Many a times, different disinfectants are used in the poultry farm for various purposes. To have some knowledge about the most commonly used disinfectants, few information are provided at Table 33 as disinfectant guide.

Styles of Poultry Houses

The style of the poultry house makes little difference as long as the birds are provided. There are several styles of poultry houses with reference to types of roofs.

Shed types. They are the simplest of poultry house and by far the most useful and practical type of house that can be used under different climatic conditions and for different systems of poultry keeping. The slope of the roof needs only be slight in the plains, while in the hills where snowfall is heavy or in heavy rainfall, it ought to be sufficiently steep. The shed-roof types of houses may be either portable or stationary. The portable house is generally a small one, not exceeding 8' × 6' while the stationary types can be made of any dimensions.

Gable type. This type requires more material and labour for construction. Some poultry-men put a ceiling floor in gable roof houses and use the space in the gable for storage. The type is more suitable in rainfall areas. Here, again gable type may be stationary or portable.

Table 33 Disinfectant Guide

Kind of Disinfectant	Usefulness	Strength	Limitations and Comments
Alcohol (elhyl-ethanol, isopropyl, methanol)	Primarily as skin disinfectants and tor emergency purposes on instruments	70% alcohol–the content usually found in rubbing alcohol	They aro too costly for general disinfection. They are ineffective against bacterial spores
Boric acid[1]	As a wash for eyes and other sensitive parts of the body	1 or in 1 pt water (about 6% solution)	It is a weak antiseptic. It may cause harm to the nervous system if absorbed into the body in large amounts. For this and other reasons, antibiotic solutions and saline solutions are fast replacing it.
Chlorines (sodium hypochlorite chlormine-T)	Used (1) for egg dipping and washing, (2) in processing plants and (3) for sanitising poultry drinking water. Chlorines will kill all kinds of bacteria, fungi, and viruses, providing the concentration is sufficiently high	Generally used at aboul 200 ppm for disinfection and 50 ppm for sanitizing	They are corrosive to metals and neutralized by organic materials. Not effective against TB organisms and spores.
Cresols (many commercial products available)	Recommended for disinfecting houses, equipment, and footbaths. Cresols in fuel oil are the best disinfectants for dirt floors. Effective against tuberculosis and the red mite.	Cresol is usually used as a 2 to 4% solution (1 cup to 2 gal of water makes a 4% solution) Cresols can be incorporated in water, kerosene, or fuel oil	Cannot be used where odor may be absorbed
Formaldeh (may be used as a gas or as a liquid)	Effective against viruses, bacteria, and fungi. It is often used fo disinfect buildings following a disease outbreak.	As a liquid disinfectant, it is usually used as a 1 to 2% solution. As a gaseous disinfectant (fumigant), use 1½ lb	It has a disagreeable odor, destroys living tissue, and can be extremely poisonous. The bactericidal effectiveness of the gas is dependent upon having the

Table 33 (Continued)

Kind of Disinfectant	Usefulness	Strength	Limitations and Comments
	It is commonly used in fumigating hatchery eggs, prior to and during incubation	potassium permanganate plus 3 pt of formaldehyde. Also, gas may be released by heating paraformaldehyde.	proper relative humidity (above 75%) and temperature (about 70°F)
Heat (by steam, hot water, burning or boiling)	In the burning of rubbish or articles of litter, bag and in disposing of infectd body discharges. The steam "Jenny" is effective for disinfection (example poultry equipment) if properly employed, particularly if used in conjunction with a phenolic germicide	10 minutes' exposure to boiling water is usually sufficient	Exposure to boiling water will destroy all ordinary disease germs but sometimes fails to kill the spores of such diseases as anthrax and tetanus. Moist heat is preferred to dry heat, and steam under pressure is the most effective Heat may be impractical or too expensive.
Iodlne[1] (tincture)	Extensively used as skin disinfectant, for minor cuts and bruises	Generally used as tincture of iodine, either 2% or 7%	Never cover with a bandage. Clean skin before applying iodine. It is corrosive to metals.
Iodophor ("tamed" iodine)	Effective against all bacteria (both Gram-negative and Gram-positive), fungi. and most viruses Used for (1) egg dipping, (2) hatchery or poultry house disinfection, and (3) sanitizing processing plants, footbaths, and poultry drinking water	Usually used as disinfectants at concentrations of 50 to 75 ppm titratable iodine, and as sanitizers at levels of 12.5 to 25 ppm. At 12.5 ppm titratable iodine, they can be used as an antiseptic in drinking water	They are inhibited in their activity by organic matter. They are quite expensive When the characteristic iodine color fades, effectiveness is gone.
Lime (quicklime, burnt lime, calcium oxide)	As a deodorant when sprinkled on manure and animal discharges, or as a disinfectant when sprin-kled on the floor or used as a newly made "milk of lime" or as a whitewash.	Use as a dust, as "milk of lime," or as a whitewash, but use fresh	Not effective against spores Wear goggles when adding water to quicklime

Table 33 (Continued)

Kind of Disinfectant	Usefulness	Strength	Limitations and Comments
Lye (sodium hydroxide, caustic soda)	On concrete floors	Lye is usually used as either a 2% or 5% solution.	Damages fabrics, aluminum, and painted surfaces. Be careful, for it will burn the hands and face. Not effective against organism of TB. Lye solution are most effective when used hot Diluted vinegar can be used to neutralize lye
Lysol (the brand name of a product of cresol plus soap)	For disinfecting surgical instru -ments Useful as a skin disinfectant and for use on the hands before Surgery	0.5 to 2.0%	Has a disagreeable odor Does not mix well with hard water Less costly than phenol
Phenol (carbolic acid) 1. Phenolics—coal -tar derivatives 2. Synthetic phenols	Commonly used for (1) egg dipping, (2) disinfection of hatcheries, poultry houses, and equipments, and (3) footbath solutions Effective against bacteria and fungi	Both phenolics (coaltar) and synthetic phenols vary widely in efficacy from one compound to another. So, note and follow manufacturer's directions. Generally used at 100 ppm for disinfecting and 50 ppm for sanitizing.	Organic materials have a diluting effect, but do not inactivate them Ineffective against viruses
Quaternary Ammonium Compounds (QAC) "quats"	Effective against bacteria and fungi. Used for (1) egg washing and dipping, (2) disinfecting hatch- eries, poultry houses, and equipments, and (3) sanitizing poultry drinking water	For sanitizing, use 200 ppm. For disinfecting, use 400 to 800 ppm.	They can corrode metal. Adversely affected by organic matter Not very potent in combatting viruses Not effective against TB organisms and spores Inactivated by soaps, calcium, magnesium, iron, and aluminum salts

Table 33 (Continued)

Kind of Disinfectant	Usefulness	Strength	Limitations and Comments
Sal Soda	It may be used in place of lye against certain diseases.	10½% solution (13½ oz to 1 gal water).	—
Sal Soda and soda ash (or sodium carbonate)	They may be used in place of lye.	4% solution (1 lb to 3 gal. water) Most effective in hot solution.	Commonly used as cleaning agents, but have disinfectant properties, especially when used as a hot solution.
Soap	Its power to kill germs is very limited. Greatest usefulness is in cleansing and dissolving coatings from various surfaces, including the skin, prior to application of a good disinfectant.	As commercially prepared	Although indispensable for sanitizing surfaces, soaps should not be used as disinfectants. They are not regularly effective, staphylococci and the organisms which cause diarrheal diseases are resistant

[1]Sometimes loosely classed as a disinfectant but actually an antiseptic and practically useful only on living tissue.

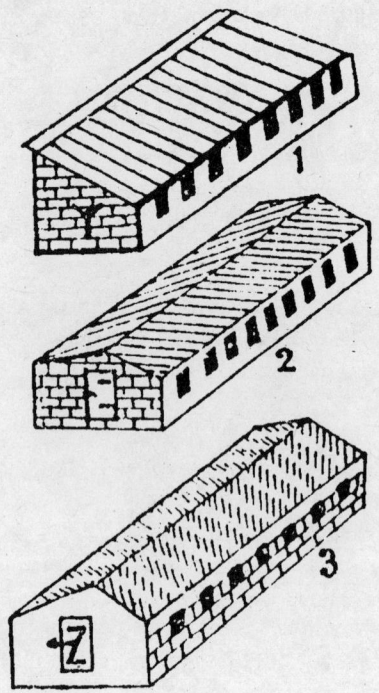
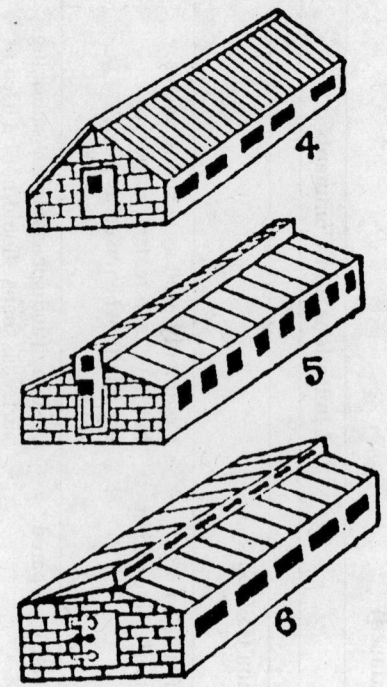

Figure 30 Types of roofs for poultry houses. (1) Shed type, (2) Combination. (3) Gable, (A) 'A' shaped, (5) Monitor type and (6) Semi monitor type.

Combination type. Such houses have double pitch roofs in which the ridge between the two slopes is not midway from front to back. Most of the houses have the long slope to the rear. Like the gable type, the combination roof requires more material and labour than the shed roof.

House Construction

Roofs. In India the cement-asbestos sheeting, corrugated iron and zinc sheets are commonly used as roofing material. Cement-asbestos sheeting although very satisfactory and durable is expensive. Corrugated iron and zinc sheets are equally satisfactory and the cost is lower than cement-asbestos. Figure 30 shows the types of roofs for poultry houses.

Floors. The floor of a laying house should be free from dampness, with a smooth surface with out cracks, easy to clean and disinfect, rat proof and durable.

Concrete floor. A well laid concrete floor is the safest way to meet these requirements and is recommended in preference to any other kind of a floor. Concrete floors laid on the ground conserve warmth from the earth in winter.

Wire mesh floor. Wire mesh floor or preferably mesh of expanded metal is the best for portable houses. The expanded metal although more expensive is stronger, more durable and does not sag like the wire mesh. The expanded metal having ½" × ½" mesh, nailed to the bottom of the house makes excellent flooring through which all the excreta drop out ensuring best sanitary condition.

Katcha floor. The poor village farmer sometimes prefer this sort of floor due to low cost, but it is difficult to keep clean. The floor usually becomes foul, harbours disease germs and vermin, and provides favourable conditions for the onset and spread of diseases.

Whatever be the kind of flooring, it is desirable to provide dry clean litter as bedding.

Walls. The walls should be water-tight, wind-proof, and finished with interior surfaces that are easy to clean and disinfect. Except for the hills, where summer is cool and winter very cold, open type houses with necessary adaptions prove quite suitable.

In plains, where safeguarding is assured from enemies, the walls may be of expanded metal wire mesh on all the sides and the roof will be on some special iron frame. In winter, it will be necessary to cover those mesh with gunny bags. etc.

Ventilation. If built of brick, the south side of the house ought to be enclosed with half-inch mesh wire netting; on the north, east and west, high up near the roof, there should be some openings, 12" × 6", covered with the same kind of wire netting. This will afford perfect ventilation at all seasons, and the house will not be too warm in the summer or too cold in the winter.

Door. The door of the house must be on the south, and made of an angle iron frame covered with ½" mesh wire netting. The size of the room should be always large enough to allow a man to conveniently get through.

Windows. At least 1½ square feet openings for each 10 square feet of floor space is recommended for the plain areas of India. In the hill regions where it becomes cold in winter and not too warm in summer, this size may be reduced to half. All openings should be covered with 1" wire netting. Equal openings on opposite sides of the house or even on all four walls are desirable. Be sure to make the roof overhang at least 18", preferably 36" out from the wall to cut down radiation through the window opening.

POULTRY HOUSE EQUIPMENT

The poultry house should be equipped with roosts, nests, feed hoppers, water containers and other items which are essential for satisfactory production. It should be simple in construction, cheap, movable, easily cleaned and disinfected whenever necessary.

Perches or roosts. Chickens start roosting when they are eight weeks old. Apart from catering to the natural instinct or desire of the chickens to get above ihe ground at night, perches help materially to keep the bird's feet and plumage clean.

Make perches from long wooden bars of two square inches rounded at the top and flat at the bottom. Fix these perches about 16 inches above the ground and near about the walls in such a way that they can be removed for disinfection. Give at least a 12-inch space between two perches. Each bird will need about 8 inches of the perch to roost.

The rear perches should rest a little higher than those at the front, if they are arranged to be horizontal with the length of the house. This will encourage some of the birds that like to roost high to go to the back perches. Paint the perches occasionally with creosote to prevent insects.

Nest boxes. Each pen of laying birds should be provided with nest boxes for laying eggs. It should be roomy, movable, cool and well ventilated, dark and conveniently located. Nests are usually constructed 14 inches square, 6 inches deep and with about 15 inches head room. All metal nests are preferred to wood nests because of easy cleaning and less chance of becoming infested with mites. Empty kerosene tins make excellent boxes. One nest should be provided for every 5 or 6 hens. Dark nest are desirable because they result in less scratching in the nest, less egg breakage and less egg eating. A wooden packing case 18 inches square or a wide mouthed earthen pot can be a suitable nest. Place some sand or soft hay or straw inside.

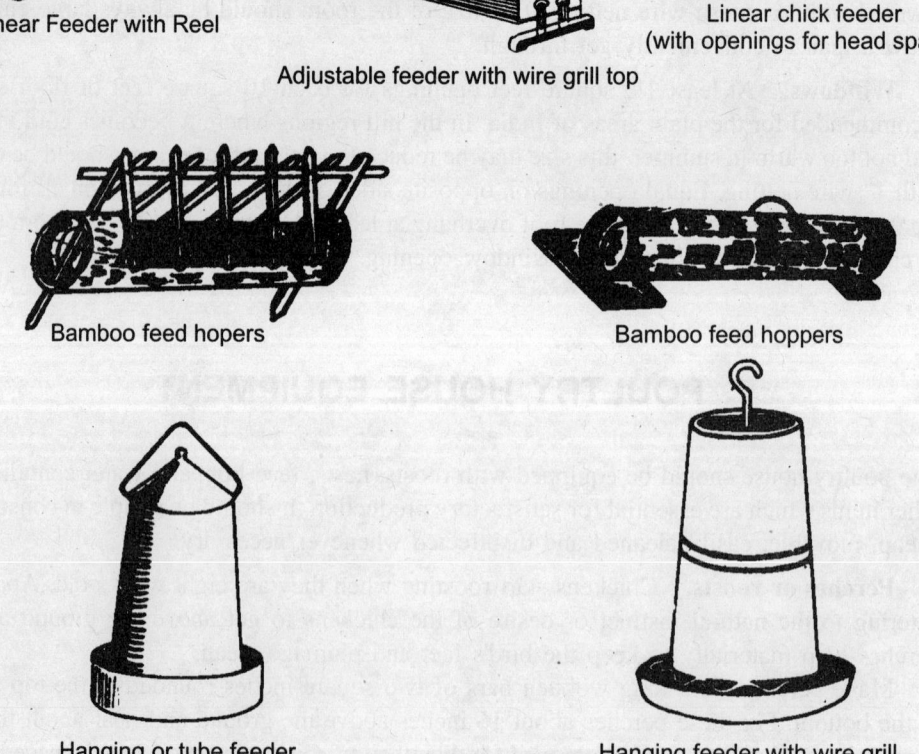

Linear Feeder with Reel

Adjustable feeder with wire grill top

Linear chick feeder
(with openings for head space)

Bamboo feed hopers

Bamboo feed hoppers

Hanging or tube feeder

Hanging feeder with wire grill

Figure 31 Types of feeders.

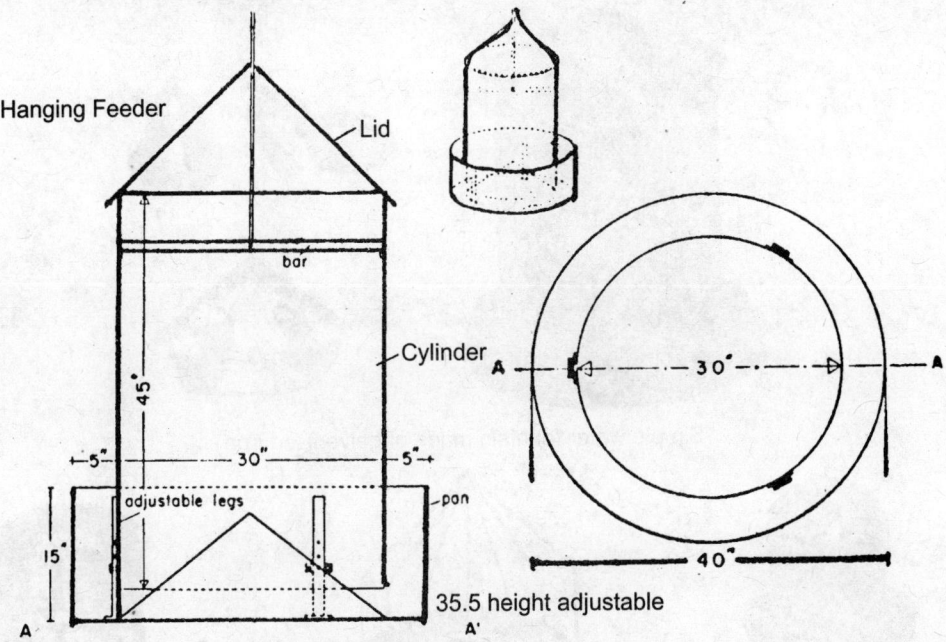

Figure 31 Types of feeders (*Contd.*)

Nests sometimes are also placed inside a run but in that case care should be taken to prevent crows, etc., by covering the top of the run with wire netting.

Trapnests.   Each nest is provided with a trap door so that when the poultryman releases the hen from the nest he can identify her and mark her leg-band number on the egg. There should be one nest for every 3 or 4 birds. Trapnests differ from regular nests in that they are provided with trap doors by which birds shut themselves in when they enter.

For convenience of the caretaker, the nests should be placed 18 to 20 inches above the floor.

Feed hoppers.   The essential features of satisfactory feed hoppers are that they (1) avoid wastage of feed, (2) prevent the birds from getting their feet into the feed and from roosting on the hopper, (3) are easy to clean, and (4) make it easy for the birds to eat from the bottom of the hopper.

Troughs, pots and pans used for feeding should be of suitable size depending on the age and size of the birds. Some of the designs are shown in the diagram (Figure 31).

Watering devices.   An ample supply of water should be made available at all times, or egg production is liable to be affected. The water container should contain clean water, kept cool in summer, and be easily cleaned because contaminated water tends to spread certain diseases from bird to bird.

A wide variety of watering utensils satisfying the above needs can be had. Some of the designs are shown in the diagram (Figure 32).

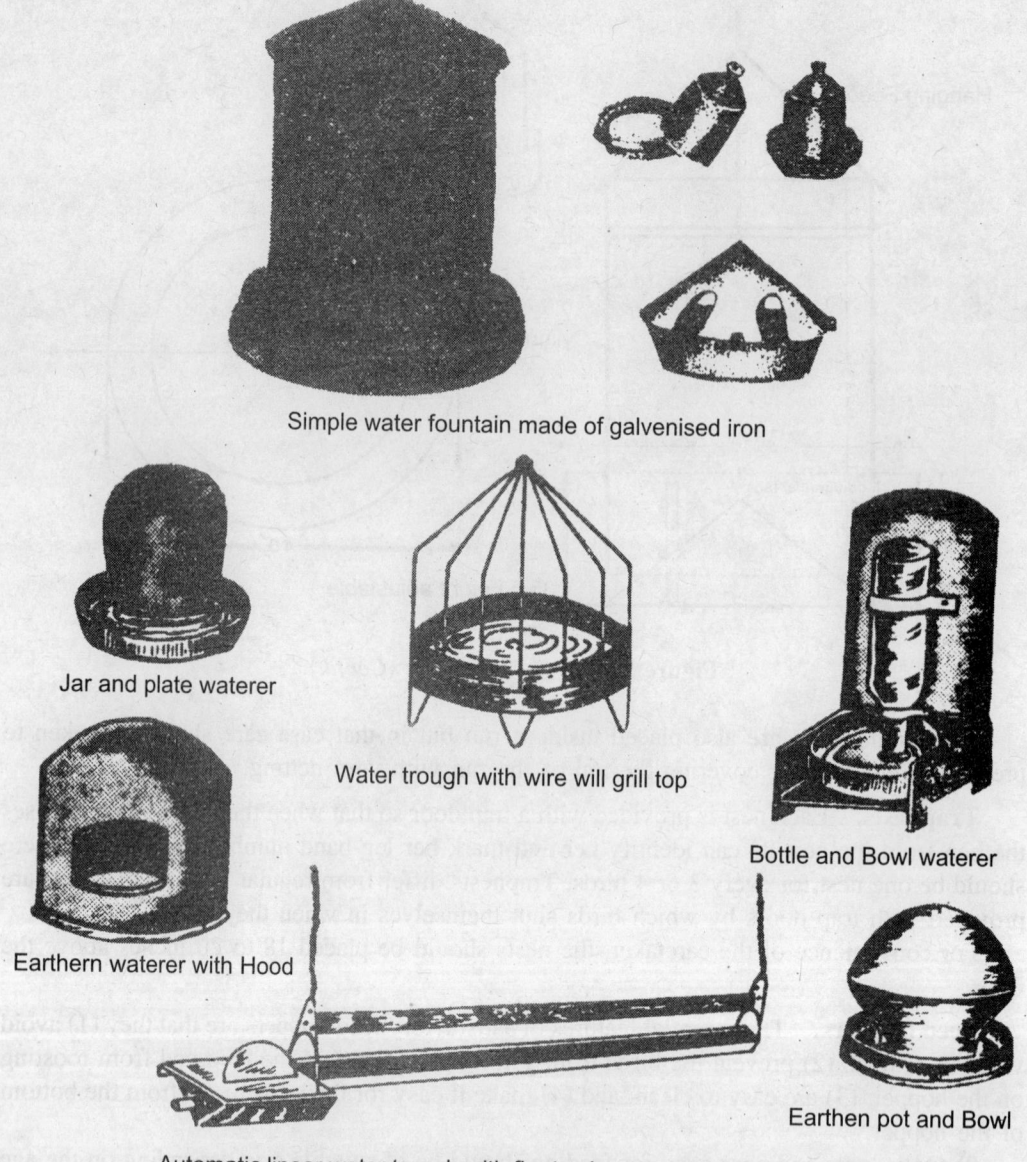

Simple water fountain made of galvenised iron

Jar and plate waterer

Water trough with wire will grill top

Bottle and Bowl waterer

Earthern waterer with Hood

Earthen pot and Bowl

Automatic linear water trough with float valve assembly

Figure 32 Types of waterers.

Grit and shell container. Ordinary hoppers made either of wood or metal can be used for oyster shells or other grit. It is advantageous to have the source of calcium for egg shell formation near the feed hopper.

Dust bath. An earthen pot or a hole in the ground, 2′ in diameter, should be filled with dry, clean, shifted earth or ashes and placed in the shed on the east side. The container should be continually refilled. Flours of sulphur should be added to the ashes, along with some dry coarse tobacco leaves. Coal ashes or cowdung cake ashes may be used alternatively.

HOUSING SYSTEMS OF POULTRY

There are four systems of housing generally found to follow among the poultry keepers. The type of housing adopted depends to a large extent on the amount of ground and the capital available.

1. Free-range or extensive system
2. Semi-intensive system
3. Folding unit system
4. Intensive system
   A. Battery system
   B. Deep litter system

Free-range system. This method is the oldest of all and has been used for centuries by general farmers, where there is no shortage of land.

This system allows great but not unlimited, space to the birds on land where they can find an appreciable amount of food in the form of herbage, seeds and insects, provided they are protected from predatory animals and infectious diseases including parasitic infestation. At present, due to advantages of intensive methods the system is almost obsolete.

Semi-intensive system. This system is adopted where the amount of free space available is limited, but it is necessary to allow the birds 20-30 square yards per bird of outside run. Wherever possible this space should be divided giving a run on either side of the house of 10-15 square yards per bird, thus enabling the birds to move onto fresh ground.

Folding-unit system. This system of housing is an innovation of recent years. In portable folding units, birds being confined to one small run, the position is changed each day, giving them fresh ground and the birds find a considerable proportion of food from the herbage are healthier and harder. For the farmer, the beneficial effects of scratching and manuring on the land is another side effect.

The disadvantages are that food and water must be carried out to the birds and eggs brought back and there is some extra labour involved in the regular moving of the fold units.

The most convenient folding unit to handle is that which is made for 25 hens. A floor space of 1 square foot should be allowed for each bird in the house, and 3 square feet in the run, so that a total floor space to the whole unit is 4 square feet per bird, as with the intensive system.

A suitable measurement for a folding house to take 25 birds is 5 feet wide and 20 feet long, the house being 5′ × 5′, one-third of the run. The part nearest the house is covered in and the remaining 10′ open with wire netting sides and top.

Intensive System

In this system the birds are confined to the house entirely, with no access to land outside, and it is usually adopted where land is limited and expensive.

This has only been made possible by admitting the direct rays of the sun on to the floor of the house so that part of the windows are removable, or either fold or slide down like windows of railway train to permit the ultraviolet rays to reach the birds. Under the intensive system, Battery (cage system) and Deep litter methods are most common.

A. Battery system. This appliance is the inventor's latest contribution to the commercial egg farmer. This is the most intensive type of poultry production and is useful to those with only a small quantity of floor space at their disposal. Now a days, in large cities hardly a poultry lover can spare open lands for rearing birds. For all such people, this system will prove worthy of keeping birds at minimum space (Plate 7 and Figure 33).

In the battery system, each hen is confined to a cage just large enough to permit very limited movement and allow her to stand and sit comfortably. The usual floor space is 14 × 16 inches and the height, 17 inches. The floor is of standard strong galvanised wire set at a slope from back to the front, so that the eggs as they are laid, roll out of the cage to a receiving gutter. Underneath is a tray for droppings. Both food and water receptacles are outside the cage.

Many small cages can be assembled together, if necessary it may be multistoried. The whole structure should be of metal so that no parasites will be harboured and thorough disinfection can be carried out as often as required. Provided the batteries of cages are set up in a place which is well ventilated, and lighted, is not too hot and is vermin proof and that the food meets all nutritional needs, this system has proved to be remarkably successful in the tropical countries. It may be that as it requires a minimum expenditure of energy from the bird, which spends all its time in the shade, it lessens the load of excess body heat. The performance of each bird can be noted and culling easily carried out. Pullets, which are more often used than birds of over one year, should be placed in the cages at least one month before they are expected to lay.

The feeding of birds in cages has to be carefully considered, as the birds are entirely dependent on the mash for maintenance and production. To supply vitamins A and D, cod-liver oil, yeast, dried milk powder are useful, and fish meal or other animal protein, and balanced minerals and some form of grit must be made available.

As in each cage there will be only pullets so one can never expect fertilised eggs, hence the vegetative eggs will be there, which can be preserved for a longer time than fertilised eggs at ordinary room temperature but can never be used for hatching purposes.

B. Deep litter system. In this system, the poultry birds are kept in large pens up to 250 birds each, on floor covered with litters like straw, saw dust or dry leaves up to depth of 8-12 inches. Deep litter resembles to dry compost. In other words, deep litter can be defined as the accumulation of the material used for litter with poultry manure until it reaches a depth of 8 to 12 inches. The build-up has to be carried out correctly to give desired results which takes very little attention.

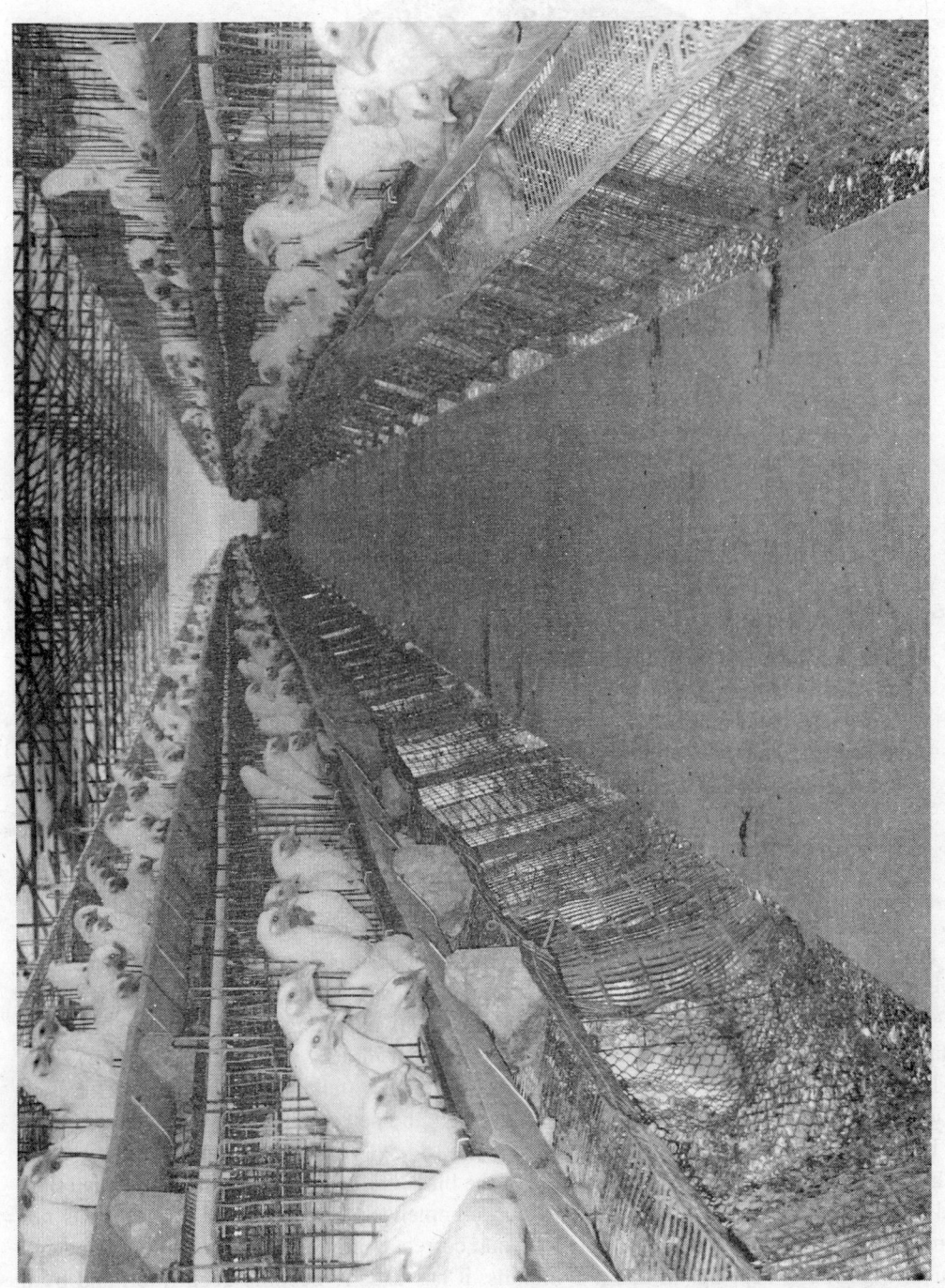

Plate 7   Modern Intensive Poultryhouse.

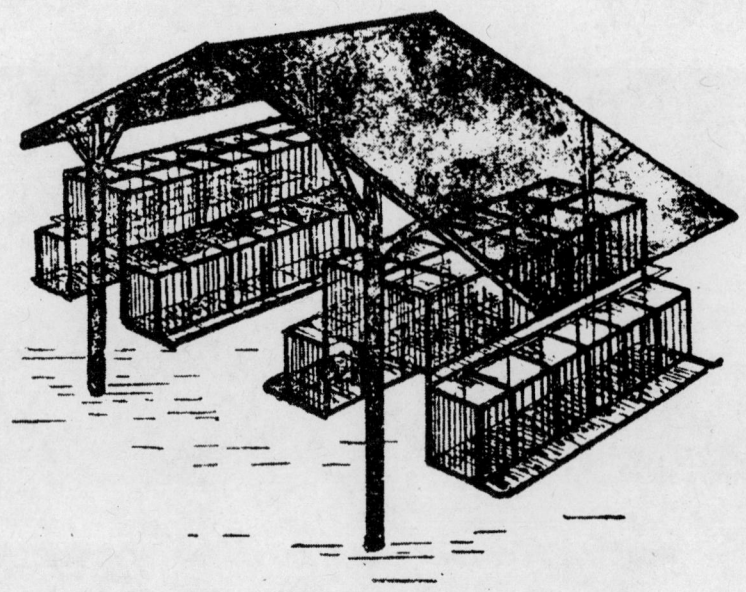

Figure 33 Battery system, Callfornian Cage

Basic Rules Needed

1. Do not have too many birds in the pen—one bird for every 3½ to 4 and preferably 5 square feet of floor space.
2. Provide sufficient ventilation to enable the litter to keep in correct condition.
3. Keep the litter dry. This is probably the master work in a deep litter system. If the litter gets soaked by leaking from roofs or from water vessels, it upsets the whole process and would have to start over again. All probable precautions should be taken to maintain the litters completely dry.
4. Stir the litter regularly. Turning the litter (just like digging in a garden) at least once weekly is very important in maintaining a correct build-up of deep litter.

How deep litter is started? For deep litter we can use many materials as a medium for starting the build-up in a pen. It can work quite well with a wide range but organic materials should always be used. The cost and ease of obtaining will be the main guide. Suitable dry organic materials like straw (needs to be cut into 2 or 3 inch lengths), saw dust, dry leaves, dry grasses, groundnut shells, broken up maize stalks and cobs, bark of trees in sufficient quantity to give a depth of about 6 inches in the pen should be used. When the litter has built up it would be very difficult for anyone to say what material was initially used. Nothing else has to be added. The droppings of the birds gradually combine with the materials used to build up the litter (the bacterial action commences as a result). When a pen is not overcrowded, these can be regularly absorbed and correct condition maintained, if stirring and even distribution is kept up. In about 2 months, it has usually become deep litter, and by 6 months it has become built-up deep litter. At about 12 months of old stage, it is fully built up. Extra litter materials can be added to maintain sufficient depth.

When to start it?   The deep litter pen should be started when the weather is dry, and is likely to remain so for about 2 months for the operation of the bacterial action which alters the composition of the litters. Start new litter with each year's pullets and continue with it for their laying period.

Deep litter in wet areas.   Laying birds can be kept quite successfully in a shed built off the ground-infact birds can be kept in houses with 2 or 3 floors one above the other. Sometimes the litters may get damp in spite of all precautions, at that time about 0.5 kg of superphosphate may be thoroughly mixed up with litters spreading in 15 square feet of floor space. When this is not available hydrated lime (but never quicklime) can be used at the same level.

Advantages of Deep Litter System

1. **Safety of birds.**   Birds on range or even in a netted yard can be taken by wild animals, flying birds, etc. When enclosed in deep litter intensive pen which has strong wire netting or expanded metal, the birds and eggs are safe.

2. **Litter as a source of food supply.**   It may come as surprise to learn that built-up deep litter also supplies some of the feed requirements of the birds. They obtain "Animal Protein Factor" from deep litter and some work indicates that this could mean that birds obtain sufficient of this to enable a suitable feed ration to be prepared with only a vegetable protein such as groundnut meal included in the feed. The level of vitamins such as riboflavin increases up to nearly three-fold, according to experiments conducted. The combination of this and the Animal Protein Factor is necessary to good hatchability of eggs and early growth of chickens.

3. **Disease control.**   Well managed deep litter kept in dry condition with no wet spots around waterer has a sterilising action. The level of coccidiosis and worm infestation is much lower with poultry kept on good deep litter than with birds (or chickens) in bare yards and bare floor sheds particularly where water spillage is allowed.

4. **Labour saving.**   This is one of the really big features of deep litter usage. Cleaning out poultry pens daily or weekly means quite a lot of work. With correct conditions observed with well managed litter there is no need to clean a pen out for a whole year; the only attention is the regular stirring and adding of some material as needed.

5. **The valuable fertiliser.**   This is a valuable economic factor with deep litter. According to McArdle and Panda, 35 laying birds can produce in one year about 1 tonne of deep litter manure. The level of nitrogen in fresh manure is about 1%, but on well built-up deep litter it may be around 3 per cent nitrogen (nearly 20% protein). It also contains about 2 per cent phosphorus and 2 per cent potash. Its value is about 3 times that of cattle manure.

6. **Hot weather safeguard.**   This is an important feature in a hot climate. The litter maintains its own constant temperature, so birds burrow into it when the air temperature is high and thereby cool themselves. Conversely, they can warm themselves in the same way when the weather is very cool. Accordingly, it is a valuable insulating agent.

BREEDING SYSTEMS

A large number of mating systems are being used in poultry breeding. There is no evidence, however, to indicate that any one system is best for all purposes. Following is a brief discussion of the procedures, advantages, disadvantages of each system.

Out-crossing. The mating of birds of the same variety but of different strains is called outbreeding. The object is to hold the good traits already in one family line and to capture the good ones from the other one. Or, it may be an attempt to get rid of the undesirable traits in one line and obtain only the good ones from another line.

Grading. This system involves the mating of superior males with successive generations of breeding hens of the same breed or variety. The system is followed until the progenies produced approach the quality of the males used. To avoid disadvantages of inbreeding one particular cock should not be used for a number of times, but different cocks of the same breed should be selected.

This method is, therefore, of great importance for improving indigenous poultry existing in our villages.

Cross breeding. The mating of pure-bred males of one breed with pure bred females of another breed is known as cross breeding. This method has been popular in livestock breeding. Cross breeding in chickens has resulted in higher hatchability, more efficient and faster gains, and lower chick mortality. Hybrid vigour resulting from cross breed utilised extensively in broiler production.

Line breeding. Line breeding is similar to inbreeding but involves the breeding of birds less closely related. The mating of cousins or grand-sire and grand-daughters are examples of line breeding. It is done to conserve and perpetuate the good traits of certain outstanding birds. It tends to produce a homozygous genetic condition.

Inbreeding. It is the mating of such closely related birds as (1) brother to sister, (2) son to dam, (3) sire to daughter. It is done primarily to intensify the degree of homozygosity. The practice has not proved satisfactory with poultry.

Bad as well as good characteristic become mixed in inbreeding.

Top crossing. This system of breeding has been used successfully in swine production and is finding its place in poultry breeding. It involves the mating of inbred males with females which are not inbred.

Tests must be made to determine the inbred lines which cross with the flock involved. The 'nicking' ability of each line must be determined.

A single inbred line in top crossing is much cheaper than a four inbred top cross. Only line has to be determined.

Single cross top crossing. This system involves the mating of single cross males to pure-bred females. Two proven inbred lines are maintained to produce the single cross males. This system has also proved desirable in swine production.

Single cross males normally demonstrate a reproductive performance far superior to that of the inbred, and equal or superior to that of pure-breds.

Methods of Mating

The methods of mating used will have a marked influence on fertility and consequently on the number of offsprings used. Most common methods of mating are flock and pen mating. Stud mating and artificial insemination are sometimes used in experimental work.

Flock mating.   It is also known as mass mating.

Other things being equal, better fertility is obtained from flock matings than from pen matings, probabiy due to the competition among males in flock mating which results in more matings and better fertility. One male is sufficient for 15 to 20 hens, but number varies with the size and age of the hens. In flock matings the percentage of chicks hatched is unknown.

Pen mating.   In pen mating a pen of hens is mated to a single male. If the birds are trap-nested and the hen's leg-band number recorded on the egg, it is possible to know the parents of every chick hatched from a pen mating. About the same number of hens are mated with a male as in the case of flock mating. Fertility is not so good in pen mating as in flock mating. This is because, certain hens may not like the cock or vice-versa.

Stud mating.   In stud mating the females are mated individually with a male kept by the owner in a coop or pen. Thus this system involves more labour than flock mating. The birds should be mated at least once each week in order to maintain good fertility.

Stud mating may be used where hens are kept in laying batteries. It is also used when a very valuable male is being used as a breeder.

Artificial insemination.   This system is not practical in poultry breeding work although it is possible to follow the system. It is used in experimental work and may be used in turkey breeding where poor fertility is encountered.

POULTRY NUTRITION

Nutrition is the process of furnishing the cells inside the animal with that portion of the external chemical environment needed for optimum functioning of the many metabolic chemical reactions involved in growth, maintenance, work, production and reproduction.

Nutrition encompasses the procurement, ingestion, digestion and absorption of the chemical elements which serve as feed. In addition, it includes the transport of these chemical elements to all cells within the animal organism in the physical and chemical forms most suitable for assimilation and use by the cells.

Principles of Poultry Feeding

Poultry feeding is one of the important branches of poultry science, since feed-cost alone accounts for 65-70 percent of the total farm expenses. It is in the interest of every poultryman to be able to get as much chicken meat or as many eggs for every rupee that he spends on the feed as possible.

The problems involved in the feeding of fowls in recent times are multifarious because of modern farming conditions such as: (i) increased cost of poultry feed; (ii) confinement rearing of poultry; (iii) inclusion of agro-industrial by-products in poultry; and (iv) increase in flock size and high flock density.

While computing ration for poultry birds, the following facts should be considered:

(i) Poultry birds have no lips or teeth, hence require a more concentrated ration.
(ii) Their digestive tract having a simple stomach is comparatively short, digestion is quite rapid. It takes about 2½ hours for feed to go from mouth to cloaca in the laying hen, and 10 hours in a non-laying hen. Therefore, the nutritive requirements of poultry are more precise.
(iii) Unlike ruminants, where micro-organisms synthesize a sizeable portion of essential amino acid, vitamin B complex, vitamin K in the stomach, the poultry completely depend upon the dietary source for all such nutrients (all essential amino acids, vitamin B complex, etc.).
(iv) Poultry birds are fed collectively rather than individually.
(v) Due to higher rate of metabolism, poultry require a more exact ration.

Nutrients-Their Nature and Functions

The term nutrient means any single class of feed, or group of like feeds, that aids in the support of life and makes it possible for birds to produce meat or eggs. Classification of nutrients by analysis have been presented in Table 34. However, they are further classified according to physical, chemical and biological properties into following groups:

1. Water
2. Proteins
3. Carbohydrates
4. Fats and oils
5. Minerals
6. Vitamins
7. Feed additives (not a nutrient, but added to enhance the quality of the nutrients)

1. **Water.** Chemically speaking, water is a compound which contains two atoms of hydrogen and one atom of oxygen. Normally here two elements which make up water are gases, but under the right conditions they form the stable compound that we know as water.

   Water is a marvellous compound. Without it, life on earth could not exist. Living things are comprised mostly of water. A very important aspect of water, especially in terms of water quality, is that many other compounds can be dissolved in it. Many times contaminants can be present at fairly high levels in water without resulting in noticeable changes in the look, odour, or taste of water. Some of the compounds which are common contaminants in water cause changes in pH, hardness or turbidity and are generally not harmful, while others, including organic and inorganic chemicals, radiological isotopes, and bacteria, have the potential for harm. All of the contaminants in water work together to reduce its quality. What about the poultry farm? Is water quality important here ? The answer is a resounding YES. There is no question that clean, fresh, high quality water is essential in poultry production to maintain maximum growth and production.

Contaminants in the drinking water of poultry can affect growth, production, quality, and health. Growing chickens from 1 to 7 weeks of age consume between 5 and 15 liters of water per 100 birds per day, while laying birds consume between 20 and 25 liters per 100 birds per day. With as much water as birds drink contamination problems can cause problems. What are some of the contaminants that poultry growers must be concerned with? They are the same that concern domestic water consumers. The most common contaminants are the dissolved mineral salts, over 30 different types, with the most common being calcium and magnesium salts. These salts make water "hard". They are found primarily in groundwater with levels varying by location and soil type. Hard water is usually not a problem unless the levels of these salts are extremely high. Another important is nitrate. High levels of nitrates in water are associated with excessive nitrogen application to the soil in the form of fertilizer or manure. The excess nitrogen in the form of nitrate either leaches through the soil into groundwater or runs off into surface water. When poultry consume high levels of nitrates, it can interfere with certain nutrient utilization or, if high enough cause acute poisoning.
Salinity can be a problem in certain areas. Excess sodium salt in poultry drinking water can result in watery droppings and eventually wet litter. It is also possible although unlikely that high salt in water combined with the salt in the feed can result in a toxic response. Disease organisms can be found in water. Coccidiosis, salmonellosis, and *E. coli* can be transmitted through the water. In cases where these organisms are found in water, treatment must be undertaken to get rid of them.

Organic and inorganic chemicals in water must always be taken seriously. Such compounds as pesticides, solvents, petroleum products and others can cause either acute toxicity of residues in eggs or meat. Contaminations of this type are rare but not unheard of. Water quality is an important topic when discussing poultry production. When dealing with an animal that is about two-thirds water, any contamination is potentially harmful.

2. **Proteins.** In poultry, the products produced consists mainly of protein. On a dry weight basis the carcass of a 6 weeks old broiler is more than 65 per cent protein and the egg contents are about 50 per cent protein. Typical broiler rations will contain from 20 to 22 per cent protein and in layers ration the amount varies between 16-18 per cent.

From the standpoint of nutrition, the amino acids that make up the protein are really the essential nutrients rather than the protein molecule itself.

Protein synthesis in chickens are required at a very rapid rate not for compensating the broken tissues of the adult body but also for the production of eggs which contain about 12 percent protein. For efficient synthesis, it is not only necessary that all the essential amino acids should be available through diet but those also should be in right proportions. Any excess of even a single amino acid which might cause imbalance

108

Table 34   Classification of Nutrients by Analysis

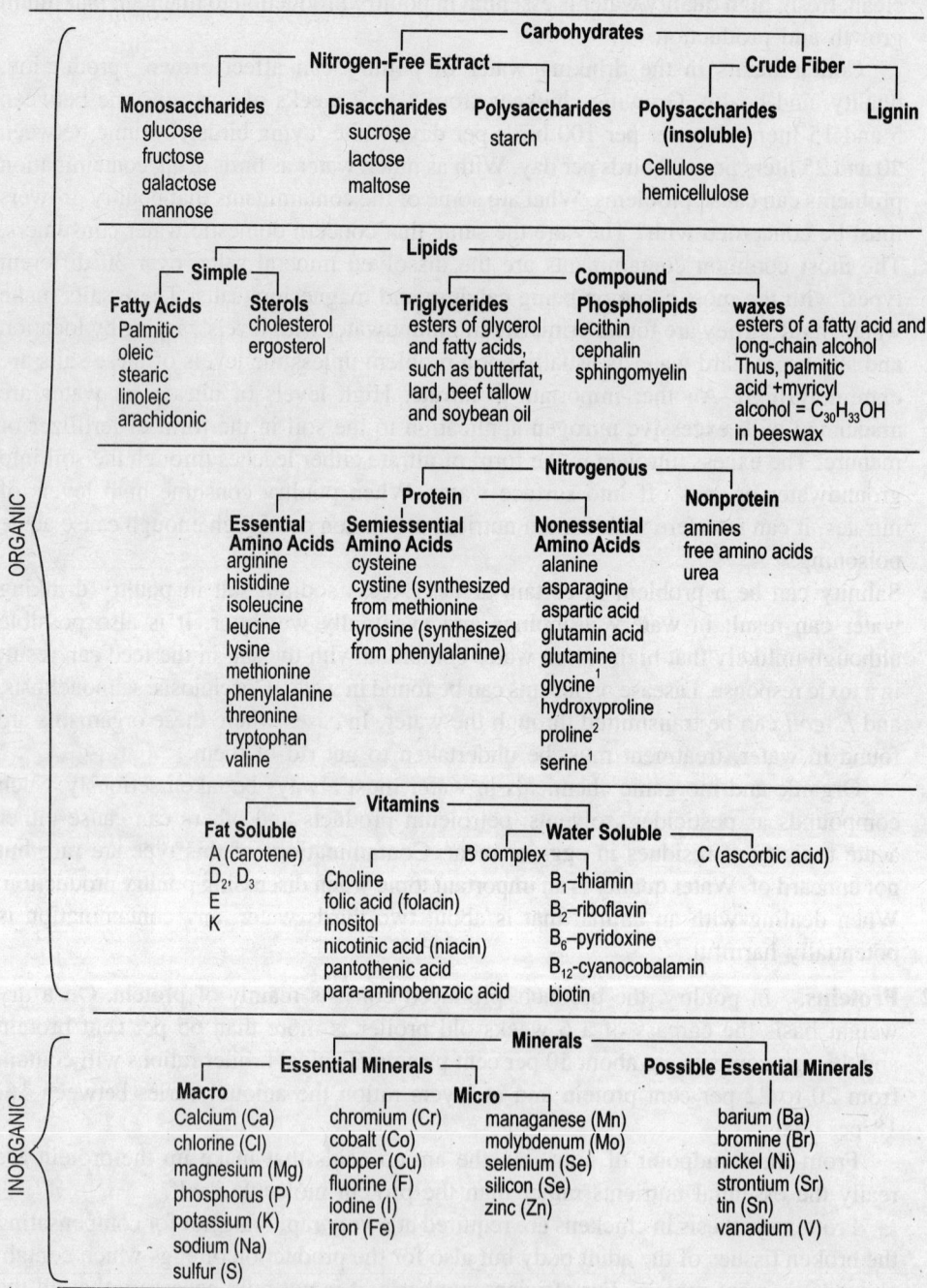

ORGANIC

Carbohydrates

Nitrogen-Free Extract

Monosaccharides
glucose
fructose
galactose
mannose

Disaccharides
sucrose
lactose
maltose

Polysaccharides
starch

Crude Fiber

Polysaccharides (insoluble)
Cellulose
hemicellulose

Lignin

Lipids

Simple

Fatty Acids
Palmitic
oleic
stearic
linoleic
arachidonic

Sterols
cholesterol
ergosterol

Compound

Triglycerides
esters of glycerol
and fatty acids,
such as butterfat,
lard, beef tallow
and soybean oil

Phospholipids
lecithin
cephalin
sphingomyelin

waxes
esters of a fatty acid and
long-chain alcohol
Thus, palmitic
acid +myricyl
alcohol = $C_{30}H_{33}OH$
in beeswax

Nitrogenous

Protein

Essential Amino Acids
arginine
histidine
isoleucine
leucine
lysine
methionine
phenylalanine
threonine
tryptophan
valine

Semiessential Amino Acids
cysteine
cystine (synthesized from methionine)
tyrosine (synthesized from phenylalanine)

Nonessential Amino Acids
alanine
asparagine
aspartic acid
glutamin acid
glutamine
glycine[1]
hydroxyproline
proline[2]
serine[1]

Nonprotein
amines
free amino acids
urea

Vitamins

Fat Soluble
A (carotene)
D_2, D_3
E
K

B complex
Choline
folic acid (folacin)
inositol
nicotinic acid (niacin)
pantothenic acid
para-aminobenzoic acid

Water Soluble

B_1–thiamin
B_2–riboflavin
B_6–pyridoxine
B_{12}-cyanocobalamin
biotin

C (ascorbic acid)

INORGANIC

Minerals

Essential Minerals

Macro
Calcium (Ca)
chlorine (Cl)
magnesium (Mg)
phosphorus (P)
potassium (K)
sodium (Na)
sulfur (S)

Micro
chromium (Cr)
cobalt (Co)
copper (Cu)
fluorine (F)
iodine (I)
iron (Fe)

managanese (Mn)
molybdenum (Mo)
selenium (Se)
silicon (Se)
zinc (Zn)

Possible Essential Minerals
barium (Ba)
bromine (Br)
nickel (Ni)
strontium (Sr)
tin (Sn)
vanadium (V)

[1]Under some conditions, glycine serine synthesis may not be sufficient for most rapid growth glycine or serine may need to be supplied in the diet.

[2]When diets composed of crystalline amino acids are used proline may be necessary to achieve maximum growth.

[3]Required by at least one animal species

will go as waste owing to what is called 'time factor' in protein synthesis. Thus from the standpoint of poultry nutrition, the amino acids that make up proteins are really the essential nutrients, rather than the protein molecule itself. Hence protein content as a measure of the nutritional value of a feed is becoming less important and each amino acid is being considered individually. Biological function of protein have been presented in Table 35.

The energy content of the diet must be considered in formulating to meet the desired intake of all essential nutrients other than energy itself, including the intake of the essential amino acids. The protein calorie ratio is thus a most important factor in poultry nutrition.

In practice, the amino acid requirement of growing chickens and of laying hens, (Table 36) are met by proteins from plant and animal sources. Usually it is necessary to choose more than one source of dietary protein, (i.e. animal and vegetable sources) then combine them in such a way that the amino acid composition of the mixture meets the requirements of the bird.

Table 35 Biological Functions of Proteins

Protein function	Role
Structural	
collagen	fibrous connective tissue
elastin	elastic connective tissue
glycoproteins	cell walls
α-keratin	skin, nails, feathers, hoofs
Contractile	
actin	thin filaments in muscles
myosin	thick filaments in muscles
dynein	involved in movement of cilia and flagella
Transport	
hemoglobin	transports oxygen in blood
myoglobin	transports oxygen in muscle
serum albumin	transports fatty acids in blood
transferrin	transports iron in blood
Hormones	
adrenocorticotropic hormone	regulates corticosteroid synthesis
growth hormone	stimulates growth of skeletal structure
insulin	regulates metabolism of glucose
Storage	
casein	milk protein
gliadin	stores amino acids in wheat
ovalbumin	protein in egg white
zein	stores amino acids in corn
Protection	
antibodies	react with foreign proteins
fibrinogen	involved in blood clotting
thrombin	involved in blood clotting

Table 36 Requirement for each individual amino acid when all other amino acids of nutritive importance are provided (figures are % of total diet except for human which are in (g/kg body weight/day)

Amino acids	Growing pigs[2]	Human[2]			Young rat[2]	Fish	Growing chickens[1]			Layers
		Infants (4-6 mths)	Child (10-12 yrs)	Adult			0-6 weeks	6-14 weeks	14-20 weeks	
Isoleucine	0.63	83	28	12	0.5	0.9	0.6	0.5	0.4	0.5
Leucine	0.75	135	42	16	0.75	1.6	1	0.83	0.67	0.73
Lysine	0.95	99	44	12	0.7	2	0.85	0.6	0.45	0.64
Methionine+ Cystine	0.56[4]	49[5]	22[5]	10[5]	0.6[4]	1.6	0.60[4]	0.50[4]	0.40[4]	0.55[4]
Phenylalanine + Tyrosine	0.88[4]	141	22[7]	16[7]	0.86[6]	2.1	1.00[6]	0.83[6]	0.67	0.80[6]
Threonine	0.56	68	28	8	0.5	0.9	0.68	0.57	0.37	0.45
Tryptophan	0.15	21	4	3	0.15	0.2	0.17	0.14	0.11	0.14
Valine	0.63	92	25	14	0.6	1.3	0.62	0.52	0.41	0.55
Histidine	—	33	NA	NA	0.3	0.7	0.26	0.22	0.17	0.16
Arginine	—	—	—	—	0.6	2.4	1	0.83	0.67	0.68
Glycine & serine	—	—	—	—	—	—	0.7	0.58	0.47	0.5
No. of Essential amino acids	8	9	9	9	10	10	11	11	11	11
Total Protein requirement	16-20%	gm per kg body weight			20%	40%	20%	16%	14%	15%
		2.0	1.5	0.8						

1. Data for chickens obtained from 1984 NRC publication on Poultry.
2. Data for rats and pigs obtained from 1972 and 1978 NRC Publication respectively. On the basis of recent findings regarding sufficient synthesis of Histidine and Arginine by the pig, data given for pig in original source have been neglected.
3. Food and Nutrition Board: Recommended Dietary allowances, 9th ed. National Academy of Sciences-NRC, 1980.
4. About 1/2 of the requirements can be met by cystine.
5. About 3/4 of the requirement can be met by cystine.
6. About 1/3 to 1/2 of the requirement can be met by tyrosine.
7. About 3/4 of the requirement can be met by tyrosine.
NA Not available.

Some high-protein feedstufifs may contain toxic compounds. For example, cottonseed meal may contain gossypol, which discolours the yolks in stored eggs. Certain strains of rapeseed meal contain high enough levels of goitrogenic compounds to be toxic. Even soyabean meal contains a number of harmful substances including trypsin inhibitor, but these are destroyed by proper heating.

Any excess protein consumed by the bird can be burned in the body to yield energy in somewhat the same manner as carbohydrates and fats. However, in practical feeding of poultry, it is seldom wise to use excessive protein because carbohydrates and fats are generally more economical sources of energy.

In addition to dietary energy concentration, the following factors affect the amino acid requirements :

1. *The rate of growth or intensity of egg production*
   The more rapid the growth and the higher the egg production, the higher the amino acid requirements.

2. *The strains*
   Even within species of like body size, growth rate, or egg production, there may be differences in requirements among strains.

3. *The protein level*
   The amino acid requirements tend to increase with dietary protein.

4. *The amino acid relationships*, specifically,
   (a) *Methionine-cystine.* The requirement for methionine can be met only by methionine, while the requirement for cystine may be met by cystine or methionine. This is because methionine is readily converted to cystine metabolically, while the reverse is not possible.
   (b) *Phenylalanine-tyrosine.* The requirement for phenylalanine is met by phenylalanine, while the requirement of tyrosine may be met by tyrosine or phenylalanine.
   (c) *Glycine-serine.* Glycine and serine can be used interchangeably in poultry diets.

5. *Antagonisms*
   There are specific antagonisms among amino acids that may be structurally related, e.g., valine-leucine-isoleucine and arginine-lysine. Increasing one or two of such a group may raise the need for another of the same group.

6. *Imbalances*
   In supplementing diets with *limited amino acids*, it is important to supplement first with the most limiting one, followed by the second most limiting one. Oversupplementation with only the second most limiting one may create an imbalance and accentuate the primary deficiency.

7. *Conversion of certain amino acids to vitamins*
   High levels of methionine may partly compensate for a deficiency of choline or vitamin B_{12} by providing needed methyl groups, and high levels of tryptophan may alleviate a niacin deficiency through metabolic conversion to niacin.

Limiting amino acid

The essential amino acids (Table 37 and 38) of a protein that shows the greatest percentage deficit in comparison to amino acids contained in the same quantity of any standard protein, viz., egg or milk.

Table 37 Limiting amino acids

Ingredients	Order of limitations				
	First	**Second**	**Third**	**Fourth**	**Fifth**
Soyabean	Methionine	Threonine	Valine	Lysine	Isoleucine
Meat and bone	Tryptophan	Methionine	Isoleucine	Threonine	Histidine
Maize	Lysine	Tryptophan	Isoleucine	Threonine	Valine
Milo	Lysine	Threonine	Methionine	Isoleucine	Tryptopan

Table 38 Amino acids

Name	% in egg protein	% in wheat Protein	% deficiency in wheat
Arginine	6.4	4.2	−34
Histidine	2.1	2.1	0
Lysine	7.2	2.7	−63
Tyrosine	4.5	4.4	−2
Tryptophan	1.5	1.2	−20
Phenylalanine	6.3	5.7	−10
Cystine	2.4	1.8	−25
Methionine	4.1	2.5	−39
Cystine + Methionine	6.5	4.3	−34
Threonine	4.9	3.3	−33
Leucine	9.2	6.8	−26
Isoleucine	8.0	3.6	−55
Valine	7.3	4.5	−38

Here lysine is the first order and isoleucine is the second order limited amino acids.

Amino acid availability

The usual assumption that amino acids are 80 to 90 percent available is not necessarily valid. For example, feathers or blood are either indigestible in native form or made indigestible by overheating in processing, respectively.

The consequences of a protein or amino acid deficiency vary with the degree of the deficiency. *A borderline deficiency* is characterised by poor growth and feathering, reduced egg size, poor egg production (but hatchability is not affected), tendency toward greater deposition of carcass and liverfat, poor feed conversion into eggs or meat, and lack of melanin pigment in black or reddish-coloured feathers with low lysine. A *severe protein deficiency* is marked by stopping of feed intake, stopping of egg production, loss of body weight, resorption of ova, a tongue deformity with leucine, isoleucine, and phenylalanine deficiency, stasis of the digestive tract, and death.

Of the essential amino acids, listed above, lysine, methionine, arginine, glycine and tryptophan are referred as "critical" amino acids, since these are usually deficient in ordinary practical poultry ration. This is because cereal grains are usually low in critical amino acids which make up a large proportion of a usual poultry ration. It is thus a must to include a good proportion of animal protein like fish meal, etc., in poultry ration to ensure the inclusion of all critical amino acids

3. Carbohydrates. The main function of carbohydrates in the diet is to provide energy to the animal. The polysaccharides of major importance are starch, cellulose, pentosans and several other complex carbohydrates. Although cellulose and starch are composed of glucose units, chickens possess enzymes that can hydrolyse only starch. Cellulose, therefore, is completely indigestible. Cereal grains and their by-products are excellent source of starch and thus constitutes a bulk of poultry ration.

4. Fats. Fats make up over 40 per cent of the dry egg and about 17 per cent of the dry weight of a broiler. Although fats supply concentrated form of energy (2.25 times more energy than carbohydrate and protein) their inclusion as true fats or oils in the ration is seldom practised because of high cost and the risk of rancidity which develops on prolong exposure to air, heat, sunlight, etc. Most feed ingredients (maize, barley, safflower, milo, wheat, rice bran, etc.) contain 2-5 per cent fat and that is enough for the inclusion of one essential fatty acid (Linoleic acid), which must be present in the young growing chicks or they will grow poorly, have an accumulation of liver fat and be more susceptible for respiratory infection. Laying hens with diets deficient in linoleic acid will lay very small eggs that will not hatch well.

Saturated Acids:

$$CH_3-CH_2-CH_2-CH_2-CH_2-CH_2-CH_2-CH_2-CH_2-CH_2-CH_2-CH_2-CH_2-COOH$$
$$C_{13}H_{27}-COOH$$

Myristic acid

$$CH_3-CH_2-CH_2-CH_2-CH_2-CH_2-CH_2-CH_2-CH_2-CH_2-CH_2-CH_2-CH_2-CH_2-CH_2-COOH$$
$$C_{15}H_{31}-COOH$$

Palmitic acid

$$CH_3-CH_2-CH_2-CH_2-CH_2-CH_2-CH_2-CH_2-CH_2-CH_2-CH_2-CH_2-CH_2-CH_2-CH_2-CH_2-CH_2-COOH$$
$$C_{17}H_{35}-COOH$$

Stearic acid

Unsaturated Acids:

$$CH_3-CH_2-CH_2-CH_2-CH_2-CH_2-CH_2-CH_2-CH=CH-CH_2-CH_2-CH_2-CH_2-CH_2-CH_2-CH_2-COOH$$
$$C_{17}H_{33}-COOH$$

Oleic acid; 9-octadecenoic acid

$$CH_3-CH_2-CH_2-CH_2-CH_2-CH_2-CH_2-CH_2-CH=CH-CH_2-CH=CH-CH_2-CH_2-CH_2-CH_2-COOH$$

$$C_{17}H_{31}-COOH$$

Linoleic acid; 9,12-octadecadienoic acid

$$CH_3-CH_2-CH_2-CH_2-CH_2-CH_2-CH_2-CH_2-CH=CH-CH_2-CH=CH-CH_2-CH=CH-CH_2-COOH$$

$$C_{17}H_{29}-COOH$$

Linolenic acid; 9,12,15-octadecatrienoic acid

$$CH_3-CH_2-CH_2-CH_2-CH=CH-CH_2-CH=CH-CH_2-CH=CH-CH_2-CH=CH-CH_2-CH_2-CH_2-CH_2-COOH$$

$$C_{19}H_{31}-COOH$$

Arachidonic acid; 5,8,11,14-eicosatetraenoic acid

(a)

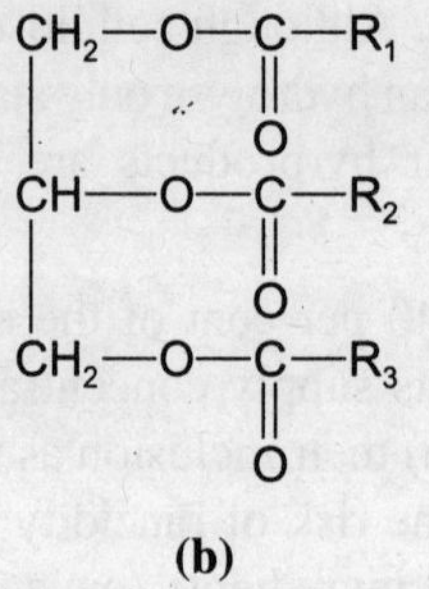

(b)

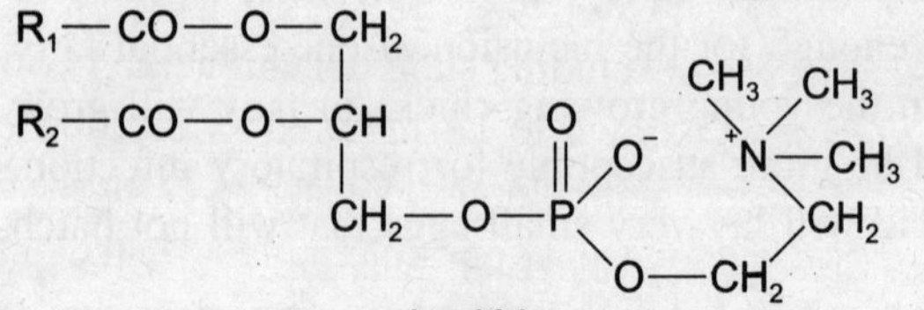

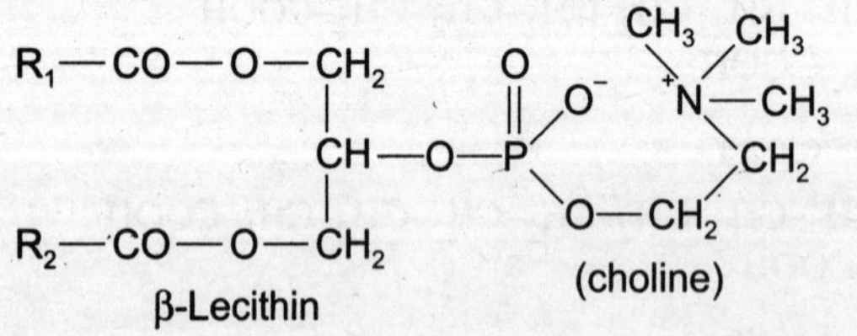

α-Lecithin

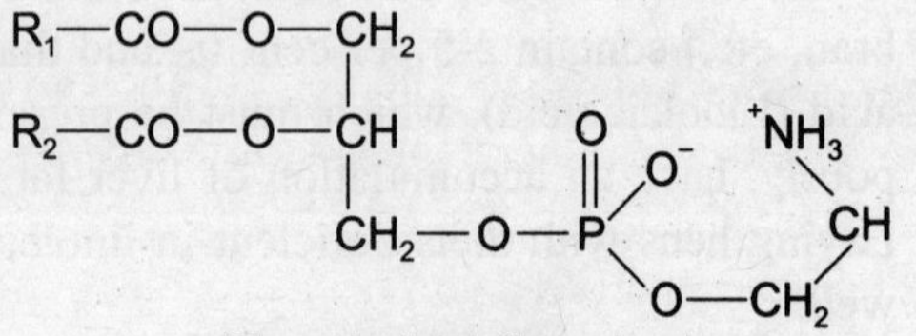

Phosphatidylethanolamine
(cephalin)

β-Lecithin

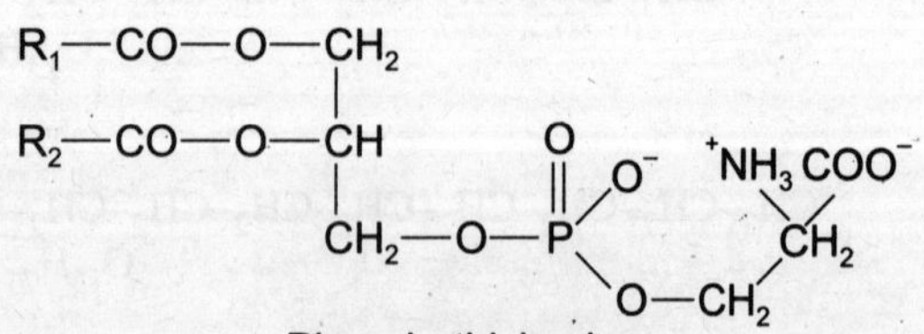

(choline)

Phosphatidylserine

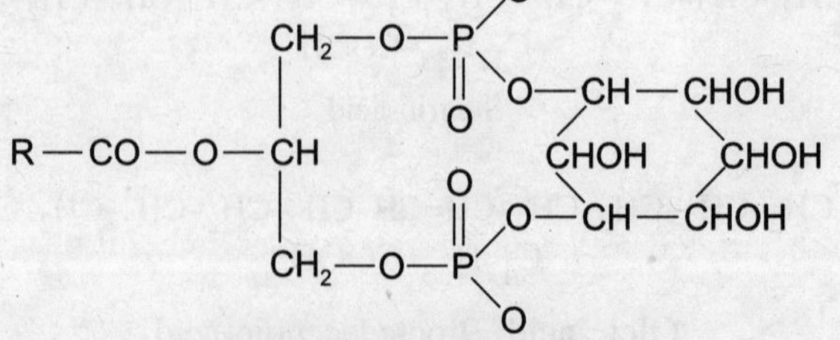

Diphosphoinositide

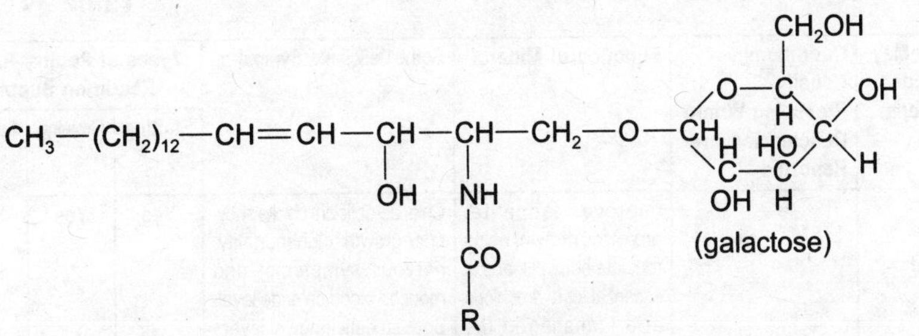
CH₂OH
O—C
OH
H
CH₃—(CH₂)₁₂—CH=CH—CH—CH—CH₂—O—CH
H HO
C
H
C—C
OH
NH
OH H
(galactose)
CO
R

Cerebroside

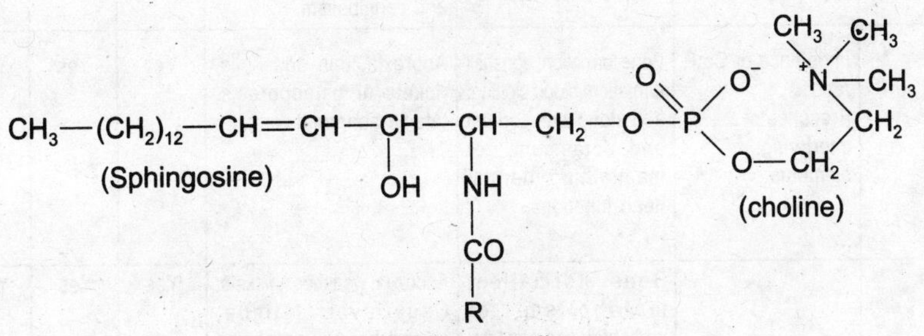
CH₃ CH₃
O
O⁻
N—CH₃
CH₃—(CH₂)₁₂—CH=CH—CH—CH—CH₂—O—P
CH₂
(Sphingosine)
O—CH₂
OH
NH
(choline)
CO
R

Sphingomyelin

(c)

5. Minerals. The body of the chicken and the egg excluding shell contain nearly 4 and 1 per cent mineral matter respectively. The elements known to be required in the diet of poultry are calcium, phosphorus, sodium, potassium, magnesium, chlorine, iodine, iron, manganese, copper, molybdenum, zinc and selenium. Usually the grains and vegetable protein ingredients are relatively poor in mineral contents when compared with those of animal protein feed stuffs. The common mineral supplements in poultry feed are as follows:

(i) Limestone
(ii) Bone meal
(iii) Oyster shell
(iv) Sodium chloride
(v) Dicalcium phosphate
(vi) Manganese sulphate
(vii) Potassium iodide
(viii) Superphosphate.

Details about the functions, deficiency symptoms and other informations about different minerals have been presented in Table 39 as "Poultry mineral chart."

Table 39   POULTRY

Minerals Which May Be Deficient Under Normal Conditions	Conditions Usually Prevailing Where Deficiencies Are Reported	Function of Mineral	Some Deficiency Symptoms	Types of Poultry Rations Usually Requiring Supplementation			
				Starting	Growing	Laying	Breeding
Major or macro minerals: **Salt** (sodium and chlorine) NaCl		Improves appetite, promotes growth, helps regulate body pH, and is essential for hydrochloric acid formation in the stomach.	Chloride-deficient chicks show poor growth, high mortality, nervous symptoms, and reduced blood chloride level. Sodium deficiency in layers results in decreased egg production, poor growth, and cannibalism.	Yes	Yes	Yes	Yes
Calcium (Ca)	Imbalance of Ca:P ratio. Presence of interfering elements	Bone formation; eggshell formation; blood clotting; and along with sodium and potassium, for maintaining normal heart function.	Anorexia, thin eggshells, rickets or osteoporosis, tetany, abnormal walk.	Yes	Yes	Yes	Yes
Phosphorus (P)		Bone formation; metabolism of carbohydrates and fats; a component of all living cells; maintenance of the acid-base balance of the body; and calcium transport in egg formation.	Anorexia, weakness, rickets. Cage-layer fatigue, characterized by birds being paralized and unable to rise from a recumbent position. But there is evidence that this condition is not due to this factor alone.	Yes	Yes	Yes	Yes
Magnesium (Mg)	Diets containing high levels of Ca and P.	Essential for normal skeletal development, as a constituent of bone, enzyme activator, primarily in glycolytic system	Decreased egg production, depressed growth and lethargy, convulsions.	Yes	Yes	Yes	Yes
Potassium (K)		Major cation of intracellular fluid where it is involved in osmotic pressure and acid-base balance. Muscle activity. Required in enzyme reaction involving phosporylation of creatine. Influences carbohydrate metabolism.	Chicks. Retarded growth and high mortality.	No	No	No	No
Trace or micro minerals: **Copper (Cu)**		Essential element in a number of enzyme systems and necessary for synthesizing hemoglobin and preventing nutritional anemia.	Anemia, depigmentation of feathers, digestive disordcrs. *Poults* : Marked cardiac hypertrophy	Yes	Yes	Yes	Yes

MINERAL CHART

Mineral Requirements[1]				
Minerals/Bird/Day	Mineral Content of Ration	Recommended Allowances[1]	Practical Sources of the Mineral	Comments
Variable according to class, age, and weight of poultry	Variable according to class, age, and weight of poultry.	0.2-0.5% of the diet.	Common table salt	Sodium level is sometimes reduced to minimal to control the moisture level of the feces.
Variable according to class, age, and weight of poultry.	Variable according to class, age, and weight of poultry.	The calcium allowance should vary with level of production and temperature. A minimum of 3.25% is believed to be optimum for layers in moderate climates. Growing rations should contain 0.8-0.9% of Ca and 0.4-0.7% of P.	Oystershell. Limestone. Dicalcium phosphate.	For young poultry, the Ca:P ratio should be about 1.2:1. For the laying bird, the ratio must be wider (4:1 or more) An excess of calcium interferes with the utilization of magnesium, manganese, and zinc.
Variable according to class, age, and weight of poultry.	Variable according to class, age, and weight of poultry.	Dependent on production Laying hens require diets containing at least 3% Ca and 3% P. Growing rations should contain 0.8-0.9% of Ca and 0.4-0.7% of P.	Dicalcium phosphate. Defluorinated phosphate. Steamed bone meal. Monosodium phosphate. Phosphoric acid.	Organic phosphorus (present in plants) is poorly utilized by growing birds, but is satisfactory for adult birds. Only about 30% of the phosphorus in plant products is available to the young chick, poult, or duckling.
Variable according to class, age, and weight of poultry.	Variable according to class, age, and weight of poultry.	500 ppm in the ration should suffice.	Magnesium oxide or magnesium sulfate.	Requirements are affected by Ca and P levels in the diet Not normally deficient in poultry rations.
Variable according to class, age. and weight of poultry.	Variable according to class, age, and weight of poultry.		Corn contains 0.27% potassium, and other cereals contain 0.42-0.49% potassium.	Potassium is not deficient in normal rations, due to large amounts of plant products in poultry feeds.
	Variable according to class, age, and weight of poultry.	Rations containing 6 ppm of copper should be adequate.	Copper sulfate, copper carbonate, and copper oxide are about equally effective.	

Table 39

Minerals Which May Be Deficient Under Normal Conditions	Conditions Usually Prevailing Where Deficiencies Are Reported	Function of Mineral	Some Deficiency Symptoms	Types of Poultry Rations Usually Requiring Supplementation			
				Starting	Growing	Laying	Breeding
Iodine (I)	Feeds produced on iron deficient soils.	Needed by the thyroid gland for making thyroxin, an iodine-containing hormone which controls the rate of body metabolism or heat production.	Enlarged thyroid. Eggs produced from deficient breeder hens have a lowered hatchability, prolonged hatching time, and a subsequent retardation of yolk-sac absorption.	Yes	Yes	Yes	Yes
Iron (Fe)		Necessary for formation of hemoglobin, an iron-containing compound which enables the blood to carry oxygen. Iron is also important to certain enzyme systems.	*Chicks and poults* Microcytic, hypochromic anemia. In red-feathered chickens, complete depigmentation of the feathers occurs.	Yes	Yes	Yes	Yes
Manganese (Mn)		Necessary for growth, bone structure, and reproduction	Chicks and poults: Perosis, shortened leg bones, skull deformation, parrot beak. Poor egg production, shell quality, and hatchability.	Yes	Yes	Yes	Yes
Selenium (Se)	Feed that are grown in selenium deficient areas	Not completely known But involved in vitamin E absorption and/or retention Also, a required nutrient in its own right. Involved in the destruction of peroxides within the cell as a constituent of glutathione peroxidase.	Exudative diathesis Pancreatic fibrosis. Steatitis Muscular dystrophy. With a severe selenium deficiency, growth rate is reduced and mortality is increased *Turkeys*: Myopathics of the gizzard and heart. A zinc deficiency in breeder diets reduces egg production and hatchability.	Yes	Yes	Yes Feeds with selenium supplementation cannot he fed to hens laying eggs for human consumption	Yes
Zinc (Zn)		Zinc is a component of several enzyme systems, including peptidases and carbonic anhydrase. Also, zinc is required for normal protein synthesis and metabolism and is a component of insulin	Bone problems, poor feathering (feather fraying occurs near the ends of the feathers), retarded growth, and loss of appetite	Yes	Yes	Yes	Yes

1. As used herein the distinction between "mineral requirement" and "recommended allowances" is as follows. In mineral requirements no margins of safety are included intentionally, whereas in recommended allowances, margins of safety are provided in order to compensate for variations in feed composition, environment and possible losses during shorage or processing.

(Continued)

Mineral Requirements[1]				
Minerals/Bird/Day	Mineral Content of Ration	Recommended Allowances[1]	Practical Sources of the Mineral	Comments
Variable according to class, age, and weight of poultry.	Variable according to class, age. and weight of poultry.	Growing chicks require feed containing 350 ppb. Laying hens require feed containing 300 ppb.	Stabilized iodized salt containing 0.007% iodine. Trace mineral mixes.	
	Variable according to class, age, and weight of poultry.	Rations should contain about 80 ppm of iron.	Meal, liver, and fish meals. Alfalfa meal.	Iron salts are used as a means of detoxifying gossypol from cottonseed meal.
Variable according to class, age. and weight of poultry	Variable according to class, age, and weight of poultry.	Rations should contain at least 55 ppm.	Alfalfa meal, distillers' solubles, or grain by products Manganese sulfate, manganous chloride, mnngannus carbonate, and manganous dioxide.	
	Variable according to class, age, and weight of poultry		Sodium selenite or sodium selenate Fish meal and brewers' dried yeast.	Selenium can pose toxicity problems Hence, care should be taken when adding it to poultry rations. In 1974, FDA approved the addition of Se in either sodium selenite or sodium selenate at the rate of 0.1 ppm to complete rations for growing chickens to 16 weeks of age, breeder hens producing hatching eggs; and at the rate of 0 2 ppm in complete rations for turkeys.
	Variable according to class, age, and weight of poultry		Zinc carbonate or zinc sulfate.	

6. Vitamins. Vitamins most commonly function as coenzymes and regulators of metabolism. The 13 vitamins required by poultry have been summarised in tabular form (Table 40) whereas Table 41 shows the conversion of beta-carotene to vitamin A for different species. Apart from natural sources, commercial vitamin mixture suitable for poultry are also available. One point to remember, of course, is that the natural vitamins are likely to have other factors associated with them. These may be other recognised nutrients or they may be unidentified factors. Diets continuously deficient in any one of the required vitamins will seriously affect initially upon the egg production and then the life of the chickens.

7. Feed additives. A full discussion including importance of various feed additives has been made separately.

Table 40 Vitamin deficiency symptoms in poultry and the principal natural sources of these vitamins

Vitamin	Deficiency symptoms	Principal natural source
Vitamin A	Retarded growth, general weakness, emaciation, staggering gait, ruffled feathers, mortality, watery or sticky eyelids, xerophthalmia, creamy white pustules on roof of mouth and along esophagus, ureates in kidney tubules and ureters. In young and adult birds a cheesy exudate from eye and sticky discharge from nostrils is often observed. Egg production and hatchability are markedly reduced.	Cod-liver and other fish oils, animal liver meals, green grasses, yellow corn, lucerne green or dried, maize gluten meal, leaf meals from tropical legumes.
Vitamin D	Rickets-leg weakness, stiff legged gait, crooked keels, beaded ribs, swollen hocks, soft bones, ungainly manner of balancing body, appear unthrifty, depigmentation of feathers, and mortality; in adults, fragile bones, thin-shelled eggs, reduced egg production and hatchability.	Cod-liver oils and certain other fish oils or concentrates. Deactivated animal sterol. Sunshine by irradiation of sterols under the skin, ultraviolet ray lights by similar irradiation.
Vitamin E (α-tocopherol)	Encephalomacia ("Crazy chick" disease) inco-ordination of movement, frequently unable to stand, turns in circle, edema beneath skin and hemorrhage in cerebellum. In turkeys, enlarged hock disorder and dystrophy of smooth muscle of gizzard lining reported. In ducks, dystrophy of skeletal muscle. In adults, reduced hatchability in chickens and turkeys.	Green forage, vegetable oils, whole and sprouted grains, lucerne meal.

Table 40 (*Continued*)

Vitamin	Deficiency symptoms	Principal natural source
Vitamin K	Prolonged blood clotting time. Haemorrhages develop internally and subcutaneously on the legs, breast, abdomen, neck, under the wings, and in the intestinal tract.	Lucerne, kale, green leafy vegetables, meat scraps, fish meal.
Vitamin B_1 (thiamine)	Polyneuritis-retracted head, retarded growth, reduced appetite, extreme weakness, ataxia, emaciation, impairment of digestion, convulsions, and death.	Whole grain, wheat by-products, yeast, liver meal, groundnut meal, molasses, grasses, lucerne, rice by-products.
Vitamin B_2 (riboflavin)	"Curled toe" paralysis (toes curl inward) and paralysis of legs, retarded growth, diarrhoea, tendency to walk on hocks, hypertrophy and softening of brachial and sciatic nerves and dry scaly skin, severe dermatitis in poults at corners of mouth, vent, eyelids and footpads. In adults, reduction in egg production and hatchability, dwarfed embroys showing edema, degeneration of Wolffian bodies, and 'clubbed down' condition. Embryo motality peak at about the eleventh day of incubation.	Liver meal, yeast, milk by-products. Concentrates made from fermentation residues, lucerne leaf meal, young grasses, kidney, some fish meals, distillers' solubles.
Vitamin B_6 (pyridoxine)	Retarded growth, hyper-excitability, tend to run aimlessly, flapping their wings with head down, repeated convulsions with distended or twisted neck, complete exhaustion and death. In adults, loss of appetite, reduced egg production and hatchability, loss of weight and death.	Liver meal, yeast, rice bran, meat (muscle tissue and glands), cane molasses, fish, wheat and rice by-products, lucerne.
Vitamin B_{12} (cyanocoba-lamine)	Reduced growth, poor feathering and mortality in young chicks. In adult hens, poor hatchability of fertile eggs. Chicks that do hatch have low "carryover" and show high early mortality unless injected with or fed, high levels of vitamin B_{12}	Fish meal, liver, whey, soybean oil meal, cow manure, egg yolk, egg white, various fermentation products.
Pantothenic acid	Retarded growth, ragged feather development, dermatitis lesions on eyelids, at corners of mouth, around vent and sometimes on top of the feet,	Liver meal, yeast, cane molasses, groundnut meal, milk by-products, wheat bran, rice bran, soybean meal, lucerne leaf meal, kale cabbage,

Table 40 (*Continued*)

Vitamin	Deficiency symptoms	Principal natural source
	liver damage and changes in spinal cord may develop. In adult fowls, lowered hatchability and impaired egg production result.	broccoli, cauliflower, cucumbers, fermentation residues, maize, distillers solubles grasses.
Nicotinic acid (niacine)	Poor growth, poor feathering inflammation of the mouth and tongue ("black tongue"), perosis, reduced feed consumption and occasionally dermatitis on skin and feet of young chicks and poults. In poults, enlarged hock disorder; in ducks and goslings, bowed legs occur. In adults, poor egg production and reduced hatchability.	Yeast, liver meal, rice bran, wheat feeds, groundnuts, greens, meat (muscle tissue), maize distillers solubles.
Folic acid (Folacin)	Retarded growth, poor feathering depigmentation of feathers in coloured chicks and poults, reduction in red blood cell numbers and haemoglobin (anemia), reduction in white blood cells, occasionally perosis, and high mortality. In poults, cervical paralysis (paralysis of neck) also observed. In adults, anemia, weight loss, reduced egg production and lowered hat-chability.	Green leafy plants, grass, spinach, lucerne, etc. Yeast, liver, kidneys. Whole grain supplies enough in poultry rations.
Biotin	Poor growth, perosis and severe dermatosis. Bottoms of feet become roughened and crack open, then dermatitic lesions also appear, at corners of mouth and on eyelids as described for pantothenic acid deficiency. In adults, impaired hatchability with embryos showing skeletal deformities including parrot beak and short legs.	Liver, yeast, potatoes, kidneys and other glands, milk, cane molasses, lucerne leaf meal, grasses. Whole grain supplies enough in the poultiy ration
Choline	Poor growth, perosis (slipped tendon), poor feed utilisation, unthrifty appearance and slight increase in liver fat. Practical rations for adult fowl appear to contain adequate levels of choline.	Liver meal, meat, fish, whole grain, wheat by-products, milk by-products, groundnut meal, soy-bean oil meal.

SOURCE: *Poultry Feeding in Tropical and Subtropical Countries*, FAO Rome, 1964.

Table 41 Conversion of beta-carotene to vitamin A for different species[1]

Species	Conversion of mg of Beta-Carotene to IU of Vitamin A		IU of Vitamin A Activity (calculated from carotene)
	(mg)	(IU)	(%)
Standard (rat)	1	1,667	100
Poultry	1	1,667	100
Beef cattle	1	400	24.0
Dairy cattle	1	400	24.0
Sheep	1	400-500	24.0-30.0
Swine	1	500	30.0
Horses:			
Growth	1	555	33.3
Pregnancy	1	333	20.0
Mink	Carotene not utilized		–
Man	1	556	33.3

[1]Adapted from the Atlas of Nutritional Data on United States and Canadian Feeds. NRC-National Academy ot Science 1972 p XVI Table 6

REQUIREMENTS FOR POULTRY FEEDS

Chickens of different ages require different levels of nutrients, The Buraue of Indian Standards (BIS) has prescribed the standard specifications for broiler, starting, growing and laying chickcn feeds to serve as a guide for the feed manufacturers and poultry keepers in the country in their publication number ISI: 1374 : 2007 (Fifth revision). The nutrient requirement of chicken feeds are detailed in Table 43 whereas Table 42 shows the sources of nutrients required by poultry.

Poultry feeds are of the following three types:

1. *Starting poultry feed*: An all mash ration to be fed to chicks upto the age of 8 weeks.
2. *Growing poultry feed*: A ration to be fed to growing chickens after 8 to 20 weeks of age or until laying commences.
3. *Laying poultry feed*: A ration to be fed to laying birds after the age of 20 weeks onwards or after laying commences.

Feeding Broilers

A broiler, also known as fryer is a young chicken, which grow very fast and can be marketed after 6 weeks of age. By this time it attains about 2.0 kg live weight. It may be of either sex, tender-meated with soft, pliable, smooth, textured skin and flexible breast bone cartilage.

Broiler rations are especially formulated in such a way that they promote an early rapid growth. Usually broiler rations are prepared in such a way so that the feed contains relatively high energy and high protein when compared with the feed of chickens other than broilers. A protein per cent of 22 is fed to broilers for the first 3 weeks to obtain rapid early growth. These rations are called broiler starter rations. After this period, broilers are fed with a different type of ration having relatively less protein (20%) and more energy for fattening. Such a feed is known as broiler finisher ration. The ideal compositions of broiler rations are given in Table 45 while Table 44 show the inter-relation between nutrients in poulty rations.

Table 42 Sources of Nutrients Required by Poultry

Nutrient	Sources
Protein	Meat scraps (lysine), fish meal (lysine, methionine), poultry by-product meal (tryptophan, lysine), blood meal, liver and glandular meal, feather meal (hydrolyzed), animal tankage, milk products, cottonseed meal, peanut meal, soybean meal (lysine), corn gluten meal (methionine), saffflower meal, sesame meal, sunflower seed meal.
Carbohydrate	Corn, sorghum grains (milo). barley, rye, oats, wheat, wheat middlings, various grain by-products.
Fat	Animal tallow (beef), lard, corn oil, other vegetable oils.
Minerals	Meat scraps, fish meal, milk products, ground limestone (calcium), ground oyster shells (caicium), dicalcium phosphate (calcium, phosphorus), defluorinated rock phosphate (phosphorus, calcium), steamed bone meal (phosphorus, calcium), salt (sodium, chlorine, iodine), manganese sulfate (manganese), manganese oxide (manganese), zinc carbonate (zinc), zinc oxide (zinc).
Vitamins	Yeasts, fish solubles, distillers' solubles, liver meal, alfalfa meal, milk by-products.

Table 43 Nutrient requirements for chicken feed

Sl. No.	Characteristics	Broiler starter (0-3 weeks)	Broiler finisher (4 to 6 weeks)	Chick (0-8 weeks)	Grower (9-20 weeks)	Layer (21-72 weeks)	Breeder (21-72 weeks)
(1)	(2)	(3)	(4)	(5)	(6)	(7)	(8)
1.	Crude protein (%)**	22	20	20	16	18	17
2.	Crude fibre (%)*	5	5	7	9	9	9
3.	Ether extract (%)**	3.5	4	2	2	2	2
4.	Acid insoluble insoluble ash (%)*	2.5	2.5	4	4	4	2.5
5.	Salt (NaCl) (%) *	0.5	0.5	0.5	0.5	0.5	0.5
6.	Moisture (%)*	11	11	11	11	11	11
7.	Metabolizable energy (KCal/kg)**	3100	3200	2800	2500	2600	2600
8.	Lysine (%)**	1.2	1	1	0.7	0.7	0.7
9.	Methionine (%)**	0.5	0.45	0.4	0.35	0.35	0.4
10.	Methionine + cystine (%)**	0.9	0.85	0.7	0.6	0.6	0.6
11.	Vitamin A (IU/kg)**	11,000	10,000	9,000	8,000	8,000	15,000
12.	Vitamin D_3 (IU/kg)**	3,000	3,000	1,800	1,600	1,600	3,000

(1)	(2)	(3)	(4)	(5)	(6)	(7)	(8)
13.	Thiamine (mg/kg)**	2.5	2.5	2	1.5	1	3
14.	Riboflavin (mg/kg)**	6	6	6	5	5	6
15.	Pantothenic acid (mg/kg)**	15	15	10	9	7	25
16.	Nicotinic acid (mg/kg)**	40	40	40	20	20	50
17.	Biotin (mg/kg)**	0.15	0.15	0.1	0.1	0.1	0.2
18.	Vitamin B_{12} (mg/kg)**	0.015	0.015	0.01	0.008	0.008	0.03
19.	Folic acid (mg/kg)**	1	1	1	0.5	0.5	4
20.	Choline (mg/kg)**	500	500	500	200	400	700
21.	Vitamin E (mg/kg)**	30	30	15	10	10	50
22.	Linoleic acid (%)**	1.1	1.1	1	1	1	1
23.	Calcium (%)**	1	1	1	1	3	3.5
24.	Total phosphorus (%)**	0.7	0.7	0.7	0.65	0.65	0.6
25.	Available phosphorus (%)**	0.45	0.45	0.45	0.4	0.4	0.4
26.	Manganese (mg/kg)**	100	100	70	60	60	100
27.	Iodine (mg/kg)**	1.2	1.2	1	1	1	1.5
28.	Iron (mg/kg)**	80	80	70	60	60	80
29.	Zinc (mg/kg)**	80	80	60	60	60	80
30.	Copper (mg/kg)**	12	12	12	9	9	12

*Maximum, ** Minimum

Notes: (i) The values specified for characteristics at Sl. Nos. 1 to 5 are on dry matter basis.

(ii) Earlier the broiler cycle was for 8 weeks. It has now been reduced to 6 weeks. Further, BIS has now split 0-7 days as pre-starter; 8 to 21 days as starter and finisher feed from 22 days till finish under sophisticated management system of large farms.

(iii) Now-a-days layer stage has been splitted as phase I (21 to 45 weeks) and phase II (46 to 72 weeks) of age under sophisticated management system of large farms.

(iv) Extra calcium source in the form of shell grit / limestone at about 4-5 gm per bird per day is advised in case of laying stage (both in Phase I & II)

Source: Adopted from BIS (IS 1374:2007 Fifth Revision) with some modification.

Table 44 Inter-relations between nutrients in poultry rations

	Broilers		Replacement pullets (egg or meat type)			Laying and breeding
	0-6 weeks	6- 9 weeks	0-6 weeks	6-14 weeks	14-20 weeks	hens (egg and meat type)
Calorie: protein (C/P)	139:1	160:1	145:1	180:1	241:1	190:1
Calcium: Phosphrous	1.4:1	1.4 1	1.4:1	2:1	2:1	4.5:1
Vitamin D_3(ICU/kg)	200	200	200	200	200	200
Arginine: Lysine	1.12:1	1.09:1	1.09:1	1.05:1	1.03:1	1 6:1
•Methionine: cystine	1.15:1	1.14:1	1.14:1	1.14:1	1.14:1	1.12:1
Phenylalanine: Tyrosine	1.14:1	1.16:1	1.16:1	1.1:1	1.16:1	?
Tryptophan (%)	0.2	0.2	0.2	0.16	0.12	0.11
Niacin (mg/kg)	27	27	27	11	10	10

• Methionine content in ration should not be less than 0.46 for 0 to 6 weeks old chicks.

Table 45 Compositions of Broiler rations

Ingredients (kg/100 kg)	Broiler starter rations					
	1	2	3	4	5	6
Maize	44.25	43.75	48.17	44.12	50.88	57.10
Rice polish	10.00	10.00	10.00	15.00	10.00	–
Groundnut cake	15.00	14.00	30.00	26.00	14.00	–
Sunflower cake	15.00	14 00	–	–	8.00	15.00
Mustard cake (solvent extracted)	–	–	–	–	–	10.00
Fish meal (43% pro)[1]	6.00	10.00	10.30	7.30	8.00	6.00
Meat meal (56% pro)	6.00	–	–	–	–	7.00
Meat-cum-bone meal (54% pro)	–	–	–	–	3.00	–
Silkworm-pupae meal deoiled (70% pro)	–	–	–	5.00	5.00	3.00
Blood meal (73% pro)	–	3.50	–	–	–	–
Lysine HCl	0.15	–	0.18	0.25	0.22	–
DL-methionine	–	–	0.10	0.10	–	–
Animal fat	2.00	3.00	–	–	–	1.00
Bone meal	0.75	1.15	0.75	1.40	–	–
Limestone	0.50	–	–	–	–	–
Salt	0.25	0.50	0.40	0.30	0.40	0.50
Choline chloride	–	–	–	0.03	–	0.30
Mineral[2] and vitamin mixture[3]	0.10	0.10	0.10	0.10	0.10	0.10
Total	100.00	100.00	100.00	100.00	100.00	100.00

Ingredients (kg/100 kg)	Broiler Finisher rations					
	1	2	3	4	5	6
Maize	44.10	45.30	46.80	50.38	49.90	65.10
Rice polish	20.00	20.00	20.00	20.00	20.00	–
Groundout cake	11.00	9.50	19.00	13.00	8.00	–
Maize gluten meal	–	–	–	–	8.00	–
Sunflower cake	11.00	9.50	–	–	–	12.00
Mustard oil cake (solvent extracted)	–	–	–	–	–	10.00
Fish meal (43% pro)	5.50	9.00	13.00	10.00	10.00	5.00
Meat meal (56% pro)	5.50	–	–	–	3.00	5.00
Meat-cum-bone meal (54% pro)	–	–	–	–	–	–
Blood meal (73% pro)	–	3.00	–	–	–	–
Silkworm-pupae meal (de-oiled (70% pro)	–	–	–	5.00	–	1.20
Fat	1.25	2.00	–	–	–	–
Bone meal	0.60	1.10	0.70	1.00	0.70	0.60
Limestone	0.70	–	–	–	–	0.60
Salt	0.25	0.50	0.40	0.50	0.30	0.40
Choline chloride	–	–	–	0.02	–	–
Mineral[2] and vitamin[1] mixture	0.10	0.10	0.10	0.10	0.10	0.10
Total	100.00	100.00	100.00	100.00	100.00	100.00

1. The quantity of fish meal can be reduced if good quality fish meal is available.
2. Mineral mixture to contain : ferrous sulphate, 20 g, manganese sulphate, 25 g; zinc sulphate. 25 g; copper sulphate. 25 g; and potassium iodate, 100 mg.
3. Vitamin mixture to provide : vitamin A, 800,000 IU; vitamin D_3, 100,000 ICU; riboflavin, 400 mg; and folic acid, 100 mg.

Table 46 Recommended range of proportion of poultry feeds

Ingredients	Proportion (per cent by weight of material)	Ingredients	Proportion (per cent by weight of material)
Grain and Seeds		*Oil-cakes and meals*	
Bajra, bajri (*Pennisetum typhoides*)	10-15	Copra cake, coconut cake	5-10
Barley (*Hordeum vulgare*)	5-10	Cottonseed oil-cake	Up to 5%
Black-gram (*Phaseolus mungo*)	10-15	(decorticated)	by weight
Chinna, cheena (*Panicum miliaceum*)	10-15	Groundnut oil-cake (decorticated)	15-30
Kulthi or horse-gram	10-20	Guar (*Cyamopsis*	Up to 5%
(*Dolichos biflorus*)		*tetragonoloba*) meal	by weight
Jowar, Cholam (*Sorghum vulgare*)	10-15	Safflower (*Carthamus*	10-15
Oat (*Avena sativa*)	5-20	*tinctorious*) cake	
Arhar (*Cassia tora*)	5-10	Mustard cake: Expeller	10-20
Ragi (*Eleusine coracana*)	10-20	Deoiled mustardcake	25-50
Yellow maize	15-50	Salseed cake (*Shorea robusta*)	0-5
Tapioca flour	5-15	Sesamum (*Sesamum indicum*	
Corn (*Maize yellow*)	0-55	*orientale*) cake	10-20
		Soybean meal	10-20
		Karanja deoiled cake (*Pongamia*	
		glabra)	7-8
Grain by-products		*Tubers and roots*	
Arhar chuni	10-15	Tapioca flour	10-25
		Greens	
Gram chuni	10-15	Berseem (*Trifolium alexan-*	
Black-gram chuni	10-15	*drinum*) leaf-meal	3-5
Maize grit	10-15	Lucerne (*Medicago sativa*)	
Maize-gluten meal	10-20	leaf-meal	3-5
Rice bran	10-20		
Wheat bran	10-15		
Rice polish	10-30		
Minerals, Vitamins and antibiotics		*Waste materials and industrial by-products*	
Common salt	0.3-0.5	Brewers' grains	2-5
Dicalcium phosphate (fluorine		Dried yeast and yeast sludge	2-5
content not exceeding 0.5 per cent)	1-2	Mango-seed kernel	5-10
Limestone	1-3	Molasses	5-10
Oyster shells	1-3	Penicillin mycelium residue	5-15
Vitamins (mineral stabilised)	As recommended by the manufacturer	Silkworm pupae (freed from membranous covering)	5-10
		Bloodmeal	3-5
Manganese sulphate	0.02-0.3		
Antibiotic feed supplement	0.1-0.5	*Animal products*	
		Fiih-meal	5-10
		Liver residue meal	5-10
		Meat-meal and meat-scarp	5-10
		Skim milk (dried)	5-10
		Blood meal	3-5
		Bone meal	1.5-2.5
		Hatehery waste	0-3

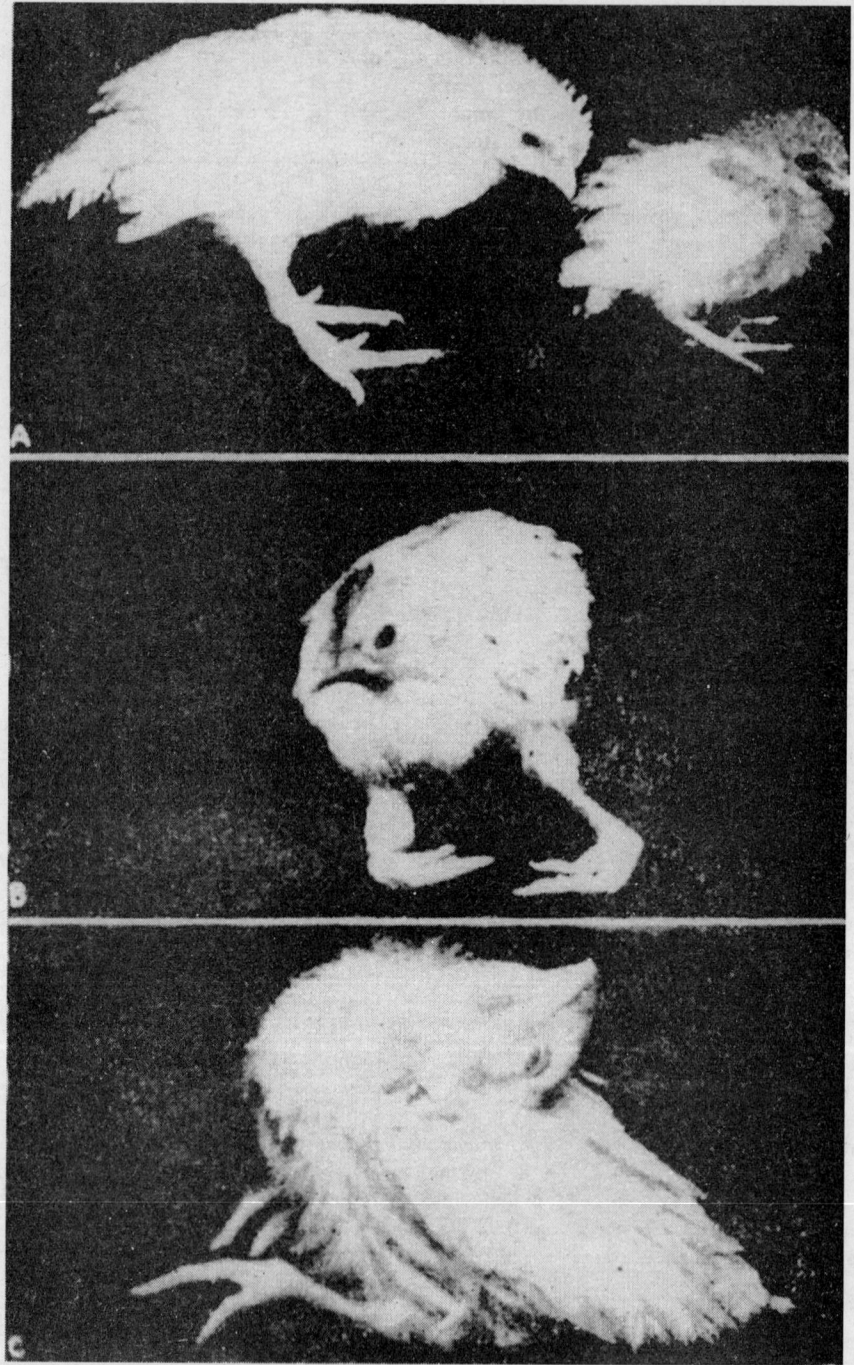

Plate 8. Effects of vitamin deficiencies. A. Effect of nicotinic acid deficiency on chick growth. B. Riboflavin deficiency in a young chick. Note the curled toes and the tendency to squat on the hocks. C. Head retraction caused by a deficiency of thiamin.

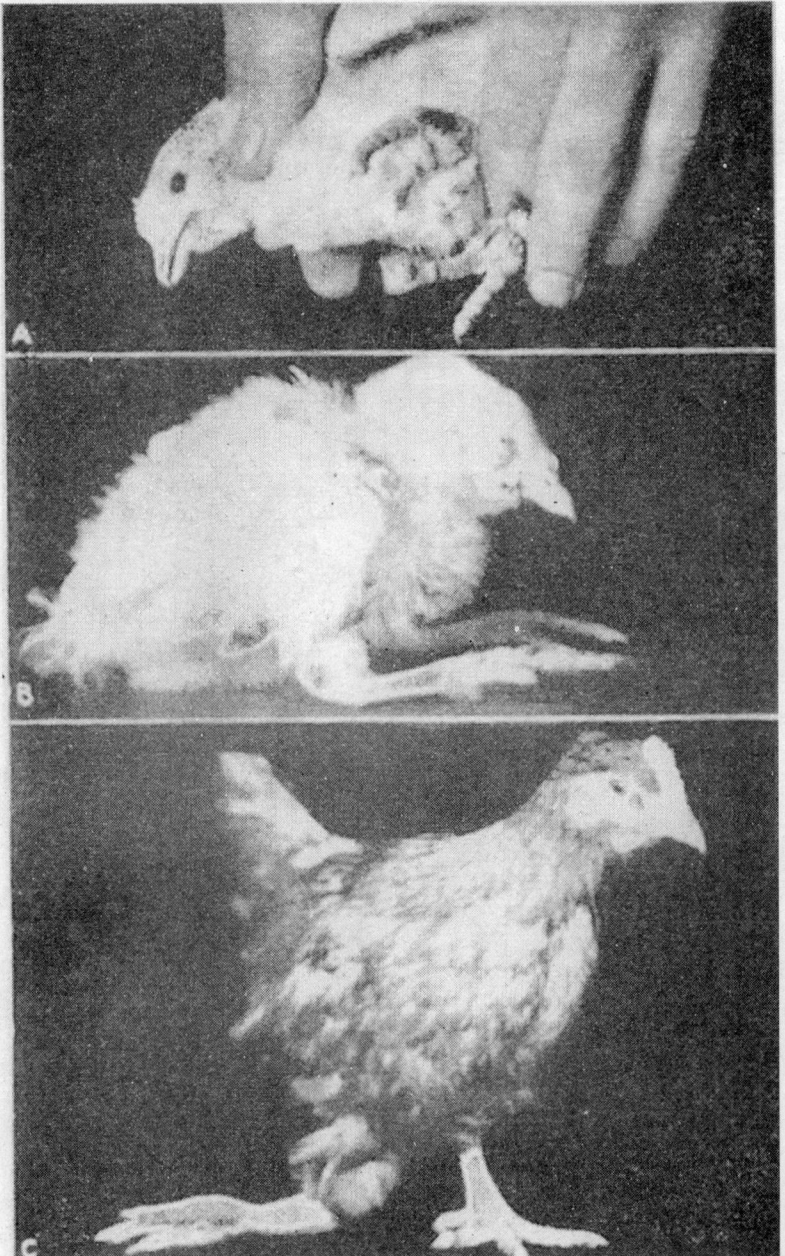

Plate 9.   Effect of vitamin deficiencies. A. Biotin deficiency, Note the severe lesions on the bottom of the feet, and the lesions at the corner of the mouth, B. An advanced stage of pantothenic acid deficiency. Note the lesions at the corner of the mouth, and on the eyelids and feet. C. Perosis or slipped tendon resulting from a deficiency of manganese. This condition may also be caused by a deficiency of choline, blotin, nicotinic or folic acid.

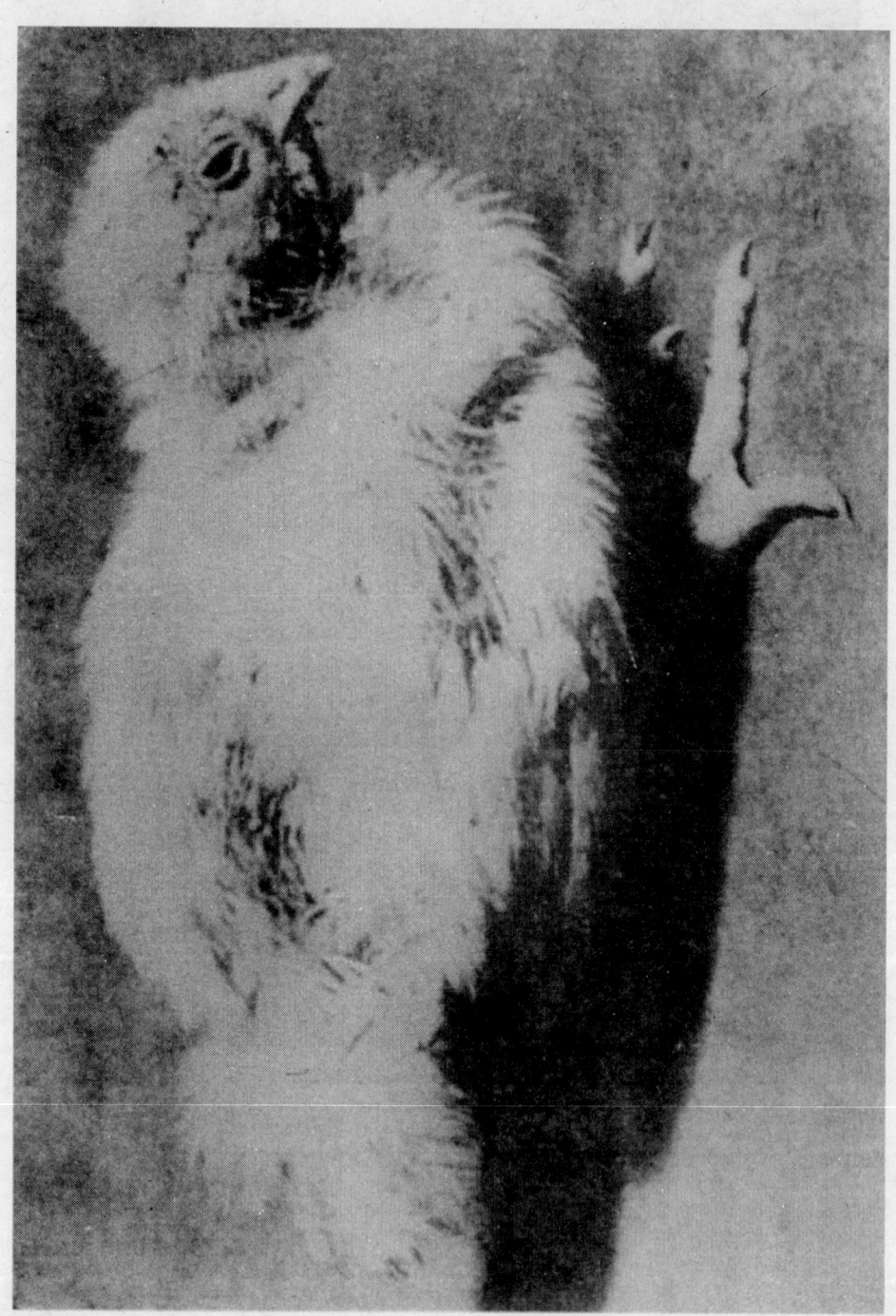

Plate 10.   Exudative diathesis (blood serum oozed into the tissues) in the chick.
Note the oedema of the neck. The condition develops due to lack of either Vit. E or Selenium.

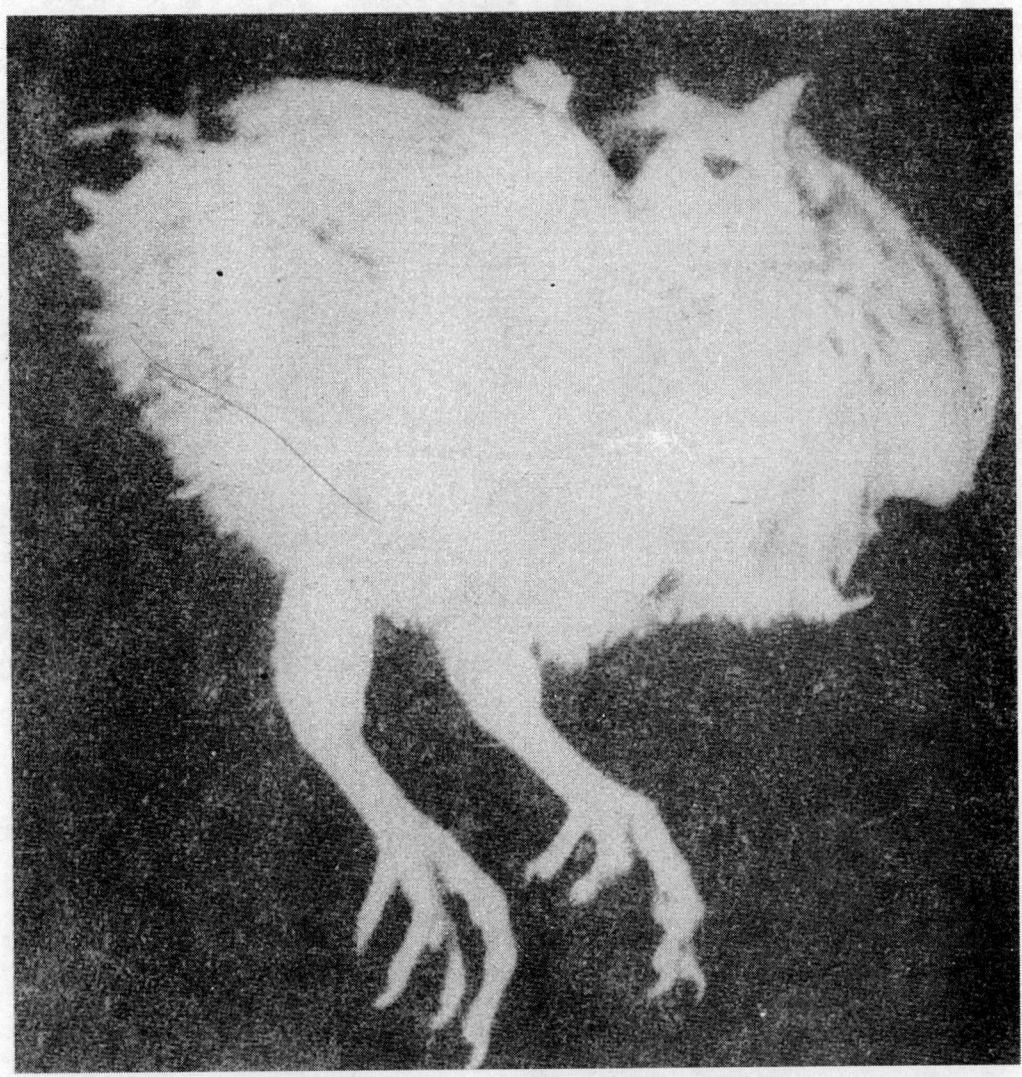

Plate 11. A chick with Nutritional Encephalomalacia, due to lack of Vitamin E. Note head retraction and loss of control of legs.

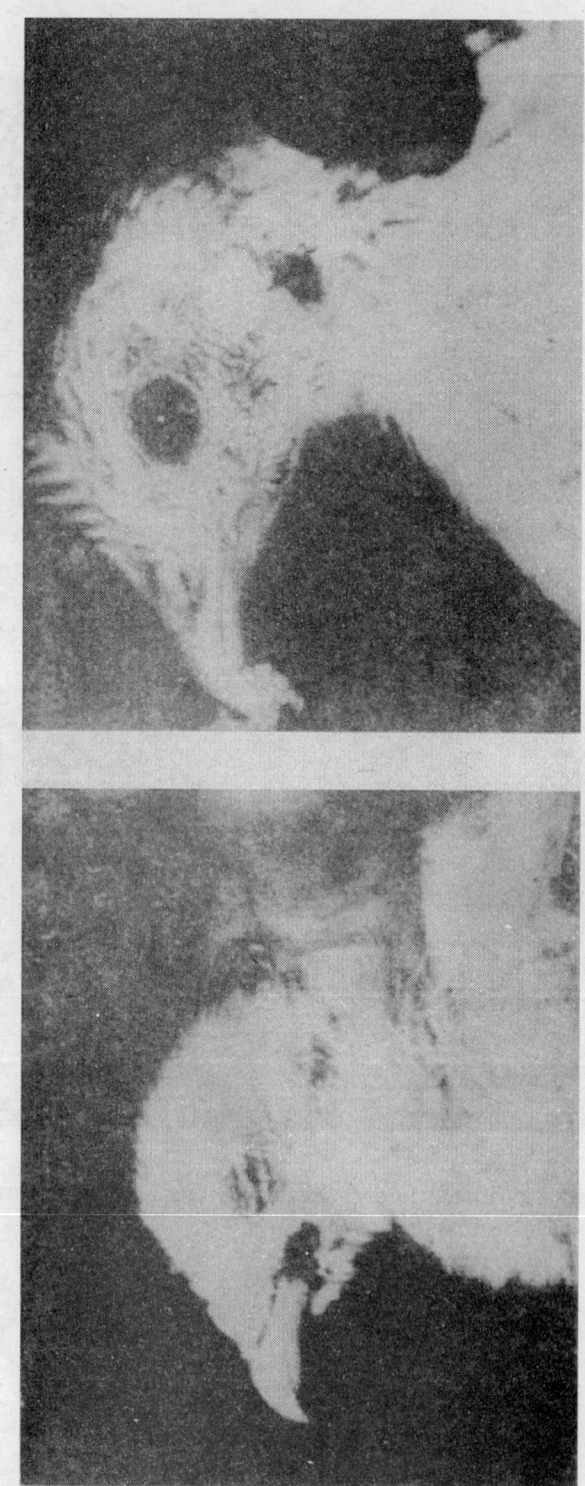

Plate 12. Pantothenic acid deficiency in the chick. The eyelids, corners of the mouth, and adjacent skin areas are involved. Feathering is retarded and rough (left). The same bird (right) after receiving Calcium pantothenate for 3 weeks.

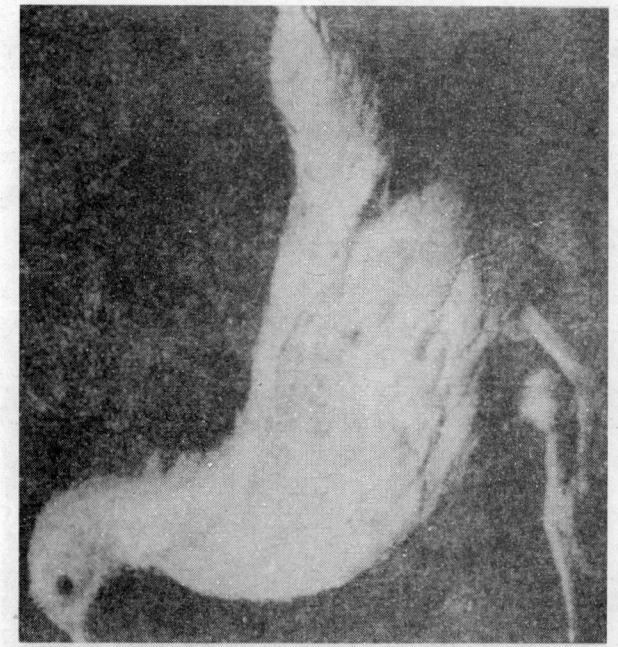

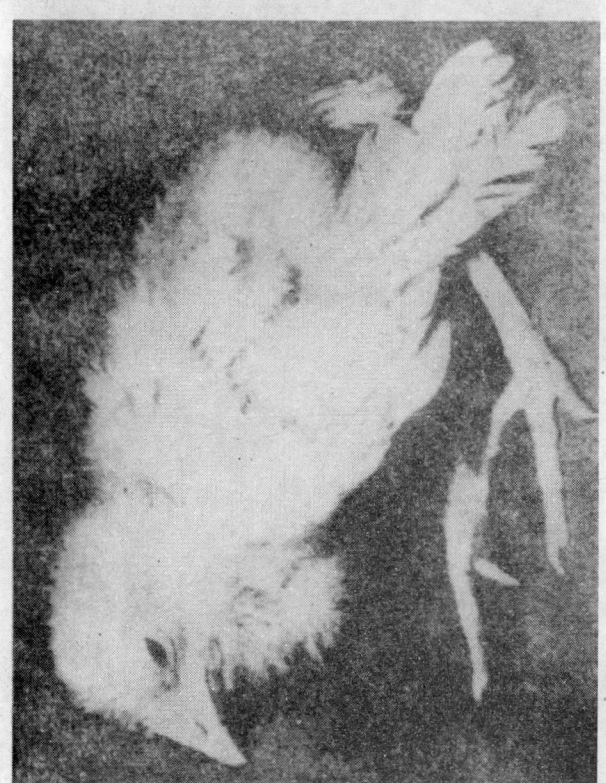

Plate 13. Fotic acid–deficient chick (left) is stunted, poorly feathered, and severely anemic. The healthy chick (right) received the same ration supplemented with 100 mg of folic acid per 100 g. of ration. Both are 4 weeks old.

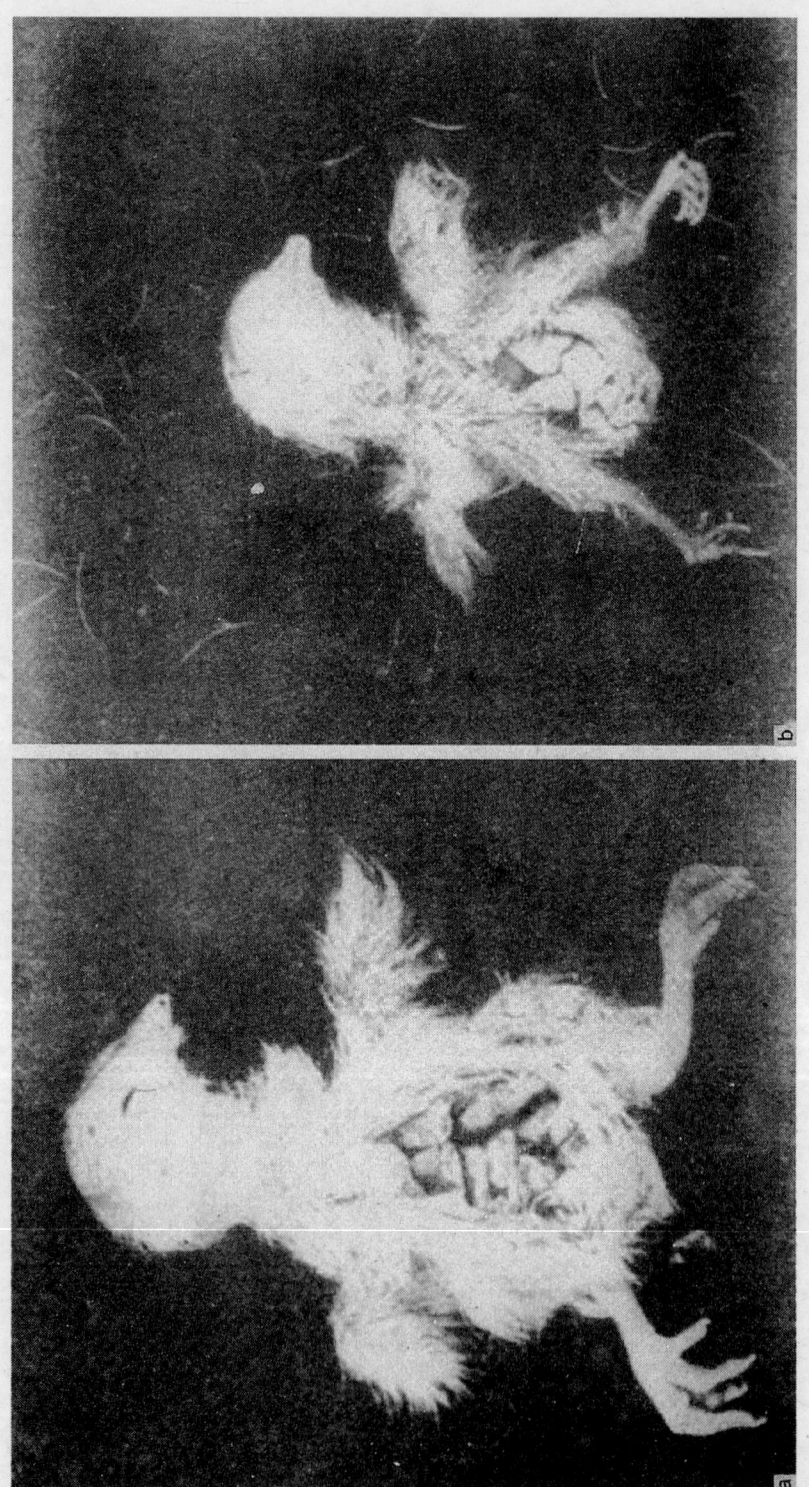

Plate 14. Chick embryos, with yolk sec removed, at the 18th day of incubation (a) from a normal hen, (b) from a hen deprived of vitamin B_{12}; note the small size, myoatrophy of the legs, pale fatty liver and detached feathers.

Table 47 Classification and composition table for poultry feed ingredients*

Feed ingredient	ME (kcal/kg)	D.M.	C.P.	C.F.	E.E.	N.F.E.	Total ash	Acid Insol. Ash	Ca	P.	Lys.	Met.	Tryp.
Energy feeds:													
Bajra grain	2642	89.6	12.7	2.2	4.9	78.2	2.0	1.50	0.13	0.72	0.42	0.24	0.18
Cashew bran	–	94.4	16.9	6.9	27.1	45.4	3.7	0.10	0.45	0.40	–	–	–
Cashew kurna	–	95.7	18.4	9.5	52.9	15.6	3.6	0.40	0.50	0.60	–	–	–
Jower	2645	87.3	10.3	3.6	46	78.1	3.4	—	0.18	0.32	0.32	0.28	0.08
Lentils dehusked	–	94.2	24.6	0.7	1.0	71.1	2.6	0.36	0.20	0.83	0.97	0.32	0.26
Maize bran	–	93.7	8.5	14.9	1.4	73.8	1.4	—	0.07	0.13	–	0.03	0.06
Maize damage	–	89.7	10.1	2.8	3.9	80.1	1.7	0.39	0.25	0.40	0.21	0.18	0.16
Maize grit	2742	90.8	13.6	5.3	2.1	76.1	2.9	1.23	0.22	0.35	1.01	1.20	1.35
Maize opaque–2	–	–	9.9	–	–	–	–	–	–	–	0.34	–	–
Metha	–	92.1	20.6	8.6	6.1	60.9	3.8	0.45	0.35	0.80	–	–	–
Molasses	2400	73.6	2.8	–	–	86.3	10.9	0.44	1.51	0.66	–	–	–
Mowha flour	–	80.0	6.0	8.7	0.3	78.7	6.3	–	–	–	–	–	–
Oak kernels	–	–	5.4	2.1	10.2	79.4	2.9	–	0.13	0.15	–	–	–
Oats	–	91.7	14.7	13.5	4.6	60.8	6.4	—	0.11	0.41	0.38	0.23	0.10
Rice deoiled	2235	92.3	14.1	13.8	1.7	53.4	17.0	8.37	0.37	1.80	0.45	0.44	0.15
Rice kani	2345	90.7	7.9	1.4	1.7	87.1	1.9	0.66	0.11	0.48	0.06	–	–
Rice polish	2937	91.8	12.7	11.2	13.9	48.6	13.6	6.77	0.27	1.37	0.40	0.38	0.25
Salseed cake	3096	90.4	10.4	3.4	2.9	79.6	3.7	2.16	0.24	0.16	0.60	6.38	0.41
Starch	3938	89.4	10.6	0.03	0.09	99.4	0.28	0.04	–	–	–	–	–
Tapioca flour	3000	–	2.9	10.9	0.7	77.0	8.5	–	0.58	0.12	0.06	0.006	0.005

Table 47 *(Continued)*

Feed ingredient	ME (kcal / kg)	D.M.	CP.	C.F.	E.E.	N.F.E.	Total ash	Acid Insol. Ash	Ca	P.	Lys.	Met.	Tryp.
Tapioca waste	–	90.4	4.1	15.9	1.5	72.5	6.0	–	0.58	0.19	–	–	–
Wheat bran	1069	88.9	14.7	11.3	3.8	62.3	7.9	–	0.19	1.12	0.50	0.16	0.18
Wheat damaged	–	89.9	9.5	2.3	2.3	81.9	4.0	1.66	0.08	0.41	–	–	–
Wheat dust	–	92.1	12.3	18.3	2.3	57.3	9.6	–	0.52	0.33	0.37	–	–
Protein Supplements:													
Blood meal	1420	88.8	73.4	0.7	–	–	6.0	3.0	0.32	0.31	4.79	0.66	0.88
Liver residue meal	–	90.9	65.4	1.3	15.8	11.9	5.6	–	–	–	3.85	0.89	0.50
Meat meal	2319	92.5	56.2	2.2	11.9	8.7	21.0	9.17	2.68	2.06	3.73	0.80	0.60
Poultry by-product meal	–	93.0	56.4	0.9	17.8	7.6	17.3	2.20	3.95	1.73	–	–	–
Casein	–	95.6	80.2	–	–	–	–	–	–	–	–	–	–
Coconut cake	1190	91.0	22.6	12.5	8.7	49.4	6.8	–	–	–	0.70	0.32	0.32
Cotton seed cake	1556	92.3	25.9	25.4	8.6	33.7	6.4	0.79	0.52	0.86	0.76	0.45	0.35
Dhaincha	–	91.2	28.3	11.0	5.8	50.7	4.2	0.10	0.30	0.55	2.30	0.60	0.67
Fish meal	1834	93.8	43.1	3.6	4.3	11.5	37.5	22.85	7.16	1.67	3.01	1.19	0.80
Frog meal	–	97.4	68.2	0.4	4.9	2.4	24.1	–	11.75	5.38	–	–	–
Gram baked dry	–	94.5	38.8	10.7	6.6	38.1	5.8	–	–	–	–	–	–
Bengal gram	2496	65.1	14.0	6.5	5.7	68.2	5.6	–	0.20	0.28	0.31	0.29	0.20
Black gram	2614	92.4	20.8	6.1	6.4	60.8	5.9	0.19	0.34	0.51	0.29	–	–
Gram chuni	2320	87.6	29.2	12.1	7.0	45.7	6.0	–	1.30	1.30	0.94	0.23	0.18
Gram red dehusked (Arhar)	–	93.1	21.7	0.9	1.9	71.0	4.5	0.08	0.19	0.92	0.69	0.74	0.14
Gram green (Mung)	–	93.5	19.7	5.2	1.3	70.1	3.7	0.32	0.25	0.84	–	0.41	0.13
Gram Horse (Kullhi)	2614	93.6	20.1	8.3	5.7	63.1	2.8	0.12	0.35	0.53	–	–	–
Groundnut cake (expeller)	2596	91.5	40.9	8.9	7.9	36.4	5.9	0.86	0.23	0.59	1.50	0.42	0.53
Groundnut cake(deoiled)	2328	93.3	57.9	11.2	2.2	27.2	10.8	2.24	0.31	0.67	1.51	0.43	0.71
Guar dal	–	89.7	48.0	5.3	7.4	23.7	5.7	–	0.26	0.79	–	–	–
Guar meal	–	91.0	42.6	10.9	6.2	35.1	5.8	0.59	0.54	0.70	2.94	–	0.59
Meat scrap with shell	–	89.7	55.2	1.0	14.5	11.9	17.4	–	–	–	–	–	–

Table 47 (Continued)

Feed ingredient	ME (kcal /kg)	D.M.	CP.	C.F.	E.E.	N.F.E.	Total ash	Acid Insol. Ash	Ca	P.	Lys.	Met.	Tryp.
Linseed oil cake	–	94.0	29.6	11.1	10.4	42.6	6.3	–	–	–	0.94	0.51	0.44
Maize gluten feed	2315	92.3	26.9	5.1	4.8	59.6	2.3	–	–	–	–	–	–
Maize grit	2742	90.8	13.6	5.3	2.1	76.1	2.9	0.21	0.31	0.15	0.33	0.26	0.07
Mustard oil cake	2373	91.3	35.1	8.2	14.1	33.4	9.2	1.20	0.89	1.78	0.99	0.72	0.68
Mustard cake (deoiled)	–	–	41.96	11.68	1.43	35.91	9.02	–	1.01	1.11	2.25	0.79	0.18
Neem seed cake	2817	–	34.0	27.4	2.8	29.2	6.6	5.60	0.74	0.57	–	–	–
Ramtil cake	–	96.6	36.0	18.6	8.9	28.3	8.2	1.85	0.62	0.96	1.37	–	–
Rape seed cake	–	87.6	36.0	10.4	12.8	31.4	9.4	–	1.12	1.05	–	–	–
Rubber seed cake	–	85.9	25.4	25.0	9.7	50.3	9.6	–	0.37	0.33	–	–	–
Safflower oil cake (decorticated)	–	92.8	42.2	8.5	8.2	32.2	8.9	–	0.40	0.51	–	–	–
Safflower oil cake (undecorticated)	–	95.0	23.1	29.9	5.5	36.9	4.6	–	–	–	–	–	–
Sesame cake	1882	90.7	39.1	4.7	9.3	34.3	12.6	1.50	2.46	1.42	1.04	0.84	0.72
Spent coffee cake powder	–	90.8	19.4	17.7	1.2	56.2	5.5	–	–	–	–	–	–
Sunflower cake	2230	89.1	37.2	11.6	10.9	32.6	7.7	0.62	0.43	1.14	–	–	–
Sunhemp meal	–	91.1	40.0	9.3	5.4	40.3	5.0	0.36	0.47	0.68	2.1	0.52	0.57
Taramira cake	–	96.9	40.5	8.0	9.5	35.9	6.1	1.04	0.57	0.71	0.97	–	0.55
Yeast sludge	–	94.8	32.1	1.8	1.3	46.3	18.5	–	6.05	0.41	–	–	–
Mineral supplements:													
Egg shell meal	–	98.2	5.8	–	0.3	1.4	92.5	–	33.63	–	–	–	–
Limestone	–	99.9	–	–	–	–	99.6	–	34.42	0.02	–	–	–
Feed additives:													
Penicillin mycelium residue	–	–	17.9	5.6	5.5	35.8	35.2	–	3.80	0.17	–	–	–
Penicillium mycelium waste	–	91.8	31.9	8.4	6.7	34.5	18.5	–	3.97	1.12	1.24	0.46	0.37
Terramycin waste	–	96.6	31.7	7.2	4.1	15.4	41.6	–	–	–	0.73	0.84	1.05
Dry Roughage:													
Agathi leaf meal	–	–	32.3	6.7	6.1	45.1	9.5	–	3.26	0.22	–	–	–

138

Table 47 (*Contd.*)

Feed ingredient	ME (kcal / kg)	D.M.	CP.	C.F.	E.E.	N.F.E.	Total ash	Acid Insol. Ash	Ca	P.	Lys.	Met.	Tryp.
Berseem leaf meal (dehydrated)	–	89.7	15.3	23.5	3.7	42.8	14.7	–	–	–	0.66	0.30	0.29
Cowpea leaf meal	–	21.2	21.1	17.7	9.4	36.1	15.7	3.53	4.45	0.46	–	–	–
Guar leaf meal	–	14.2	22.5	9.7	3.5	49.9	14.4	2.36	3.98	0.33	0.52	–	–
Groundnut plant meal	1812	92.1	14.4	32.5	3.1	37.4	12.6	–	1.69	0.34	–	–	–
Lucerne leaf meal	–	95.6	20.3	16.0	4.0	51.1	9.6	0.23	2.25	0.35	–	–	–
Lucerne dehydrated	–	91.0	19.1	21.6	2.8	42.1	14.4	–	1.83	0.45	–	–	–
Maize husk	1512	92.3	9.7	13.7	2.0	70.5	4.1	3.17	0.63	0.12	0.43	0.26	0.13
Mowha residue	–	–	14.5	30.9	5.4	31.0	1.3	–	–	–	0.76	–	0.55
Sugarcane bagasse	–	–	2.5	33.1	3.7	46.4	14.3	–	0.74	0.07	–	–	–
Sunhemp leaves	–	–	34.7	13.6	10.2	30.4	11.1	–	2.17	0.36	–	–	–
Tapioca leaf meal	–	90.9	15.4	22.8	12.2	41.1	8.5	–	1.43	0.25	–	–	–
Miscellaneous :													
Linseed	–	97.9	28.9	6.3	40.5	21.4	2.9	0.03	0.44	0.53	–	–	–
Potato peelings	–	16.9	10.0	2.4	2.1	81.5	4.0	–	0.21	0.32	–	–	–
Salseed	2827	92.0	8.1	3.2	16.4	69.0	3.3	0.96	0.19	0.17	9.48	0.33	0.36
Soybean meal	–	89.9	41.7	6.3	21.2	26.0	4.8	–	0.36	0.90	2.31	0.51	0.72

Abbreviations

M.E. = Metabolisable energy, D.M. = Dry matter, Ca = Calcium, P = Phosphorus, *Lys* = Lysine, Met = Methionine.
C.P. = Crude protein, C.F. = Crude fibre, Tryp = Tryptophan.
E.E. = Eiher extact, N.F.E. = Nitrogen free extract Except M.E. & D.M. all parameters are expressed in % on D.M. basis
* *Compiled by* – The Division of Poultry Research, Indian Veterinary Research Institute, Izatnagar, Bareilly, U.P.

Table 48 Amino-acid contents of feed ingredients (g/kg)

Feed ingredients	Arginine	Cystine	Glycine	Histidine	Leucine	Isoleucine	Lysine	Methionine	Phenylalanine	Threonine	Tryptophan	Tyrosine	Valine	Serine
Barley	6.8	2.1	4.8	2.4	7.8	4.2	4.2	2.1	5.3	4.2	1.5	3.5	5.6	4.4
Naked barley	6.4	2.1	4.6	2.6	8.3	4.2	4.8	1.0	6.7	4.2	1.7	4.8	5.9	4.9
Malt culms	11.2	—	—	4.8	14.7	9.8	12.2	3.5	8.2	9.1	3.7	5.8	13.1	—
Brewer's dried grains	12.7	3.0	9.8	6.4	24.9	13.2	10.6	5.2	14.0	10.3	3.0	15.7	15.5	—
Malt distillers' dried solubles	4.5	0.8	11.2	4.3	20.8	15.2	11.9	3.7	7.0	9.7	0.7	2.1	15.2	
Dried dreg	11.9	4.3	1.1	8.4	4.3	14.2	7.8	10.4	24.1	12.3	0.8	8.8	16.5	-
Maize	4.3	1.9	3.2	2.6	10.6	3.2	2.7	1.8	4.2	3.2	0.5	3.6	4.0	4.0
Maize germ meal	9.7	5.1	6.9	3.8	10.4	3.6	6.7	2.8	5.4	4.7	2.1	4.1	6.5	6.2
Maize germ meal (Ocrim process)	11.2	5.7	7.7	4.2	10.9	4.9	7.6	3.3	6.1	6.3	1.6	5.4	7.4	6.8
Maize gluten feed	11.2	5.3	9.5	7.6	19.5	6.2	6.9	5.6	7.4	7.9	2.4	7.1	10.3	9.5
Maize gluten meal	13.0	8.9	15.2	8.4	62.8	17.3	7.1	9.6	28.4	15.2	2.7	16.5	21.8	—
Millet	3.5	0.8	3.2	2.3	12.3	4.9	2.5	3.0	5.9	4.4	1.7	2.7	6.2	9.9
Oats	8.0	2.2	5.5	2.6	8.3	4.4	4.7	1.7	5.6	4.0	1.2	3.7	5.6	5.2
Naked oats	8.2	2.6	5.7	2.2	7.7	5.0	4.1	1.8	5.9	4.1	1.4	4.3	6.3	5.4
Rice, rough	6.5	1.4	8.1	1.8	6.2	3.6	3.1	-1.8	3.8	2.8	1.3	4.0	5.0	2.6
Rice, brown	13.0	1.8	3.7	3.5	12.6	7.0	7.0	3.5	7.6	5.4	2.4	5.4	10.0	4.0
Rice, bran	12.5	1.6	7.9	4.1	10.4	6.4	7.8	2.8	6.8	5.7	2.8	5.4	8.8	—
Rice polishings	11.7	1.7	7.4	3.6	9.1	5.0	7.2	2.4	5.4	5.1	2.1	4.6	8.4	—
Rye	6.2	1.1	4.8	3.2	6.5	3.9	3.4	1.3	6.0	4.0	1.4	3.1	5.1	4.6
Sorghum (milo)	4.0	2.5	3.0	2.3	12.2	3.8	2.4	1.7	4.7	3.9	1.3	3.3	5.5	4.3
Triticalc	8.0	1.7	5.6	3.5	9.2	5.0	4.3	2.0	7.0	4.6	2.8	4.3	6.1	6.5
Wheat	5.4	2.2	3.8	2.7	7.2	4.1	3.8	1.8	5.2	3.2	1.0	3.1	4.4	3.4
Wheat germ meal	18.3	3.5	12.4	5.7	14.7	8.6	16.3	4.1	9.8	9.8	2.6	7.3	12.4	11.2
Wheat middlings	10.4	3.5	7.9	3.8	8.7	4.5	5.9	2.4	5.8	4.6	2.0	4.5	6.6	6.6

139

Table 48 (Continued)

Feed ingredients	Arginine	Cystine	Glycine	Histidine	Leucine	Isoleucine	Lysine	Methionine	Phenylalanine	Threonine	Tryptophan	Tyrosine	Valine	Serine
Wheat fine middlings	11.3	3.3	4.1	5.0	10.8	6.6	7.1	3.2	6.8	6.2	2.8	5.0	9.1	7.6
Wheat bran	5.5	2.1	8.6	2.9	10.2	5.9	3.1	2.2	6.6	4.0	2.2	1.5	6.3	7.6
Bean meal, *Vicia faba* (Spring)	23.2	1.4	11.5	5.9	19.9	10.7	16.2	1.5	11.6	10.2	2.5	9.6	12.2	14.9
Bean meal, *Vicia faba* (Autumn)	17.6	1.0	10.0	5.1	16.6	8.9	14.1	1.7	9.2	8.7	2.0	8.2	10.3	14.9
Coconut meal	22.3	3.7	9.1	3.3	12.3	7.8	6.0	3.1	8.3	7.4	1.8	4.8	10.7	10.4
Cottonseed meal, dec., exp.	41.8	8.3	23.0	10.2	23.5	15.2	16.0	5.6	20.0	13.2	6.0	12.1	18.9	17.3
Groundnut meal, dec., exp.	46.0	6.6	25.3	10.9	28.9	14.7	14.4	5.0	23.3	12.2	3.9	17.1	19.7	22.7
Linseed meal, exp.	31.7	3.1	2.3	6.1	20.4	15.6	12.3	5.7	15.4	12.9	6.0	7.5	19.0	17.6
Palm kernel meal, ext.	23.6	2.8	8.1	3.2	11.9	6.4	5.4	3.3	7.9	6.1	2.0	4.7	8.2	–
Pea meal	20.6	2.4	11.0	6.5	18.6	18.1	20.9	4.9	11.7	10.6	2.2	9.8	11.4	7.4
Rapeseed meal	20.5	4.3	18.0	9.8	24.9	13.6	20.7	7.0	14.0	15.8	4.4	8.1	17.8	15.8
Safflower meal, dec, exp.	27.5	7.0	20.6	9.1	24.4	16.0	10.4	7.9	17.5	13.6	6.8	9.5	21.5	25.8
Sesame meal, exp.	46.4	9.4	23.1	10.0	29.6	16.9	10.2	11.4	19.0	15.8	3.0	15.6	19.3	–
Soybean meal (44 per cent pr.)	37.6	6.9	19.4	11.6	36.1	20.2	29.9	6.4	24.7	18.9	5.1	18.5	21.0	25.1
Sunflower meal, dec.	26.5	2.6	18.0	7.3	19.5	11.8	10.4	4.1	14.6	11.6	4.1	8.6	14.5	13.5
Blood meal	33.7	15.0	39.5	42.5	111.0	9.9	38.7	12.8	58.0	43.4	11.7	22.1	77.6	45.7

Table 48 (Continued)

Feed ingredients	Argi-nine	Cystine	Glycine	Histi-dine	Leucine	Iso-leucine	Lysine	Methio-nine	Pheny-lalanine	Thre-onine	Tryp-tophan	Ty-rosine	Valine	Serine
Feather meal	67.3	30.0	69.2	5.8	72.3	45.7	18.0	5.0	42.1	45.0	10.3	23.4	68.4	98.2
Fish meal (white)	42.6	5.9	56.4	12.1	44.6	26.2	49.0	18.8	19.7	25.6	5.9	20.6	30.2	27.6
Fish meal (anchovy)	37.1	6.2	40.6	13.7	49.4	28.0	53.3	19.5	26.0	28.6	7.8	20.4	37.1	28.0
Fish meal (pilchard)	37.0	8.0	41.6	19.5	46.8	28.0	52.0	20.0	28.0	27.3	6.5	19.5	35.1	28.6
Herring meal	39.0	6.9	45.0	15.3	54.0	34.0	58.8	21.9	29.5	31.4	8.0	21.9	41.0	31.6
Fish solubles	7.4	1.1	20.0	2.9	14.1	6.5	12.1	7.0	5.1	6.7	1.3	2.1	10.7	24.2
Liver and lung meal	35.2	10.5	30.1	14.4	52.3	30.2	43.6	10.9	30.0	23.3	5.3	16.2	35.3	31.5
Meat meal	52.5	31.8	68.7	9.4	68.8	39.4	25.7	7.4	39.5	38.8	5.7	22.3	61.7	17.8
Meat-and-bone meal	41.5	4.4	78.2	11.9	36.9	13.5	30.7	6.8	20.2	18.4	3.5	13.9	24.1	23.9
Milk, dried, skim	10.0	2.3	60.7	10.7	30.7	24.0	24.0	7.3	16.7	14.0	3.4	7.3	20.0	14.8
Poultry dressing-plant by-products meal	45.5	31.5	62.2	11.5	58.5	32.4	29.3	14.9	32.9	30.4	7.6	21.5	49.3	44.5
Whey, dried	1.6	3.2	3.8	1.6	9.6	8.0	7.2	0.8	3.8	5.9	0.8	0.8	5.6	–
Buttermilk, dried	10.3	2.0	2.0	8.7	31.7	25.0	22.3	7.0	13.7	14.7	4.3	9.3	25.7	–
Grass, dried	7.5	1.9	7.4	2.7	12.1	5.6	7.1	3.1	7.1	6.2	3.1	4.5	7.0	6.3
Lucerne, dried	5.1	2.5	5.2	2.2	6.2	11.5	6.1	1.9	5.9	7.3	2.2	2.6	7.1	6.3
Potato meal	3.8	1.5	1.9	1.5	9.8	3.2	4.3	1.4	4.7	3.2	0.7	0.6	4.2	3.2
Yeast, brewers' dried	19.5	8.9	23.8	9.5	33.7	22.4	33.5	5.9	22.5	21.8	3.8	15.1	28.2	22.6
Yeast, paraffin grown	32.0	6.0	30.6	14.0	51.0	34.0	51.0	10.4	31.0	35.0	8.5	26.0	38.0	34.1

Table 49 Mineral contents of feed ingredients

Feed ingredients	Major minerals (g/kg)					Minor minerals (mg/kg)			
	Ca	Total P	Available P	Chloride	Na	Mn	Zn	K	Se
(1)	(2)	(3)	(4)	(5)	(6)	(7)	(8)	(9)	(10)
Barley	0.4	4		1.2	0.05	12	38	3.6	0.4
Naked barley	0.3	2			0.05	10	28	3.7	
Malt culms	2.2	7				49	99	15.0	0.6
Brewers' dried grains	3.0	7	2	1.5	0.4	25	64	1.3	0.6
Malt distillers, dried solubles	46.0					21	26		
Dried distillery concentrate (malt)	1.0				0.6	8	28	0.6	
Dried distillery concentrate (grain)	0.3	14	12	2.6	3.0	16	64	18.0	
Dried dreg	0.3				4.0	5	26	10.0	
Maize	0.1	3	1	0.7	0.1	3	20	3.4	1.3
Maize germ meal	0.7	4	1	0.5	9.0	6	43	1.3	0.1
Maize germ meal (Ocrim process)	3.0	5	1.5	0.5	0.01	28	128	13.2	0.3
Maize gluten feed	0.7	3	1	0.4	1.0	17	72	6.7	1.0
Maize gluten meal	0.4	4	2	0.7	0.1	8	34	1.5	0.1
Millet	1.4	3		0.2		35	20	4.3	0.7
Oats	1.0	3	1	0.7	0.6	44	32	4.5	0.1
Naked oats	0.8	4	1			32	35	3.9	
Rice, rough	0.7	2		0.3		40	12	3.4	
Rice, brown	0.7	11	1			26	25	3.4	
Rice bran	1.0	18	2	0.7	0.7	124	57	17.4	
Rice polishings	0.4	11	1	0.7	07			11.7	
Rye	0.5	4		0.2	0.2	17	21	5.0	
Sorghum (milo)	0.3	3	1	0.8	0.1	13	48	3.4	
Triticale	0.3	3			0.03	41	31	3.6	
Wheat	0 4	4	1	0.8	0.6	21	20	5.0	0.2
Wheat germ meal	0.7	10	3	0.7	0.5	151	146	3.0	0.8
Wheat middlings	0.7	9	4	0.3	0.2	84	106	11.0	0.8
Wheat fine middlings	0.5	7	2	0.6	0.5	95	68	6.0	0.8
Wheat bran	1.4	13	3	0.9	0.6	122	162	12.5	0.6
Bean meal, *Vicia faba* (Spring)	0.9	4	1	0.3	0.4	16	45	10.0	

Table 49 (Continued)

(1)	(2)	(3)	(4)	(5)	(6)	(7)	(8)	(9)	(10)
Bean meal, *Vicia faba* (Autumn)	1.3	6	2	0.3	0.4	16	40	10.0	
Coconut meal	4.0	7	2	0.3	0.4	68	89	16.6	
Cottonseed meal, dec., exp.	3.0	11	4	0.4	0.6	24	55	15.6	1.0
Groundnut meal, dec, exp.	1.4	13	5	0.3	0.8	52	75	12	1.0
Linseed meal, exp.	4.0	7		0.9	1.0	37	70	12.5	1.1
Palm kernel meal, ext.	2.1	5		1.6	0.2	205	60	6.7	
Pea meal	0.7	9	4	0.4	0.4	14	40	14.0	
Rapeseed meal	6.0	9	3		0.7	73	70	10.4	1.0
Safflower meal, dec. exp.	2.6	18	5		0.5	40	42	7.0	
Sesame meal	20	16	3	0.3	0.4	31	70	12.0	
Soybean meal, (50 per cent pr.)	2.0	6			3.4	22	67	20	0.6
Soybean meal, (44 per cent pr.)	2.2	6	3	0.3	2.9	31	61	20	0.6
Sunflower meal, dec.	2.0	10	2	1.9	0.2	23	98	12.3	
Blood meal	0.4	3	3	8.5	3.2	1	19	2.3	
Feather meal	2.0	8	6			5	89		
Fish meal (white)	66.0	35	35		5	7	92	5.9	1.8
Fish meal (anchovy)	45.0	25	25	3.0	8.0	22	110	5.0	
Fish meal (pilchard)	43.0	25	25	8.0	2.0	9		3.0	
Herring meal	20.0	15	15	10.0	5.0	8	94	4.5	3.6
Fish solubles	2	9	8					19	2
Liver and lung meal	4	9	9		1.1	8	50	4	
Meat meal	3	44	44	2.7	7	32	104	5.5	0 4
Meat and bone meal	75	42	42	14	7	21	95	5.5	0.6
Milk, dried, skim	13	11	11	12	5	1	45	15	0.1
Poultry dressing-plant by-products meal	29	5	5	4	4	5	76	6	1.5
Whey, dried	9	8	8	17.1	4.8	1	9	25	0.1
Buttermilk dried	14	8	8	19.7	4.8	3	23	17	
Grass, diicd	12	8	8	8	0.8	53	19	1	
Lucerne, dried	19	8	6	3.5	1.8	46	28	20	0.2
Molasses	9	t	1	20.6	1.2	50	15	41.3	
Potato meal	10	2	1	1.2	0.1	6	9	20	
Tapioca root-flour (cassava)	2	1	1	0.2		16			
Yeast, brewers dried	3	16	15	0.3	0.7	5	96	15	1.7
Yeast, paraffin grown	0.1	8			0.2	250	1300	12.8	

SOURCE: *Poultry Nutrition* by W. Bolton and R. Blair, Published by Ministry of Agriculture, Fisheries and Food, Bulletin No. 174, Her Majesty's Stationery Office, London, 1974.

Table 50 Vitamin contents of feed ingredients

Feed ingredients	Vitamin A potency IU/g	Vitamin E IU/kg	Choline mg/kg	Nicotinic acid mg/kg	Ribo-flavin mg/kg	Vitamin B_{12} µg/kg	Biotin mg/kg	Folic acid mg/kg
Barley	0.7	5	1110	52	1.3	3.3	0.15	0.6
Naked barley							0.07	0.6
Malt culms		4	1580	55	8.6			0.2
Brewers' dried grains	0.5		1550	33	0.9		0.0	9.7
Malt distillers' dried solubles			2000	510	21.0		1.5	1.0
Dried distillery-concentrate (malt)			1000	270	15.0			
Dried distillery concentrate (grain)			1300	40	6.6			
Dried dreg			400	34	2.7			
Maize	5.0	4	1110	21	1.1	0.2	0.05	0.3
Maize germ meal		87	1550	31	3.3		3.00	0.2
Maize gluten feed	2.2	40	780	78	2.2		0.30	0.3
Maize gluten meal	26.6	24	1660.	44	1.6		0.15	0.2
Millet	0.5	12	490	22	1.0			0.2
Oats	0.6	5	930	16	1.1	3.3	0.11	0.5
Naked oats			1240	17	1.1		0.11	0.6
Rice, rough				19	1.3		0.10	0.3
Rice, brown		12	780	15	0.4		0.10	0-2
Rice bran		60	990	275	2.6		0.42	
Rice polishings		90	1000	660	2.2		0.62	
Rye	0.2	17		16	1.6		0.06	0.7
Sorghum (milo)	0.7	12	440	66	1.1		0.18	0.2
Wheat	0.4	16	730	58	1.1		0.11	0.4
Wheat germ meal	0.4	130	2660	51	4.9		0.22	1.9
Wheat middlings	0.5	20	1110	100	2.2		0.37	1.1
Wheat fine middlings	0.4	57	1170	95	2.4		0.37	1.1
Wheat bran	0.4	1	1020	188	2.9		0.48	1.7
Bean meal, *Vicia faba* (Spring)		1	1110	29	3.1		0.11	1.3
Bean meal, *Vicia faba* (Autumn)		1	1110	29	3.1		0.11	1.3

Table 50 (*Continued*)

Feed ingredients	Vitamin A potency IU/g	Vitamin E IU/kg	Choline mg/kg	Nicotinic acid mg/kg	Ribo-flavin mg/kg	Vitamin B_{12} μg/kg	Biotin mg/kg	Folic acid mg/kg
Coconut meal		16	1110	27	3.3		0.06	1.3
Cottonseed meal, dec, exp.	0.3	19	2610	33	4.9		0.10	3.7
Groundnut meal, dec, exp.	0.3	3	1880	166	2.2		0.39	0.4
Linseed meal, exp.	0.4		1660	40	3.5			
Pea meal	0.5	3	2210	24	1.8		0.11	0.3
Rapeseed meal		19	660	155	3.7			0.2
Safflower meal, dec., exp.		1	2570	22	4		1.40	0.4
Sesame meal		1	1440	30	3.1			
Soybean meal, (50 per cent pr.)		1	2900	38	4.2		0.32	3.6
Soybean meal, (44 per cent pr.)		1	2840	32	4.0		0.32	3.6
Sunflower meal, dec		6	1200	250	4.0			
Blood meal		0	1100	33	2.2			
Feather meal			900	18	2.0	70.8		
Fish meal (white)		21	3100	62	6.6	100	0.26	0.2
Fish meal (anchovy)		34	3700	64	6.6	100	0.28	0.2
Fish meal (pilchard)		9	2200	55	9.5	100	0.26	0.2
Herring meal		27	4000	89	9	240	0.59	0.5
Fish solubles	4.0		2660	321	22.1	143.8	0.26	
Liver and lung meal	49.6		7540	157	47.8	283.6	0.8	4.0
Meat meal		5	2430	55	5.5	55.3	0.26	0.1
Meat and bone meal		5	2210	51	5.3	44	0.14	0.1
Milk, dried, skim	0.3	1	1060	12	21	55.3	0.33	0.0
Poultry dressing-plant by-products meal			600	40	11.0	0.3	0.3	1.0
Whey, dried		–	1550	11	26.6	22.1	0.25	0.6
Buttermilk dried	0.4	–	1000	11	28.8	88.5	0.3	0.4
Grass, dried	327.5	150	890	74	15.5		0.17	
Lucerne, dried	267	200	1110	43	16.6	2.7	0.33	3 5
Molasses			640	44	2.2	–	0.11	0.7
Potato meal			260	33	0.7		0.1	0.6
Yeast, brewers dried		0	3260	487	45.2		1.3	12
Yeast, paraffin grown			6225	430	18	1.0		6 4

Table 51 Amount of metabolisable energy provided by given weights of oils and fats

Weight of fat added kg (lb)	Metabolisable energy	
	kcal	MJ
Vegetable oils		
0.45(1)	4150	17.36
1.36 (3)	12,440	52.05
2.27 (5)	20,530	85.90
3.18(7)	28,740	120.25
4.08(9)	36,570	153.01
Animal fats		
0.45 (1)	4220	17.66
1.36(3)	12,140	50.80
2.27 (5)	19,160	80.17
3.18(7)	25,010	104.64
4.08(9)	29,840	124.85

Table 52 Nitrogen and crude protein contents of amino-acids

Amino-acid	Formula	Molecular weight	N content per cent	N × 6.25 per cent crude protein
Alanine	$C_3H_7O_2N$	89.10	15.71	98.19
Arginine	$C_6H_{14}O_2N_4$	174.17	32.51	200.94
Arginine HC (1)	$C_6H_{14}O_2N_4HC$ (1)	210.67	26.58	166.13
Aspartic acid	$C_4H_7O_4N$	133.11	10.52	65.75
Glutamic acid	$C_5H_9O_4N$	147.13	9.52	59.50
Glycine	$C_2H_5O_2N$	75.07	18.65	116.56
Histidine	$C_6H_9O_2N_3$	155.12	27.08	169.25
Histidine HC (1) H_2O	$C_6H_9O_2N_3HC(l)H_2O$	209.63	20.04	125.15
Isoleucine	$C_6H_{13}O_2N$	131.18	10.67	66.69
Leucine	$C_6H_{13}O_2N$	131.18	10.67	66.69
Lysine HC(1)	$C_6H_{14}O_2N_2HC$ (1)	182.65	15.33	95.81
Methionine	$C_5H_{11}O_2NS$	149.21	9.38	58.63
Methionine hydroxy analogue	$(C_5H_9O_3S)_2Ca$	338.00		
Cystine	$C_6H_{12}O_4N_2S_2$	240.30	11.65	72.81
Phenylalanine	$C_9H_{11}O_2N$	165.19	8.48	53.00
Tyrosine	$C_9H_{11}O_3N$	181.19	7.73	48.31
Proline	$C_5H_9O_2N$	115.13	12.16	76.00
Serine	$C_3H_7O_3N$	105.01	13.34	83.39
Threonine	$C_4H_9O_3N$	119.12	11.75	73.44
Tryptophan	$C_{11}H_{12}O_2N_2$	204.23	13.71	85.69
Valine	$C_6H_{11}O_2N$	117.15	11.95	74.69

Table 53 Elemental composition of salts used in mineral mixture

Salt (1)	Formula (2)	Elements in salt per cent (3)
Calcium		
Calcium carbonate	$CaCO_3$	40.05 Ca 59.95 CO_3
Dicalcium phosphate, anhydrous	$CaHPO_4$	29.46 Ca 22.77 P
Dicalcium phosphate, dihydrate	$CaHPO_4.2H_2O$	23.29 Ca 18.01 P
Tricalcium phosphate	$Ca_3(PO_4)_2$	38.76 Ca 19.97 P
Calcium sulphate	$CaSO_4$	29.43 Ca 70.57 SO_4
Bone meal		30.00 Ca 15.00 P
Oyster shell grit		38.00 Ca
Ground limestone		38.00 Ca
Chloride		
Sodium chloride	$NaCl$	60.65 Cl 38.35 Na
Potassium chloride	KCl	47.56 Cl 52.44 K
Chromium		
Chrome alum	$Cr_2K_2(SO_4)_4.24 H_2O$	10.42 Cr 38.49 SO_4
Chromic chloride	$CrCl_2$	32.82 Cr 67.18 Cl
Cobalt		
Cobaltous chloride, pentahydrate	$CoCl_2.5H_2O$	26.80 Co 32.28 Cl
Cobaltous chloride, hexahydrate	$CoCl_2.6H_2O$	24.77 Co 29,84 Cl
Copper		
Cupric sulphate	$CuSO_4$	39.81 Cu 60.19 SO_4
Cupric sulphate, pentahydrate	$CuSO_4.5H_2O$	25.46 Cu 38.49 SO_4
Cupric chloride	$CuCl_2$	47.27 Cu 52.73 Cl
Fluorine		
Potassium fluoride, dihydrate	$KF.2H_2O$	20.17 F 41.54 K
Sodium fluoride	NaF	
Iodine		
Potassium iodide	KI	76.45 I 23.55 K
Potassium iodate	KIO_3	59.31 I 18.27 K
Calcium iodate	$Ca(IO_2)_2$	65.09 I 10.28 Ca
Sodium iodide	NaI	84.68 I 15.32 Na
Iron		
Ferrous sulphate, heptahydrate	$FeSO_4.7H_2O$	20.09 Fe 34.59 SO_4
Ferrous acetate, tetrahydrate	$Fe(C_2H_2O_2)_2.4H_2O$	
Magnesium		
Magnesium carbonate	$MgCO_3$	28.84 Mg 71.16 CO_3
Magnesium sulphate	$MgSO_4$	20.19Mg 79.81 SO_4
Magnesium sulphate, heptahydrate	$MgSO_4 7H_2O$	9.87 Mg 39.01 SO_4
Manganese		
Manganese dioxide	MnO_2	63.19 Mn
Manganous carbonate	$MnCO_3$	47.79 Mn 52.21 CO_3
Manganous chloride, tetrahydrata	$MnCl_2.4H_2O$	27.76 Mn 35.86 Cl

Table 53 (Continued)

(1)	(2)	(3)
Manganous sulphate	$MnSO_4$	36.36 Mn 63.64 SO_4
Manganous sulphate hydrate	$MnSO_4.H_2O$	32.49 Mn 56.86 SO_4
Manganous sulphate tetrahydrate	$MnSO_4.4H_2O$	24.63 Mn 43.10 SO_4
Molybdenum		
Sodium molybdate, dibydrate	$Na_2MoO_4.2H_2O$	39.66 Mo 19.01 Na
Sodium molybdate, pentahydrate	$NaMoO_4.5H_2O$	35.15 Mo 8.43 Na
Nickel		
Nickel chloride	$NiCl_2$	45.26 Ni 54.74 Cl
Phosphorus		
Orthophosphoric acid	H_3PO_4	31.61 P
Potassium orthophosphate	K_2HPO_4	17.79 P 44.90 K
Potassium dihydrogen orthophosphate	KH_2PO_4	22.76 P 28.73 K
Sodium hydrogen orthophosphate	Na_2HPO_4	21.82 P 32.40 Na
Sodium dihydrogen orthophosphate, hydrate	$NaH_3PO_4.H_2O$	22.45 P 16.67 Na
Sodium dihydrogen orthophosphate, dihydrate	$NaH_3PO_4. 2H_2O$	19.86 P 14.74 Na
Ammonium phosphate	$(NH_2)_2 HPO_4$	23.46 P
Potassium		
Potassium chloride	KCl	52.44 K 47.56 Cl
Potassium carbonate	K_2CO_3	56.58 K 43.42 CO_3
Potassium bicarbonate	$KHCO_3$	39.05 K 60.95 HCO
Potassium acetate	$KC_2H_2O_2$	39.84 K 60.16 Acetate
Potassium orthophosphate	K_3PO_4	55.25 K 14.59 P
Potassium sulphate	K_2SO_4	44 87 K 55.13 SO_4
Selenium		
Sodium selenite	Na_2SeO_3	45.65 Se 26.60 Na
Sodium selenate	$NaSeO_4$	41.79 Se 24.34 Na
Sodium		
Sodium chloride	$NaCl$	39.35 Na 60.65 Cl
Sodium bicarbonate	$NaHCO_3$	27.38 Na 72.62 HCO_3
Sodium sulphate	Na_2SO_4	32.38 Na 67.61 SO_4
Tin		
Stannic sulphate	$Sn (SO_4)_2.2H_2O$	34.22 Sn 55.36 SO_4
Vanadium		
Sodium orthovanadate	Na_3VO_4	27.69 V 37.51 Na
Zinc		
Zinc carbonate	$ZnCO_3$	52.14 Zn 47.86 CO_3
Zinc chloride	$ZnCl_2$	47.97 Zn 52.03 Cl
Zinc oxide	ZnO	80.35 Zn
Zinc sulphate	$ZnSO_4$	40.47 Zn 59.33 SO_4
Zinc sulphate hydrate	$ZnSO_4.H_2O$	36.42 Zn 53.55 SO_4

SOURCE: *Poultry Nutrition*, by W. Bolton and R. Blair, Published by Ministry of Agriculture, Fisheries and Food, U.K., 1974, Bulletin No. 174.

METHODS OF FEEDING

A well balanced ration improperly fed will not give the most satisfactory results unless a satisfactory method is followed. Some of the popular methods of feeding are as follows:

1. **Whole grain feeding system.** By this method birds are allowed to have their required ingredients kept before them in separate containers. The system though permit birds to balance their ration according to individual needs, however, it appears doubtful. This old and abandoned system offers no particular advantage. While it entails the use of several feed hoppers and a considerable amount of time to keep them filled.

2. **Grain and mash method.** This method is slightly better than the previous one. It involves feeding of grain mixture along with balanced mash. By this, one can increase or decrease the protein level as desired. Unless the poultryman is exceptionally skilled, the method will lead to bad performances.

3. **All mash method.** In this method of feeding, all the feed ingredients are ground, mixed in required proportion and fed as a single balanced mixture. This method is desirable for all types of poultry grown under litter and cage system. By this, birds, cannot have the opportunity to have selective eating and moreover the quality of eggs produced are of uniform quality. However, ground feeds are not so palatable and do not retain their nutritive value so well as unground feeds.

4. **Pellet method.** Pellets are made of dry-mash under high pressure. These are quite hard and cylindrical shape and is being extensively used in Western countries. The greatest advantage in using pellets is that there is little waste in feeding. The disadvantage is that pellets are expensive-about 10 per cent more expensive than that of feeds not pelleted.

5. **Restricted or controlled feeding.** The method involves restrictions of feeding pullets during 6-20 weeks of age instead of *ad libitum* feeding as is practiced at present in most poultry farm. Reduction in feed cost, delayed sexual maturity but improved egg production curve, along with a reduction in the number of small eggs laid are some of the advantages of this system.

Feed restrictions to birds can be made by a number of ways, viz., (1) Skip a-day programme; (2) alternate day feeding, (3) restriction of feeding time, etc. Before adopting this practice, the readers should gather further information in this aspect to suit his particular condition as none of the methods are suitable for all conditions.

Ten Principal Points for Consideration of Poultry Feed Formulation

(1) Feeds must contain all essential nutrients in right amount and proportion required for the purpose for which it is fed.

(2) Chickens of different ages require different level of nutrients, hence only the accepted standards as per age should be followed accordingly.

(3) Ingredients chosen for preparation of poultry mashes must be palatable.

(4) While selecting ingredients for preparation of poultry mashes, nutritional value of each ingredient should be evaluated *vis-a-vis* cost.

(5) Chickens have no teeth to grind grains or oil cakes, hence these ingredients should be crushed into proper sizes in keeping with age of the chicken.

(6) Micro-nutrients and non-nutrient feed additives should be carefully chosen and mixed up meticuously for effective results.

(7) Include agro-industrial by-products to minimise cost and select a variety of ingredients to make good deficiency of one by the other.

(8) While selecting an ingredient care should be exercised to judge its optimum level of inclusion as many of the ingredients are likely to be deleterious at higher level.

(9) Fungal infested ingredients should always be avoided.

(10) Care should be taken to select optimum C/P ratio for the purpose for which feeds are compounded.

Table 54 Formulae of some economic poultry rations (in percent)

I. Starter Rations (0-8 weeks)

Ingredients ↓ / Ration →	1	2	3	4	5	6	7	8	9
Yellow maize	–	–	–	–	–	16	17	16	10
Rice polish (10% oil)	31	46	51	60	40	40	40	40	40
Deoiled rice polish	–	–	–	–	20	–	–	–	–
Wheat bran	10	–	–	–	–	10	10	10	10
Maize grit	20	15	–	–	–	–	–	–	10
Maize gluten feed	15	15	10	–	10	–	–	–	–
Maize gluten meal	–	–	10	10	–	–	–	–	–
Groundnut cake	10	10	15	16	16	20	20	10	10
Maize steep fluid (on dry basis)	–	–	–	–	–	–	–	10	10
Fish meal (or) meat meal	10	10	10	5	5	10	5	10	5
Silk worm pupae meal	–	–	–	5	5	–	4	–	4
Limestone	1.5	1.5	1.5	1.5	1.5	1.5	1.5	1.5	1.5
Steamed bone meal	1.0	1.0	1.0	1.0	1.0	1.0	1.0	1.0	1.0
Common salt	0.5	0.5	0.5	0.5	0.5	0.5	0.5	0.5	0.5
Vitamin and mineral mixture*	1.0	1.0	1.0	1.0	1.0	1.0	1.0	1.0	1.0
Antibiotic	+	+	+	+	+	+	+	+	+

*Contains 22 grams $MnSO_4$. 1000,000 IU. Vitamin A, 500 mg Riboflavin & 750001.U. Vitamin D_3,

II. Grower Rations (9 weeks to 20 weeks; in percent)

Ingredients ↓ Ration →	1	2	3	4	5	6	7	8
Yellow maize	20	20	–	–	–	20	20	–
Rice polish	40	40	51	61	61	40	40	56
Wheat bran	10	10	10	10	10	6	6	10
Maize grit	–	–	10	–	–	–	–	10
Maize gluten meal	6	6	5	5	5	–	–	–
Maize steep fluid (on dry basis)	–	–	–	–	–	10	10	10
Groundnut cake	10	10	10	10	15	10	10	10
Fish meal or meat meal	10	5	10	10	5	10	5	5
Silk worm pupae meal	–	5	–	–	–	–	5	5
Limestone	1.5	1.5	1.5	1.5	1.5	1.5	1.5	1.5
Steamed bone meal	1.0	1.0	1.0	1.0	1.0	1.0	1.0	1.0
Common salt	0.5	0.5	0.5	0.5	0.5	0.5	0.5	0.5
Vitamin and mineral mixture*	1.0	1.0	1.0	1.0	1.0	1.0	1.0	1.0

*Containing 22 gms $MnSO_4$, 1000.00 I.U. Vitamin A, 500 mg Riboflavin and 75000 I.U. of Vitamin D_3.

III. Layer Rations (21 to 72 weeks; in percent)

Ingredients ↓ Ration →	1	2	3	4	5	6	7
Maize	–	–	20	20	–	10	20
Rice polish	30	30	40	50	55	50	30
Deoiled rice polish	–	–	–	–	–	–	20
Wheat bran	10	10	–	–	10	5	–
Maize grit	25	–	–	–	–	–	–
Maize gluten meal	5	–	10	–	10	5	–
Maize gluten feed	–	20	–	–	–	–	–
Groundnut cake	10	10	5	20	15	15	20
Fish meal or meat meal	–	–	–	5	5	5	5
Silk worm pupae meal	5	5	5	–	–	–	–
Molasses	10	15	15	–	–	5	–
Pencillin mycelia	–	5	–	–	–	–	–
Limestone	3	3	3	3	3	3	3
Bone meal	1	1	1	1	1	1	1
Salt	0.5	0.5	0.5	0.5	0.5	0.5	0.5
Vitamin and mineral mixture*	0.5	0.5	0.5	0.5	0.5	0.5	0.5

*Contains 25 gms $MnSO_4$, 5000 I.U. Vitamin A, 500 mg Riboflavin and 50000 1:U. Vitamin D_3.

Table 55 Expected Performance of Commercial Layer Flocks

Sl. No.	Age in Weeks	Production (Percent)	Egg/HH (Week)	Egg(HH)	Cummulative Daily Feed consumption (gm)
(1)	(2)	(3)	(4)	(5)	(6)
(i)	19	5	0.35	0.35	75
(ii)	20	15	1.05	1.40	62
(iii)	21	38	2.66	4.06	90
(iv)	22	64	4.48	8.54	93
(v)	23	83	5.60	14.34	96
(vi)	24	80	6.22	20.55	102
(vii)	25	92	5.43	26.99	104
(viii)	26	94	6.57	33.56	106
(ix)	27	94	6.56	40.12	108
(x)	28	95	6.63	46.75	108
(xi)	29	96	6.69	53.44	109
(xii)	30	97	6.76	60.20	111
(xiii)	31	97	6.76	66.96	ill
(xiv)	32	97	6.76	73.20.	115
(xv)	33	96	6.68	80.40	115
(xvi)	34	96	6.67	87.07	115
(xvii)	35	96	6.67	93.73	114
(xviii)	36	96	6.66	100.39	114
(xix)	37	95	6.58	106.98	114
(xx)	38	95	6.58	113.55	113
(xxi)	39	95	6.58	120.13	113
(x.xii)	40	95	6.58	126.69	113
(xxiii)	41	94	6.59	133.18	113
(xxiv)	42	94	6.68	139.66	113
(xxv)	43	94	6.47	146.13	113
(xxvi)	44	93	6.40	152.53	113
(xxvii)	45	93	6.39	158.92	113
(xxviii)	46	93	6.39	165.31	113
(xxix)	47	93	6.38	171.69	113
(xxx)	48	93	6.37	178.06	113
(xxxi)	49	92	6.30	184.36	113
(xxxii)	50	92	6.29	190.65	112
(xxxiii)	51	91	6.22	196.87	112
(xxxiv)	52	90	6.14	203.01	112
(xxxv)	53	89	6.07	209.06	112
(xxxvi)	54	89	6.07	215.15	112
(xxxvii)	55	89	6.06	221.21	112
(xxxviii)	56	89	6.06	227.27	112
(xxxix)	57	89	6.06	233.33	112
(xl)	58	86	5.98	239.31	112
(xli)	59	89	5.98	245.29	112

Table 55   (*Continued*)

Sl. No.	Age in Weeks	Production (Percent)	Egg/HH (Week)	Egg(HH)	Cummulative Daily Feed consumption (gm)
(xlii)	60	60	5.97	251.26	112
(xliii)	61	68	5.97	257.22	110
(xliv)	62	87	5.90	263.12	110
(xlv)	63	87	5.89	269.02	110
(xlvi)	64	86	5.82	274.84	110
(xlvii)	65	86	5.81	280.65	110
(xlviii)	66	86	5.81	285.46	110
(xlix)	67	85	5.74	292.20	110
(1)	68	84	5.66	297.86	110
(li)	69	84	5.66	303.52	110
(lii)	70	83	5.59	309.11	110
(liii)	71	82	5.52	314.63	110
(liv)	72	81	5.44	320.07	110

Note — 'Egg Yield 320 Eggs'. Feed Consumption 41.25 kg during laying period.
Source: Poultry Feeds– Specification (Fifth Revision)–IS 1374:2007

FUNGUS IN POULTRY FEEDS AND HOW TO INHIBIT THEIR GROWTH

What are Fungi?

Of all the plants no group is more fascinating than the fungi. There are varieties of fungi, differ in appearance from one another and grow in a variety of habits. Yet, they have one common feature (differing from other plants) - they do not have a green colouring pigment, chlorophyl.

Some fungi are parasites and live on living plant and animal tissue, causing disease or deformity to the host, and also create serious problems to man. Some fungi live on dead plant and animal (saprophyte) tissues and absorb proteins and complex substances from such tissues. Such fungi cause decay and such function or process (combined with the action of bacteria, worms, beetles, flies etc) arc necessary or otherwise earth would become littered with dead plants and animals,

The matter of very much concerned is the type of fungi, which grow on feed ingredients and produce poisonous toxins in the fecdstuffs. They are also known as molds.

There are thousands of different types of molds which exist in various environments, in the air, on the ground and in moist surfaces in farm buildings where molds thrive and multiply. Although majority of molds arc harmless, there are few molds causing serious economic loss to egg producers.

These usually enter the bird through the feed. Commonest harmful toxins are : - Aflatoxin, Ochratoxin, Vomitoxin, Erogotamine, and Zearalenone and T-2 toxin. Molds grow rapidly when the moisture content in the feedstuffs increases to 13% and at higher temparatures with high humidity in a poultry house.

Effects of mold toxins on poultry

Aflatoxin

Aflatoxins are common term used for a group of toxins which differ in their chemical structure and in intensity of producing toxic effects. As the various compounds of this group are produced by the fungi *Aspergillus flavus* and A. parasiticus they resemble very much to each other and are commonly termed Aflatoxins.

The aflatoxins B_1/B_2 and G_1 produce liver cell carcinomas in experimental animals. Aflatoxin B_1 is the most potent hepatocarcinogen and can produce liver cancer in rats. Malignant tumours have also been produced by B_1 in non-human primates. Although chickens appear to be fairly insensitive to acute toxic effects of the aflatoxins, outbreaks of *aflatoxicosls* have been reported where large amounts of aflatoxins have accidentally been fed to chickens. In general, the consumption of contaminated feed by an animal may result in an unhealthy situation comprising liver damage with marked bile duct proliferation and a decrease production or even in its death. However, the presence of the aflatoxins in feed can also result in deposition of these toxins or their metabolites in the animal meat or in their products (egg, milk etc). If these are consumed as human food, the presence of toxins could represent a human health problem

Table 56 Feed Ingredients with Demonstrated Natural Contamination by Aflatoxin

Corn (stored and field)	Malt sprouts
Peanut meal	Soyabean meal
Cottonseed (processed and field)	Sunflower seed meal
Copra	Safflower meal
Rye	Rapeseed
Oats	Rice bran
Sorghum	Linseed meal
Wheat	Alfalfa
Barley	Cocoa cake
Millet	Sugar scrap
Sesame cake	Palm kernel
Cassava	Pumpkin seeds
	Sheanut

Table 57 Some Examples of Dietary Aflatoxin Concentrations which have Caused Toxicosis in farm Animals

Species	Age	Aflaioxin content (mg/kg; ppm)	Duration of feeding	Effects
Calf	Weaning	0.2–2.2	16 weeks	Stunting, death. liver damage
Steer	2 years	0.2–0.7	20 weeks	Liver damage
Cow	2 years	2.4	7 months	Liver damage
Pig	Newborn	0.23	4 days	Stunting
Pig	2 weeks	0.17	23 days	Anorexia, stunting. jaundice
Pig	4-6 weeks	0.4–0.7	3-6 months	Stunting, liver damage
Chicken	1 + weeks	0.8	10 weeks	Stunting, liver damage
Duck	Unknown	0.3	6 weeks	Liver damage, death

Ochratoxin A

Ochratoxin A is a mycotoxin produced by species of the genera *Aspergillus* and *Penicillium*. The toxin affects the proximal kidney tubules, causing nephropathy in pigs and poultry. On slaughter, the kidneys are larger, lighter in colour and firmer than normal.

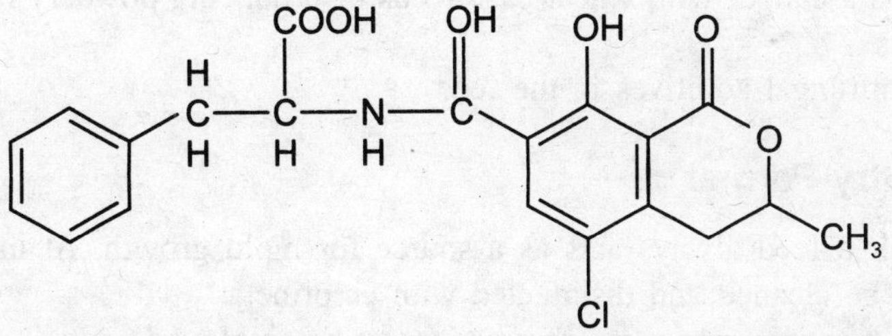

Figure 34 Structure of ochratoxin A.

Table 58 Feed ingredients found contaminated with ochratoxin A

Barley grains	Linseed meal
Oat grains	Soybean meal
Wheat grains	Rice bran
Maize grains	

Table 59 Symptoms of ochratoxin a toxicosis in chicken

Level in the feed (mg/kg)	Symptoms observed
<0.5	Diarrhoea, soiled eggs
0.5	Decreased egg production
1.0	Decreased egg size
	Decreased growth rate
2.0	Body weight reduced
4.0	High morbidity

Consumption of aflatoxin and ochratoxin A through various feedstuffs affect not only the egg production but also affect the entire physiological functions of the birds. Both feed manufacturer and the poultry farmer should take the necessary precautions in checking mold problems.

For the Feed manufacturer

1. Old feed materials eg : Maize and other grains from the bottom storage bags is more likely to be contaminated with mold. Avoid any practice which permits new feeds piled up on top of old.
2. New crop, immature grains harvested prematurely with high moisture content may also constitute a risk.
3. New sources of ingredients should be carefully checked. Keep a close watch on trade report for specific molds or toxins.
4. Avoid finely ground feed textures. Particularly where new grains are included, make sure that the screens in hammer-mills are changed to reflect the new grain types. There is a danger with wheat base feeds of producing powdery rather than granular textures.
5. Add antifungal additives in the feed.

For the Poultry Farmer

1. Old caked feed always acts as a source for mold growth. At intervals the feeders should be cleaned and disinfected with chlorine.
2. Proper hygienic management practices to be employed.
3. Prevent free tresspassing of personnel and other species of animals in the premises.
4. Avoid contamination of feed by rain and through leaky drinkers.
5. Molds grow readily on damaged grain. Avoid feeding of damaged, moldy and high moisture grain. Store grain where insect damage can be eliminated.
6. Mold growth starts where contaminated feed has a moisture content of above 13%. Once mold growth has started, it produces its own metabolic water. Therefore, even in stored feeds where moisture content is below 13% mold growth could occur provided some mold growth has started. Maintain dry litter especially near the feeders and watcrers.
7. Use mold inhibitors continuously in the feed.

Prevention is the only answer

A number of anti-fungal substances are added in milled feed to stop the fungal (mold) growth. The efficacy of these mold-inhibitors depends on its application and it must reach the sight of toxin production.

Among these mold-inhibitors, propionate salts, propionic, sorbic and ascorbic acids, mycostatin, gentian violet etc. are regularly used in the Western countries.

Acids used as mold inihibitors, do not penetrate very well into the grains of feeds when moisture levels are below 30%. They are also corrosive for handling and can cause severe burns if it comes in contact with the skin.

The best fungistatic substance is gentian violet, which inhibits the growth of molds and reduces toxin production. Gentian violet not only inhibits the fungal growth but also the growth of gram positive bacteria, which are found in the intestine of the birds. Since, gentian violet is not absorbed into the system of the bird it is very safe even at higher doses. There are also reports that addition of gentian violet at recommended levels increases egg production and feed efficiency.

USE OF AGRO-INDUSTRIAL BY-PRODUCTS IN POULTRY RATIONS

In India, the cereal grains which form the major source of energy for poultry are in short supply. They are costly and are required by people who are mostly vegetarians. Animal proteins are also in short supply and costly. Most of the Indian works on poultry nutrition have been concentrated upon investigations to utilise farm and industrial by-products as substitutes for maize, fish meal and even conventional oil cakes. With a view to compute balanced and economical rations, a brief review of some of the important ingredients is discussed.

A. Protein Supplements

1. *Mustard cake*.   Complete replacement of groundnut cake with mustard cake is not possible. Work done at I. V.R.I, and other places showed that mustard cake (expeller variety) could be included in chick starter or broiler diets upto 10% level. Work done at Bidhan Chandra Krishi Viswavidyalaya, West Bengal, showed that the deoiled variety of mustard cake could safely be included in chicken ration replacing groundnut cake upto the tune of 100 per cent.

2. *Mahua cake*.   Trend of research work indicates that mahua residue may be included upto 10 per cent replacing groundnut cake.

3. *Meat meal*.   Meat meal has been shown to replace 50 per cent of fish meal in chick rations. Variation in the nutritional value of meat meal is largely found to be determined by calcium and essential available amino acid contents of the meal.

4. *Blood meal.* Reports indicate that upto 3 to 5 per cent blood meal replacing fish meal, can be satisfactorily used in chick ration.

5. *Liver meal.* Results indicate that upto 10% liver meal (liver dry residue) replacing fish meal can be used in chick ration.

6. *Silk worm pupae meal.* Satisfactory growth and egg production have been obtained replacing some part of maize and the whole of fish meal with silk worm pupae meal. However, some workers found that silk worm pupae meal could only replace 50% of fish meal in chick starting ration.

7. *Guar meal.* A by-product from guar gum industry. Results indicate that raw guar meal proved detrimental to chick growth above 6.5 per cent inclusion in the rations but toasting or autoclaving or supplementation with 0.1 per cent hemiceliulase enzyme, significantly improve its nutritive value.

8. *Ram til cake.* The cake is extensively found in Maharashtra, M.P., Andhra Pradesh, Mysore and Orissa. It has been found to replace satisfactorily upto 50 per cent and 10 per cent of groundnut cake in the chick and layer rations respectively.

9. *Cotton seed cake.* It can replace groundnut cake upto 15 per cent. However, in layers continued use of this cake is known to cause yolk mottling on storage of eggs.

10. *Safflower oil meal.* It can replace groundnut cake upto 25 per cent.

11. *Soybean meal.* The product can easily replace groundnut.

12. *Hatchery by-product meal.* The meal is prepared from infertile eggs and dead germs, etc., and can be fed replacing 33 per cent of fish meal in the ration.

13. *Karanja cake.* The cake is one of the newer additions to the list of substitute oilseed cakes. Work conducted at Bidhan Chandra Krishi Viswavidyalaya, West Bengal showed that Karanja cake (*Pongamia glabra*) in its deoiled form can be included in chicken ration upto 8 per cent replacing other conventional oil cakes. The cake other than deoiled form is highly toxic for the chickens.

B. Energy Supplements

1. *Rice polish (bran).* The product is an excellent substitute for maize and can easily substitute maize upto 40-50 per cent in chick starter or layer ration. The deoiled form is also extensively used upto 20-35 per cent replacing ordinary rice polish.

2. *Salseed and deoiled salseed meal.* The results indicate that salseed and sal seed cake could be used in chick ration upto 5 per cent and in layer ration upto 10 per cent replacing an equal quantity of maize.

3. *Millets (Kodo, Sawan, Kanjui, etc.).* The work on Economic poultry rations scheme in U.P. showed that 10-14 per cent saving in feeding cost could be achieved by replacing maize with 24 per cent Kodo and sawan.

4. *Damaged grain.* Results obtained so far have indicated that upto 30 per cent damaged maize and 60 per cent damaged wheat could be used to replace good quality grain for chicks. However the extent of damage is to be considered first before inclusion in the chicken ration.

MODERN FEED ADDITIVES FOR POULTRY

Efforts to produce human foods from animal sources more efficiently and at lower cost have stimulated continued research for new additives. Considerable information has accumulated about the multifarious utility of various feed addilives.

Additives are never nutrients. They either singly or in combinations are added to a basic feed, usually in small quantities for the purpose of fortifying these with certain nutrients or stimulants or medicines. Often they arc called "non-nutrient" feed additives. The inclusion of most of these materials in poultry rations are controlled by law in most of the counlries. Some of the useful effects of such non-nutritive feed additives are discussed below:

A. Additives that promote Feed Intake or Selection

Like people, most of the animals have taste and aroma preferences, some feed arc more liked by them than others.

1. Antioxidants

All feeds are susceptible to spoilage, but those which are high in fat content are specially prone to antioxidation followed by rancidity. Most animals will refuse to eat spoiled feed. But when feed is limited, they may consume it with digestive disturbances resulting in many cases. To curb the oxidation of feeds, antioxidants are routinely added to many livestock feeds.

Antioxidants are compounds that prevent oxidative rancidity of polyunsaturated fats. In absence of these, there may be rancidity which also cause destruction of Vitamins A, D, and E. and several of the B complex vitamins. In some cases, the breakdown products of rancidity may react with the epsilon amino groups of lysine and thereby decrease the protein and energy values of the diet. Some common antioxidants are: BHT (Butylated hydroxytoluene); Santoquin; Ethoxyquin; BHA (Butylated hydroxyanisode); DPPD (Diphenyl paraphenyl diamine). All are added at 0.01 % level in poultry feed.

2. Flavouring Agents

These are feed additives that are supposed to increase palatability and feed intake. There is need lor flavouring agents particularly (1) when highly unpalatable medicants are being administered, (2) during attacks of diseases, (3) when animals are under stress, and (4) when a less palatable feed stuff is being incorporated in the ration.

"Poultry Nector". a flavouring agent has been studied initially at Mississippi University (U.S.A.) and proven to give consisiant improvement in performance when added at 0.05% to poultry diets particularly when less palatable ingredients are used.

3. Pellet binders and Additives that alter Feed texture

Pellet binders are products that enhance the firmness of pellets; among them, (1) sodium bentonite (clay). (2) liquid or solid by-products of the wood pulp industry, consisting mainly of hemicelluloses, or combinations of hemicellulose and lignins, (3) molasses or fat are sometimes added to feed as an aid in pelleting, as well as a concentrated source of energy, (4) guar meal is another example. All are added @ 2.5% of the diet.

B. Additives that Enhance the Colour or Quality of the Marketed Product.

Many marketing concerns have 'brain washed' consumers into believing that broilers having a deep yellow coloured shank are of top quality. A similar situation exists relative to eggs, in which deep yellow yolks are considered to be highly desirable. Consequently, Xanthophylls are routinely incorporated into broiler feeds. Another synthetic carotinoid, Canthaxanthin when added @ 2-10 grams per tonne of feed along with yellow maize and lucerne helps to produce orange-yellow colour in the shanks and skin of broilers along with yolks.

C. Additives that Facilitate Digestion and Absorption

1. Grit
Since poultry do not have teeth to facilitate grinding of feed, most grinding takes place in the thick muscled gizzard. Grit is added to supply additional surface area of the feed by grinding those inside the gizzard. Oyster shell, limestones are common grits. Gravel and pebbles have been used successfully as long lasting sources of grit.

2. Chelates
Chelating agents, such as EDTA, are sometimes used to increase the availability and absorption of certain minerals. In chicks, zink absorption is enhanced through addition of EDTA.

3. Enzymes
These are complex protein compounds produced in living cells which cause changes in other substances without being changed themselves. They are organic catalysts.

For common poultry diets, the enzymes of the digestive system cause normal hydrolysis of the dietary proteins, carbohydrates and fats. Thus, no benefit may be expected from the use of enzyme preparation as feed additives unless feed composed of higher amounts of barley, wheat, sunflower, rye, ricebran or oat grains are fed to chickens. Barley to a large extent than wheat contain compounds named beta-glucans which give viscocity to the contents of the digestive tract. Such viscous material interferes with the activity of all digestive enzymes. Very small concentration of beta-glucans, 0.75 to 1.0% can produce this effect. The beta-glucanase in the enzyme products, by breaking down the beta-glucans, reduces the viscosity of the feed in the digestive tract and thus facilitates the action of natural digestive enzymes. The cellulases in the enzyme products would act on the cellulose present in the cell walls of grain by-products like rice bran, rice polish, wheat bran and other crude fibres present in other feed ingredients in the feed and would improve availability of nutrients from these products. The enzyme preparations which are being marketed are Agrozyme, Diazyme, Zymo-pabst, Porzyme and Avizyme etc.

4. Probiotics
Probiotics are live cultures of useful bacteria along with medicine in which they were grown. The organisms used are beneficial strains of lactobacillus and streptococcus. The reasoning behind the use of probiotic is that ingestion of these organisms would lend an increase in their number in the digestive tract. Their dominance would reduce

the population of undesirable organisms like E. Coli and thus save the birds from the toxins that these undesirable organisms produce in the digestive tract.

5. Antibiotics

These are substances which are produced by living organisms (molds, bacteria, or green plants) and which have bacteriostatic or bactericidal properties.

As early as 1949, it was observed that chickens fed with vegetable protein, gain in more weight when they were fed antibiotics 5-10 mg. per kg. of feed.

The probable modes of action of antibiotics follow:

1. They may spare certain nutrients. Studies in some cases indicated that antibiotics can replace inadequate intakes of certain vitamins and amino acids.
2. They may selectively inhibit growth of nutrient-destroying organisms while promoting growth of nutrient producing organisms.
3. They increase feed and/or water intake.
4. They may inhibit growth of organisms which produce toxic waste products or toxins.
5. They may kill or inhibit pathogenic organisms (a) within the gastrointestinal tract, or (b) systemically.
6. They may improve the digestion and subsequent absorption of certain nutrients.

The normal levels of incuusion are 4 grams per tonne of feed for the narrow spectrum, viz., penicillin, streptomycin etc., and 10 grams per tonne for the broad spectrum types, viz., tetracyclines, aureomycin etc. Higher levels of antibiotics (50 to 100 grams per tonne) may be used only after the careful consideration of disease level.

D. Additives that alter Metabolism

1. Hormones:

Hormones are chemicals released by a specific area of the body and being transported to another region within the animal they elicit a physiological response.

Hormonal preparations are added in the diet of chickens with a view to bring about desirable metabolic changes so that increased egg production or carcass fat deposition in birds could be achieved. These fall into about following four categories:

(a) *Anabolic compounds* are chiefly progesterone and related steroids which may stimulate protein metabolism. The objectives are clear, but to-date results have not been promising.
(b) *Oestrogens* in the form of Diethylstilbestcrol (DES) were used for several years largely as a subcutenious implant in broiler chicken. It resulted carcass quality having more tender and tastier. However, since hormone residues remain present in carcass, its use in chicken feed is now prohibited in U.S.A.

Dienestrol diacetate is the only feed additive of this type that is currently approved at a level of 0.0023 to 0.0035 percent in the feed for the last 4-10 weeks to improve the carcass quality of broilers and roasters. The practice must be discontinued at least 48 hours before slaughter. It must not be fed to laying hens or breeding stock.
(c) *Thyroxine* and related compounds are reported to stimulate growth and to improve egg production during the later part of the laying year. They are usually given in the

form of iodinated casein at levels of 100 to 200 grams per ton (110 to 220 mg./kg.) of feed. Results from the use of iodinated casein have been variable may be due to the differing needs of individual birds. A slight excess dose may bring about moulting and drop in egg production.

E. Additives that affect Health Status

1. **Antifungal additives** are agents that destroy fungi. Fungi can affect feed intake and subsequent production through contamination at one or more of four stages in the feeding chain: (1) in the field before harvesting, (2) during storage, (3) at mixing, and (4) within the animal itself. Once contaminated, fungi can pose problems through the production of toxins, alterations of the chemical composition of the diet, or alterations of the metabolic functioning of the animal ingesting or harboring the fungus. Production of aflatoxin by *Aspergillus flavus* is a classical example which is carcinogenic (tumor producing).

   The best method of controlling fungal infestation is to dry all feeds below 12 percent moisture. Additionally, mold inhibitors should be added to high moisture feed that are exposed to air during storage. Sodium propionate, sodium benzoate, quaternary ammonium compounds, acetic acid and certain antifungal antibiotics as nystatin or copper sulfate etc. are added to concentrate feeds to prevent further growth by molds. The toxicity of aflatoxin-contaminated feed can also be reduced by irradication of ultraviolet light or exposed to anhydrous ammonia under pressure.

2. **Anticoccidial** drugs are used to control coccidial infections which is a parasitic disease caused by microscopic protozoan organisms known as coccidia, which live in the cells of the intestinal lining of livestock. At least nine species of coccidia affect chicken: *Eimeria tenella, E. necatrix, E. maxima, E. acervulina, E. brunetti, E. hagani, E. praecox, E. mites* and *E. mivati.*

   There are over two dozen coccidiostats combinations commercially available. Bifuran supplement, Amprol-25%, Embazin, Zonamix, Nitrofurazone, Furazolidone etc. are very common coccidiostats. Most of these inhibit further proliferation of parasites during their sexual cycles. Coccidia tend to develop resistance to a coccidiostat to which they are exposed over a long period of time. When resistant forms appear, a change to another coccidiostat will usually restore control of the disease.

3. **Antihelmintic Drugs.** Chickens are subject to infestation with a wide variety of parasites, external and internal. External parasites can be eliminated by use of available insecticides. Likewise intestinal worms can also be killed or expelled by feeding suitable vermifuges (wormers).

The four most common intestinal parasites are large roundworms (*Ascaris*), caecal worms (*Heterakis*), capillary worms (*Capillaria*), and tape worms (Taenia). Of these, the large round worms are more easily expelled; caecal worms, capillary worms and tape worms, in the order given, are less easily expelled.

Antihelminties generally require more than one administration. The first administration kills those worms which are present in the body; and subsequent wormings kill those worms which hatched from eggs after the initial dose.

HOW TO COMPUTE A RATION FOR CHICKEN?

A farmer interested in compounding poultry mashes should have the basic knowledge of various types of raw ingredients as to their efficacy and nutrient composition *vis-a-vis* cost to make any mash effective for his flock. A short description has already been made in regard to various feed ingredients. However, they may be broadly classified as follows:

(i) *Protein supplement*:   (Primary source of protein)
   (a) Vegetable protein supplement-e.g., groundnut, soybean cake, mustard cake, maize gluten, etc.
   (b) Animal protein supplement–Fish meal, skim milk powder, liver meal, etc.

(ii) *Energy supplement*:
   (a) Primary source of energy–Cereal grains like maize, wheat, millet grains like jowar, milo, rice polish etc.
   (b) Cereal by products (Diluents–medium energy content and sources of minerals) e.g., wheat bran, rice bran, maize grit, etc.

(iii) *Salt*,

(iv) *Minerals*,

(v) *Vitamins*

(vi) *Non-nutrient feed additives–e.g., antibiotic, antioxidants, etc.*

In the formulation of poultry ration, the farmer has to consider first protein and energy and their ratio to each other what is known as C/P ratio. Protein again should be provided so that it satisfies the requirement in terms of amino acids with particular reference to Lysine, Methionine and Cystine. Then the ration should also fulfil the requirement of minerals with particular reference to calcium and available phosphorus. It should also satisfy the requirement of both fat soluble and water soluble vitamins.

Having various points as above in mind, a poultryman desirous of compounding a poultry mash, e.g., layers mash should first find out from the Table the requirement of various nutrients of layers mash and then proceed to satisfy these requirements by selecting proper protein and energy rich ingredients supplemented with minerals, vitamins, etc. Experience suggests that if formulation is made as per following assumption, then a lay farmer can manage to prepare his own layers mash without going for meticulous calculation.

Protein rich supplement   : $\begin{cases} \text{Vegetable protein, suppl.} & : 18\text{-}22 \\ \text{Animal protein, suppl.} & : 5\text{-}8 \end{cases}$

Energy rich supplement   :   Cereals, millets : 60-65

Mineral supplement   : $\begin{cases} \text{Calcite} & 5 \\ \text{Standard mineral mixture} & 2\text{-}3 \end{cases}$

Vitamin supplement   :   Standard Vit. AB_2D_3 complex.

Example 1

To cite a concrete example in terms with above assumption a model pattern of formula for layers mash is given below which will satisfy in terms of protein (with particular reference to amino acids make up), energy, minerals and vitamins, etc.

Maize	46 parts
Wheat	20 parts
Fish meal	6 parts
Groundnut cake	15 parts
Til cake (black)	5 parts
Calcite	5 parts
Any standard mineral mix.	2.5 parts
Dicalcium phoshate/bone meal	0.5 parts
	100

Rovimix (Vit. AB_2D_3) @250 gm/qtl and if possible Rovibe (B-complex) @20 gm/qt1 should be added.

Example 2

For the sake of economy, however, the above formula may be modified in the following pattern which will be almost equal in production value as the original one:

Maize	19
Wheat	7
Tapioca chips	10
Rice polish	17
Rice bran (deoiled)	5
Molasses	5
Sal seed cake	4
Groundnut cake (deoiled)	8
Maize gluten/til cake	7
Mustard cake (deoiled)	5
Fish meal/silk worm pupae meal or liver meals	5
Calcite	5
Standard mineral mixture	2.5
Dicalcium phosphate/bone meal	0.5
	100

Rovimix (Vit. AB_2D_3) (@ 250 gm/qtl [and where possible Rovibe (B-complex vitamin) @ 20 gm/qtl should be added for better hatchability, if required].

By this way various economic rations can be formulated using agro-industrial by-products intelligently.

Table 60   Expected Performance of Broilers (Typical Body Weights, Feed Requirements and Energy Consumption of Broilers)

Sl. No.	Age (Weeks)	Body Weight (gms)			Weekly Feed Consumption (gms)			Cummulative Feed Consumption (gms)			Weekly Energy Consumption Cal ME/Bird			Cummulative Energy Consumption ME/Bird		
		Male	Female	Avg.	Male	Female	Avg.	Male	Female	Avg.	Male	Female	Avg.	Male	Female	Avg.
(1)	(2)	(3)	(4)	(5)	(6)	(7)	(8)	(9)	(10)	(11)	(12)	(13)	(14)	(15)	(16)	(17)
(i)	1	152	144	148	134	131	132.5	135	131	133	395	386	391	395	386	391
(ii)	2	376	344	360	290	273	281.5	425	404	414.5	856	805	830	1251	1 191	1221
(iii)	3	686	617	651.5	487	444	465.5	912	848	880	1437	1 310	1373	2 686	2 501	2594
(iv)	4	1085	965	1025	704	642	673	1 616	1 490	1553	2 077	1 894	1985	4765	4 341	4579
(v)	5	1576	1344	1046	960	738	849	2576	2 228	2402	2 925	2 251	2 590	7 693	6 592	7169
(vi)	6	2088	1741	1915	1 141	1 001	1 071	3 717	3 229	3 473	3 480	3 503	3 267	11173	9 645	10436
(vii)	7	2590	2134	2362	1281	1081	1181	4998	4310	4654	3907	3297	3602	15080	12972	14038

Source: Poultry Feeds–Specification (Fifth Revision)–IS 1374:2007

EVALUATION OF POULTRY FEED

Knowledge of the nutrient content, the relative nutrient availability to the birds, and the variation in composition of feed stuffs is as important as knowledge of the nutritional requirements of the animals for the successful application of the principles of nutrition to poultry feeding. The various chemical and biological methods of evaluation of poultry feeds are indispensible for any poultry nutritionist.

The value of poultry feed can be judged by various methods. These include the following:

1. *Appearance* : Very little information can be gained merely from the, appearance of the feed. Moldy or wet condition at the most can be judged.

2. *Microscopic* : The amount of fibre or bulk in a feed stuff can be estimated but when odour and appearance are added to this, a fair guidance in detecting the quality of ingredients used in feed mixture is possible.

3. *Proximate chemical analysis* : The method gives the amounts of the different groups of nutrients present. By this method the moisture, crude fibre, crude protein, ether extract, nitrogen free extract and ash content of the feed are determined. Merely knowing the percentage of nutrients present in the feed does not help to answer as actual feed value since, the question of percentage digested or retained by the animal is not solved. But in general, the method gives a fair first hand information about the quality and as such is much in use in all nutrition laboratories.

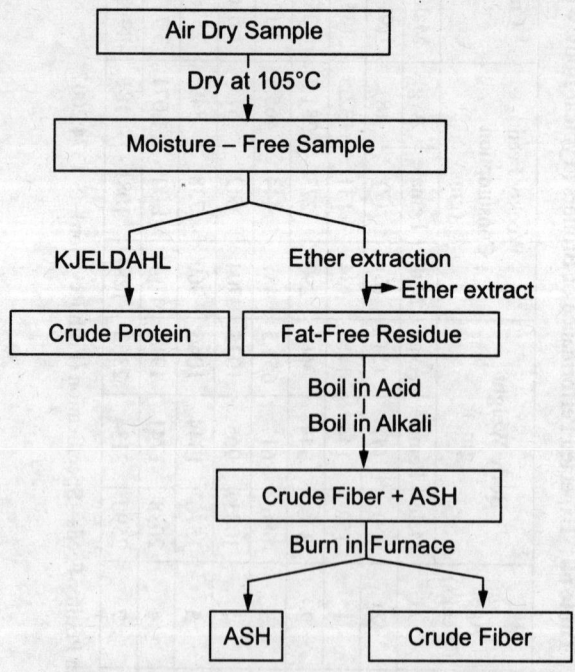

Flow diagram for the proximate analysis.

1. **Dry Matter**. That material remaining after drying a feed sample at 100°C for a given period of time.

$$\% \, DM = \frac{Dry \, weight}{Wet \, weight} \times 100$$

$$\% Moisture = \frac{Wet \, weight - dry \, weight}{Wet \, weight} \times 100$$

2. **Total Protein**. The percentage of nitrogen (N) of a sample of feed is multiplied by the factor 6.25. The factor 6.25 is used because average protein contains 16% nitrogen.

100 units of protein ÷ 16 units of nitrogen = 6.25

$$\% \, TP \, (as\text{-}fed \, basis) = \frac{6.25 \times units \, of \, N}{As\text{-}fed \, weight \, of \, sample} \times 100$$

$$\% \, TP \, (DM \, basis) = \frac{6.25 \times units \, of \, N}{Dry \, weight \, of \, sample} \times 100$$

3. **Ether Extract or Fat.** The fat and other ether-soluble substances are determined by subjecting a known amount of the dry matter of a feedstuff to an ether extraction. The ether is then evaporated and the extract weighed.

$$\% \, EE \, (as\text{-}fed \, basis) = \frac{Weight \, EE}{As\text{-}fed \, weight \, of \, sample} \times 100$$

$$\% \, EE \, (DM \, basis) = \frac{Weight \, EE}{Dry \, weight \, of \, sample} \times 100$$

Some feeds, especially coarse roughages, contain small amounts of gums, resins, and waxes that are soluble in ether and are included in the ether extract.

4. **Crude Fiber**. In the laboratory, crude fiber is measured by refluxing a dry sample in acid and then in base. The residue is filtered out of the solution, dried, and weighed. Crude fiber represents the majority of the cellulose and lignin in the feed.

$$\% \, CF \, (as\text{-}fed \, basis) = \frac{Weight \, of \, fibe \, residue}{As\text{-}fed \, weight \, of \, sample} \times 100$$

$$\% \, CF \, (DM \, basis) = \frac{Weight \, of \, fibe \, residue}{Dry \, weight \, of \, sample} \times 100$$

5. **Ash.** This represents the mineral components of a feed. A dry sample is placed in a crucible and completely combusted in a furnace at 650°C. The residue is the ash.

$$\% \, ash \, (as\text{-}fed \, basis) = \frac{Weight \, of \, ash}{As\text{-}fed \, weight \, of \, sample} \times 100$$

$$\% \, ash \, (DM \, basis) = \frac{Weight \, of \, ash}{Dry \, weight \, of \, sample} \times 100$$

6. *Nitrogen-Free Extract*.   This represents the more soluble carbohydrates such as starches and sugars. The nitrogen-free extract is determined mathematically by difference and not by actual analysis.

$$\% \text{ NFE} = 100 - (\% \text{ H}_2\text{O} + \% \text{ ash} + \% \text{ EE} + \% \text{ CP} + \% \text{ CF})$$

The coefficient of digestibility for any of the nutrients may be calculaed as follows.

$$\frac{\text{Weight of the nutrient in the feed eaten} - \text{Weight of the nutrient in the faeces}}{\text{Weight of the nutrient in the feed eaten}} \times 100$$

4. *Chemical Methods for estimation of ME* :   Of the various methods of measuring the availabie energy content of feed for poultry, the metabolizable energy (ME) value is the method of choice. The starting poultry feed and laying poultry feed should contain minimum of 2800 kilocalories and 2600 kilocalories of ME per kg of ration respectively.

The method developed by Carpenter and Clegg in 1956, used to estimate the energy value of cereals and cereal by-products, is based on proximate analysis and determination of the starch and sugar content of ingredients. The equation developed by these workers is : M.E. in kcal/kg. = 53 + 38 (% Crude protein + 2.25 x % ether extract + 1.1 x % starch + % sugar)

5. *Determination of amino acids* : Among the various essential amino acids, the declaration only for available lysine and methionine has been desired because Rao and Bose (Ind. J. Poult. Sci I(i) : 11. 1966 ; Ind. J. Nutr. Dietet. 7, 300, 1970) have observed that the poultry rations computed on the basis of economic considerations are likely to be deficient, especially, in lysine and methionine.

As regards crude protein content of feeds, it is wellknown that the measure of protein quantity indicated by chemical analysis of nitrogen content is not good enough for evaluation of protein feeds. Protien concentrates, such as, cakes, blood meal, meat meal, fish meal etc. subjected to excessive heating during processing may lose nutritive value, due to reduction in availability of lysine, an important essential amino acid without any change in the total quantity of nitrogen present. The non-availability of lysine is thought to result from the reactions of the free epsilon amino groups of lysine and other components of the substance. There are many ways of assessing the value of protein in feeding stuffs. These range from straight forward laboratory estimations of individual amino acids to elaborate biological methods in which the materials are fed to test animals under vigorously controlled conditions. The conventional methods of protein evaluation by growth assay, though highly accurate, are not convenient for routine commercial use because of the time involved. Chemical and microbiological methods are comparatively rapid and evidence is available indicating their potential value as quality predictors (Boyne, A.W., Carpenter, K. J. and Woodham, A. A. 1961. J. Sci. Fd. Agric. 12, 832-48). The most significant advance in this field has been the adaptation of the reaction between fluoro-2 : 4- dinitrobenzene and the free amino groups of lysine molecules within 'the protein chains (Carpenter, K.J. 1960. Biochem. J. 77, 604-10), In view of variable results obtained with compounded poultry rations due to production of interferring coloured compounds Ghosh and Bose (Ind. J. Anim. Sci. 43, 38-42, 1973) developed a rapid method for estimating available lysine in compounded poultry rations. The separation and estimation of available lysine were carried out by chromatography of dinitrophenyl amino acids after necessary purification and standardization of the technique of thin layer chromatography.

Biological Methods for Evaluating Feed Ingredients

Although chemical methods are useful for analysis of individual feed ingredients and of total rations, all these evaluations must be backed up by biological tests.

For most animals digestible energy is easiest to determine. With avian species, where the undigested residue and urinary wastes are excreted together, it is very difficult to find out true digestibility. It is more convenient to determine the metabolizable energy (ME) of a diet by treating the pooled excreta as a single material representing the unutilized portion of the food energy.

Determination of M.E. value of a complete ration or of any feed ingredients can be made by two conventional methods (A) Hill and Anderson method, (B) Sibbald and Slinger method. The basic principles are the same in both the cases except that in case of Hill and Anderson method the reference diet composed of mostly glucose which is costly, whereas in case of Sibbald and Slinger method the reference diet consists of practical type of feed ingredients. The procedures are described as below :

Determination of M.E. value of any poultry rations by Sibbald & Slinger method

Day-old healthy chickens are placed in a battery-brooder and fed on the experimental feed for about five to six weeks. During the last three days of the experimental period, the chickens are given requisite amount of accurately weighed experimental diet at a fixed hour in the morning. Simultaneously, the polyethylene sheets are spread on the trays for the collection of excreta. The representative samples of feed are collected for estimation of dry matter and for proximate analysis. Next day at the same hour the feed residue and the excreta are collected and weighed. The representative samples of feed residues are analysed for dry matter percentage. The difference in dry weights of feed offered and the remaining feed residues gives the amount of dry matter consumed in 24 hours. The total excreta collected for 3 days are pooled for analysis. For dry matter estimation, about 10 ml of 2 percent acetic acid is added for every 50 gm of the excreta and dried in an oven at about 80°C till constant weight is obtained. The total dry matter voided in 3 days is then determined.

Samples of feed and excreta are then analysed for crude protein, ether extract, total ash, NFE, crude fibre by official methods of analysis of the AOAC and their percentage on dry matter basis are determined.

Gross calories in feed and excreta are calculated assuming calorific value of crude protein, 5.65, ether extract, 9.40 and of total carbohydrates, 4.15 calories per 1 gm. M.E. is then calculated from the following equation :

M.E. per 1 gm feed = E diet—E excreta—N × 8.22

where   E diet = gross calories per 1 gm of feed (dry matter)

E excreta = gross calories in excreta per 1 gm of feed (dry matter) consumed.

N = nitrogen retention per gm of feed (dry matter) consumed. This is obtained by subtracting total nitrogen excreted from the total nitrogen consumed per 1 gm of the feed (dry matter).

Therefore, M.E. per kg of feed = M.E, per gm feed × 1,000

N. B. The age of birds during collection period may vary from 5-10 weeks, as this does not affect the M.E. value significantly. Chromic oxide can be used as a metabolically inert indicator at 0.3 percent in the ration to obviate total collection of the excreta.

Determination of M.E. value of any poultry feed ingredients by Sibbald and Slinger method

For this the general procedure described as above will hold good. In this case the reference

Ingredients			Percentage
Basal:			
Groundnut cake			23.0
Fish meal	–	–	10.0
Skim milk powder	–	–	5.0
Til cake (Sesame)	–	–	5.0
Maize	–	–	45.0
Rice polish	–	–	7.0
Groundnut oil	–	–	1.0
			Total: 96.0 parts
Additives :			
Dicalcium phosphate	–	–	2.080
Calcite	–	–	0.910
Sodium chloride	–	–	0.300
Nuvimin	–	–	0.500
Rovibe	–	–	0.100
Choline chloride	–	–	0.055
Trace Mineral mix.	–	–	0.055
			Total: 4.000 parts
			Grand Total: 100.00

ration should be perfectly balanced and may compose of practical type of ingredients which are locally available. An example of such ration is given below. It is absolutely necessary that while preparing the experimental diets, all the ingredients should be properly ground so that the birds are unable to sort out any particular ingredient of their choice.

For estimating the M.E. value of any test ingredient say 'Q', replace the basal part of the reference ration with Q at suitable portions say 20, 30 and 40 parts. Thus in total there will be 4 diets including reference. Chicks should randomly be placed in each dietary regime at least in duplicate.

By the procedure described as before find out first the M.E. value of all 4 diets. The method of calculating M.E. value of 'Q' is then done by solving the simultaneous equations as adopted by Sibbald and Slinger (1963).

Suppose the average M.E. value of the reference diet = 3.00... A and M.E. value of the diet at 20% level of inclusion of 'Q' = 2.91.. .B

Then,   100 R = 3.00 .... A (where R = Reference diet)

$$R = \frac{3}{100} = 0.03$$

One of the experimental diets was composed of 80 parts of basal ration and 20 parts of test ingredients. Among 80 parts there were 4 parts of additives. This 4 parts to be subtracted during calculation of M.E. value.

Then after correction :

$$96 R = 3.00$$

or $$R = \frac{3}{96} = 0.03125$$

Thus for the diet containing 80 parts basal and 20 parts test ingredient the calculation should be :

$$76 R + 20 T = 2.91 \dots (B)$$

or $$76 \times 0.03125 + 20 T = 2.91$$

or $$20 T = 2.91 - 2.375$$

or $$T = 0.0267$$

or $$100 T = 2.67$$

where T = M.E. Value of test ingredient, 'Q'.

Thus, the M.E. value of this particular test ingredient at 20% level of inclusion is 2.67. In this way the M.E. value of the same ingredient at different levels of inclusion can be found out. The average of all three will give an average M.E. value of the test ingredient (Q).

N.B.—The subtraction of additive parts (as because it does not contribute any energy) is still controversial as some workers believe that additives also contribute some amount of energy though in very negligible amounts. In that case the formula will remain as 80R + 20T = 2.91 instead of 76R + 20T = 2.91.

Determination of M.E. value of any poultry feed ingredient by Hill & Anderson method

Methods and principles are the same as described by Sibbald and Slinger method. The only difference is in the composition of reference ration which contains a high proportion of glucose. The test ingredient is substituted for part of the glucose (not the entire basal portion like that of previous case) as shown in the following example :

		Reference diet	Test diet
Glucose	–	45.7	5.7
Premix (supplies protein vitamins, minerals)	–	54.3	54.3
Ingredients studied (40% replacement)	–	–	40.0

These diets are fed to groups of chicks for the period from 14 to 28 days of age. During the last four days of the feeding period, collections of the excreta (mixed faeces and urine) are made. Samples of both diets are also analysed.

To compute ME of material substituted for glucose, the following equation applies :

$$\text{ME per gram substituted ingredient} = 3.64 - \frac{\text{ME per gm reference diet} - \text{ME per gm diet with substitute ingredient}}{\text{Proportion of substitute ingredient}}$$

The terms of this equation are derived from :

ME of reference diet = Calculated from experimental data either using proximate analysis or by using bomb calorimeter, as above.

ME of diet with ingredient = Decimal equivalent (0.40 representing 40% substitution in diet).

3.64 = Experimentally established ME per gram of glucose dry matter (Anderson, Hill and Renner, 1958).

MANAGEMENT OF BROILERS

A broiler or fryer is a young chicken of either sex of about six weeks of age weighing 1.5 to 2.0 kg body weight, with a tender meat, soft, pliable, smooth textured and flexible breast. Roaster on the other hand is also a young chicken but are much older and heavier than broiler.

Broiler Management: Object of broiler management should be to keep the broilers growing continuously as fast as possible and any possible stresses affecting growth should be avoided. For maximum profit, on a broiler farm attempts should be made through proper management right from the day old stage to keep the mortality low and growth and efficiency of feed utilization high. Skill in management of broilers can be developed through practice and long experience.

Location of the farm: A broiler farm should be located near the source of feed and chicks and also close to the final market in order to prevent shrinkage during transportation of live birds.

Broiler Chicks: Day old commercial broiler chicks of mixed sexes (straight run) should be procured from established and reputed hatcheries selling broilers of rapid and uniform growth, high disease resistance and with ability to convert feed into meat efficiently. Selection of good quality chicks should be done on the following basis. Chicks should be from healthy and disease free parents. The day old chicks should have a body weight of 38.5 to 39.5 g each. They should be of uniform size and colour. They should have been cleanly hatched, alert with good standing posture, round, bright eyes and are well feathered. Legs must be stout with bright shank. Vent should be clean and not pasty. They should have no deformity like crooked legs, defective head or eyes, crossed beak etc. In each brooder flock, at least 75% of male chicks and 78% of female chicks should be within 10% of the average body weight of each sex.

Systems of broiler production: There are two systems for producing broilers -

(a) *All in all out system*: It is most practical and convenient for efficient management. Here all the chicks are obtained at a time and after they have attained market weight, they are sold at the same time. After the sale of first crop of broilers and complete depopulation of the farm the brooder sheds are cleaned and disinfected and kept idle for nearly a fortnight before the second batch of chicks arrives. This intermittent period breaks any cycle of an infectious disease and the next batch of chicks had a clean start with no possibilities of contacting a disease from older flocks on the farms. The size and number of sheds will be according to the number of broilers to be produced in one crop. In this system, the difficulty is that large number of broilers are ready for marketing at a time and then there is a gap of nearly 6 weeks period in between the two crops when no broilers are available for sale. Hence many farmers who want a continuous and regular supply of broilers they do not adopt this system and choose the other systems.

(b) *Multiple rearing system*: In this system the chicks are obtained at regular short interval such as weekly, 10 days, fortnightly or monthly. Hence on the farm there are several batches of different age groups, which pose difficulties in the prevention of disease and makes management a little more difficult. Recent advances in isolation and disease control have made it possible to keep chicks of several age groups on the same farm but the system calls for expert management and the programme is not for the novice. The advantage of the system is that it enables the farmer to have a continuous supply of marketable broilers at regular short intervals. Usually a batch is ready for marketing in 6-7 weeks and hence the number of sheds required will depend upon the schedule of procurement of day old chicks. The following precautions must be taken in this system.

1. Adequate isolation is to be ensured by giving at least 35 ft. or more space between any two sheds. Each brooder house must be enclosed in a tight fence with gates and the locks on all entrances. Even feed and other supply vehicles should not be allowed to enter the fence unless they pass through a disinfectant.
2. No visitor should be allowed to enter the sheds unless he/she takes a shower and changes clean dress and shoes.
3. Never rear different age chicks in the same shed.
4. Never take a fresh batch of chicks on used litter.
5. Restrict the movements of workers from older chicks to younger chicks because older chicks are comparatively more resistant to diseases and even milder infection from older chicks to younger ones cause heavy mortality or at least affect growth rate and hence the profits in the younger lot.

Management procedure: Broiler management is essentially the brooding management or chick management and a broiler house is basically a brooder cum grower house. Day old

174

chicks are purchased and placed in the brooder house and reared there for 4 week. It is critical period in the life of a bird and hence full attention should be paid in rearing day old broilers. In broilers farming there is no optimum period to receive the chicks as it is a continuous operation throughout the year. For proper management, the following factors must be kept in mind.

I. *Ventilation*: The brooder house should be well ventilated but should be free from draughts. Too dusty environment causes irritation in the respiratory tract and it transmit respiratory diseases in the chicks. Too much moisture in the house causes ammonia fumes which also irritates the respiratory tract and eyes.

II. *Sanitation and hygiene*: Before a new batch of chicks is received, the brooder house should be properly cleaned and disinfected with a disinfected solution. All movable equipments like brooder hover, feeders, waterers must be removed from the shed and cleaned and disinfected. Litter should be scrapped and removed. Then the shed is cleaned by pressure cleaner and sprayed with malathion or creosote solution. New litter should be spread only after each cleaning. A foot bath may be provided at the entrance of each building. Outsiders and workers from other sheds should not be allowed to enter the enclosure unless they shower and change clothes and shoes. In one enclosure, there may be more than one brooder shed but the chicks should be of similar age and source in all such sheds with a maximum difference of one week of age and all must be vacated at a time and prepared for the next batches of chicks.

Idle periods between batches of chicks should not be less than 14 days, so that the cycle of disease is broken. The following procedure should be adopted for clearing the house.

1. Remove the litter outside the enclosure.
2. Clean and scrub the house, wires or slats and wash thoroughly with a pressure sprayer. The interior of the brooder house should be disinfected with a powerful disinfectant and allow the house to dry.
3. All equipments must be scraped, washed and disinfected. Dip the smaller items in a disinfectant solution, allow to dry outside the house in the fenced area and then moved them back in the house.
4. Fumigation may be done using 3X formalin gas (one x = 20 g KMnO4 and 40 ml of formalin per 1000 cubic ft. area). The house should be made air tight or curtains should be closed at the time of fumigation.
5. Clean and fumigate bulk feed bins.
6. Treat dirty floors with disinfectants.
7. Clean the grounds and remove all weeds and debris from the fenced area outside the house. Complete necessary road repair and spray the area with the oil and disinfectant mixture.
8. Chick delivery van or the feed truck has to enter the gate of the enclosure and hence at the gate there should be a truck dip vat filled with a suitable disinfectant through which truck must pass, so that any possible infection carried by the truck wheels is killed.

III. *Litter and litter management*: A layer of 5 cm thickness of a suitable material like paddy husk, saw dust or any available straw of not more than 6 inches length and soft in nature could be used as litter. The thickness of the litter may be increased to 7-10 cms in the course of time by gradual addition. Wet or mouldy litter material should not be used. Wet litter spots should be replaced with dry litter and the litter should be regularly stirred at least fortnightly. The moisture content of the litter must be 20-25% only. If the moisture content is less than 20%, the litter becomes dusty and if more then 25% the litter becomes hot and caked. A good litter adheres slightly and breaks up when dropped from hands. After each stress, one kg, of dry lime powder may be mixed per 100 sq. ft., area of litter to keep the litter dry and hygienic. When the litter becomes old and wet it produces ammonia fumes which are injurious for the birds. A continuous exposure of 50 ppm of ammonia fumes will reduce 7 week weight by 8%. These fumes may be controlled by super phosphate and phosphoric acid. The later is more effective. In acidic medium very little ammonia will be released but it is rapidly formed at pH 8.0 and above. The litter should be treated with phosphoric acid 1.9 litres per 10.5 ft| (lm^2) or with super phosphate 2.2 lb (1.0 kg) per 10.5 ft^2 (lm^2) of litter. Under the brooder hover before arrival of chicks several layers of waste paper (old news papers) are laid, so that the chicks are not able to eat litter material in the first few days of their life.

IV. *Temperature*: Proper temperature in the brooder house and optimum temperature under the hover brooder is most important factor to determine the comfort of chicks and the quality of management. Too high or too low a temperature slows the growth and causes mortality. Artificial heat is provided to the brooding chicks through a brooder hover mostly seen by electricity. Gas brooder or a petromax or a bukhari should also be kept as a standby for power failure. An electric brooder may have ordinarily light bulbs or heat bulbs (infrared bulbs) or heating coils. More sophisticated brooder hovers have a thermostatic control of temperature. The optimum temperature during the first week of brooding is 35°C (95°F) which may be reduced to 2.5°–3°C (5°F) per subsequent week till the temperature reaches to 21°C (70°F) in about six weeks time particularly in winter. After the sixth week, heating arrangements may not be necessary unless the chicks are not properly feathered or the ambient temperature is very low. The temperature in the cool zone (in the brooder house beyond the brooder hover) should be about 10°C less than the brooder temperature. A maximum and minimum thermometer in each house will give an idea of the difference in the cool and warm zone in the brooder house.

The best guide of temperature prevailing under a brooder hover is the sitting behaviour of chicks. When the temperature is higher than needed the chicks encircle the source of heat at a distance but when the temperature is lower than needed the chicks huddle down in the centre of the hover, resulting in death of several chicks under the pressure of the upper ones. When the temperature is optimum, the chicks spread out evenly throughout the brooder should be measured at 2 inches (5.1 cm) above the surface of the litter and about 2 inches within the brim of the brooder hover with the help of a thermometer. In the first 2 weeks, the temperature should not be allowed to go below 30°C (86°F). When infra red bulbs are used, a 250 watt bulb is sufficient for 100 chicks. When the chicks in a brooder house are more than 100, more than one infrared bulbs are to be used, there should be a distance of 18″–20″ (45 – 50 cms) between two bulbs.

When the weather is excessively chilly, in the middle of brooder house a limited area is enclosed by plastic curtains and brooding of chicks is done within it. In this system it is easy to control the temperature and it saves lot of fuel or energy.

V. *Space Requirement*: Growth, feathering, mortality and feed conversion are invariably proportional to floor space per bird which is evident from the fact in an experiment when 1 sq. ft. (0.093 sq. m) floor space was provided, the body weight per bird was 4.35 lbs (1.88 kg), mortality was 2%, poorly feathered birds were 0.2% and there was a feed conversion ratio of 1.73 but the weight of birds raised per unit of floor space (4.35 lbs or 1.88 kg) increased to 9.65 lb (4.37 kg) of body weight per unit of floor space when only 0.4 sq. ft. (0.03 sq. m.) area per bird was provided but then the body weight per bird becomes only 3.86 lbs (1.75 kg) with 4.5 % mortality, 14.1% poorly feathered birds and a feed conversion ratio of 1.98. Hence, sometimes when the farmer wants more turnover of live weight from a specified floor space available, he takes a risk of overcrowding the stock even when he knows that average body weight per bird will decrease, mortality and percentage of poorly feathered birds will increase and efficiency of feed utilization will deteriorate but what is the minimum floor space per bird necessary to provide the greatest return or invest should be worked out in the specific circumstances of a farm. This space should be more for larger birds than smaller birds and should be less in winters than the summers. Overcrowding results in poor growth, higher incidence of cannibalism and other diseases.

VI. *Brooder guards*: Chick guards are provided to check straying of baby chick from the source of heat and to prevent floor draughts. These guards are placed at an average of 0.9 to 1.2 meters away from the edge of the hover (30 inches in winter and 36 inches in summer). This distance is increased slowly each day to maximum of 1.5 meters. Usually it is not needed after 7-14 days.

VII. *Supply of water to chicks*: Plenty of clean and fresh water should be made available to chicks during brooding period. As soon as chicks arrive, they be made to drink sugared water (8% sugar solution). At least for 4-5 days, water must be provided from automatic chick fountains. Dissolve 1362 g of sugar to 11.3 litres of water to obtain 8% sugar solution. For the first 3-4 days, soluble vitamins, electrolytes and antibiotics may also be added to the drinking water to take care of transient stress and disease in chicks. Some disinfectant may be added to the water to kill the microorganism and to prevent mouldy growth afterwards. Sometimes some water sanitizers are used in drinking water provided no vaccines are to be used through drinking water.

Sufficient light be provided for easy location of waterers and feeders at least in the first 2 days of brooding.

VIII. *Supply of feed to chicks*: Feed should be freshly prepared form quality ingredients and should be perfectly balanced. Most farmers do not compound it themselves and purchase it from tested and reputed firms. The feed supplies should be received weekly. In the first few days, feed is provided in the chick's box lids or unused egg trays. One chick box lid or two egg trays are sufficient for 100 chicks. The feed is offered after 3 hours of arrival and of drinking water. Feed is sprinkled in the entire area of the tray uniformly. Plenty of light must be available to chicks for easy location of feeders and waterers. Feeders or lids must be placed outside the canopy of the brooder. Watch-out for starved chicks whose crops are empty. Try to feed them individually and find its reason and remove the problem. To prevent vent picking, give some cracked corn or jowar as part of their first sprinkled on the top of the regular broiler starter feed. The cracked grains are fed only first 2 days @ 5 kg per 1000 chicks. After two days, regular feeders are placed.

About 3-6% of feed may be wasted per chick during the 6 week period, if proper precautions are not taken. Even if the level of feed in the feeders is 2/3rd, about 10% feed will be wasted; if ½ full, the wastage is 3% and if 1/3rd full, the wastage is only 1%. Hence after a few days, the level of feed in the feeders should be kept low (less than 1/3rd) to reduce the wastage.

As age and body weight increase, feed consumption and water consumption per bird increase and the cumulative feed conversion at the end of each week, also increases but with an increase in the house temperature, feed consumption decreases and water consumption increases at all ages.

Broilers are usually fed with two types of rations, broiler starter and broiler finisher (Table 45). The former ration is fed upto 3 weeks of age and the latter is continued till marketing.

IX. *Light management of broilers*:   The amount of light needed by a growing broiler is only that amount which is necessary to enable the bird to move about and see to eat and drink. Activity is to be reduced to a minimum.

Continuous light in open sided house start with 48 hours of continuous light with an intensity of 3.5 foot candle at floor level, then supply dim artificial light during all the dark hours except 1 hour during mid night for training the birds in getting accustomed to darkness so that there is no panic when power fails. One 150 watt bulb for each 1000 sq. ft. (93 sq. m.) of floor space will provide 0.50 foot candle light at floor level. This is the minimum light needed by the birds.

X. *Some important points regarding growth, feed consumption and efficiency of feed conversion in broilers*:
  (i) With an increase in body weight with age, feed consumption and water consumption increases per bird.
  (ii) With an increase in the ambient temperature, water consumption increases and feed consumption decreases.
  (iii) Feed conversion is best at 70°F (21.1°C).
  (iv) Most commercial growers produce straight run broilers of nearly 2.00 kg in about 45 days on an average year round basis for marketing but optimum marketable broiler weight is around 1.8 kg. Whereas roasters are weighing 2.7 kg and over. Good quality chick with well balanced feed and correct management will attain a

body weight of 1.88 kg at the end of 6th week with a feed conversion ratio of 1.75.

(v) A study on the weekly gain has shown that maximum weight gain occurs during 6th week and then it starts declining but feed conversion goes on increasing and hence it is most economical to sell the birds where maximum gains occur and hence the best age of marketing a broiler appears to be at the end of 6th week except for coloured broilers which are marketed after 8th week.

(vi) Males are generally heavier than the females, at marketing weight males are 17% heavier than females. At roaster weights males are about 25% heavier than females.

(vii) Males convert feed to meat more efficiently than females. Hence feed conversion varies according to the age, sex and weight of the birds. Females take 43.3 days to attain a weight of 1.81 kg and the males will attain this weight about 39.3 days old only. Hence males attain the same weight about four days earlier. Accordingly one can manage the males and females separately for broiler production.

XI. *Broiler Health Programme*:   A health programme is fundamental to successful broiler production. A suggested disease prevention and control programme follows:
  (i) Start with disease-free chicks.
  (ii) Vaccine chicks against Raniket and Marek's disease at the hatchery.
  (iii) Use effective drugs in the feed, or a vaccination programme to prevent coccidiosis.
  (iv) Keep feed free from aflatoxin.
  (v) Do not allow visitors or attendants inside the broiler house unless they wear disinfected boots and clean clothing.
  (vi) When there are several age groups on the farm, always care for the youngest birds first while performing daily routine works.
  (vii) Rework built-up litter. When built-up litter is used, all caked and wet litter should be removed and replaced with fresh, clean litter before chicks arrive.
  (viii) Cover floor with clean litter at least 3 inches deep after each clean out, wood shavings, rice hulls, straws cut into small pieces are suitable litter materials.

XII. *Marketing Broilers*:   Most broilers are marketed when they are 6 week of age. For the most part, marketing involves moving the birds from the house in which they are produced to the consumer's house. Improper handling of broilers immediately prior to and during shipment will result in excess bruises, and lowered quality. Such losses may be minimized as follows:
  (i) Discontinue grit feeding at least 2 weeks prior to marketing (usually grit is not fed after 5 weeks of age).
  (ii) Let the feeders became empty about 2 hours before catching and remove the waterers to prevent bruises during catching.
  (iii) Catch and load properly by: (a) using an experienced attendant, (b) working under a dim blue light at night, (c) corralling them in small groups, (d) grasping them by shanks with no more than 4 or 5 being carried at a time.
  (iv) Protect the in-transit birds from extremes in weather. In hot weather, protect against overheating in shipment by using open crates and avoiding lengthy stops in route.

Broiler Flock Performance Standard: Facts pertinent to an understanding of broiler performances are -

1. At any given age, males are heavier than females.
2. Weekly increases in weight are not uniform, gains increases each week until reaching a maximum at about sixth week for straight-run (both sexes together) flocks.
3. Weekly feed consumption increases as weight increases; each week the birds eat more feed than they did the week before.
4. Generally, the more feed consumption, the better the feed conversion at a given age.
5. Fast gains are efficient gains, as weekly gains increase, feed efficiency increases, also
6. Healthy birds consume more feed and have better feed conversion than sick birds.
7. The greater the activity, the lower the feed efficiency.
8. Cannibalism results in lowered feed consumption, growth and feed conversion.
9. Changes in temperature causes changes in feed consumption, broilers eat about 1% more feed for each 1°F decrease in temperature and they eat about 1% less feed for each 1 °F rise in temperature. Very high temperatures drastically reduce feed consumption and cause poor feed conversion. During very cold weather, growth and feed conversion are poorer because a greater portion of the feed is used to maintain body temperature.
10. Flocks are not uniform, with the result that all birds are not of the same weight at market time. The males are heavier than the females. But neither sex is uniform, there are large, medium and small cocks and pullets. When approximately 75% of the birds are within extremes of 10% of the average weight of each sex within a given flock, the flock is of acceptable uniformity. Expected performance of broilers have been presented in Table 60.

Summary of management practices

Good management practices are herein summarised:

1. Start with quality chicks; get healthy chicks from reliable sources.
2. Debeak chicks whenever necessary.
3. Clean quarters before having birds and keep houses and equipment clean.
4. Keep litter clean, dry and free from mold.
5. Brood birds carefully; have good sanitary management.
6. Supply adequate heat and ventilation.
7. Provide enough floor space.
8. Give adequate space for feed and water, have feed delivered to bin outside house.
9. Keep the feed levels low in feeders in order to lessen wastage, but do not let feeders became empty. With full feeders, as much as 10% of the feed may be wasted.
10. Use all-night lights, except for a hour of darkness.
11. Adapt vaccination schedule to local needs.
12. Watch for disease; get prompt diagnosis when disease occurs; remove diseased birds from flock.
13. Dispose off dead birds promptly; have satisfactory disposal facilities.
14. Keep visitor's out of houses; lock doors.

The above management practices have a lot of little details, all of which add upto to make broiler management of great economic importance.

CARE OF THE CHICKENS DURING SUMMER

The overall performances of chickens either for meat or for egg is definitely governed by the interaction of two important factors, viz. (1) genetic constitution and (2) environment.

Summer heat is one of the major important environmental factors that all bird owners of the tropical countries experience among their flocks.

Effects of Summer heat on Chicken

1. Reduced feed intake along with increased water intake
2. Poor feed conversion and growth (weight gain)
3. Drop in egg production
4. Egg size diminishes significantly
5. Increase in cracked eggs and poor shell quality
6. Very fast breathing (panting) along with high pulse rate and metabolic counts.
7. Body temperature is raised and birds try to regulate in absence of sweat glands, by evaporation of moisture from lungs (panting)
8. Reduced resistance to diseases
9. Prostration due to heat stroke and possible mortality resulting from this.

Environmental temperature vis-a-vis chickens reaction

65°F to 80°F—The desirable temperature under which chicken feels comfortable and functions normally.

81 °F to 85°F—Feed consumption drops, irregular variation in egg production, shell quality and feed conversion.

86°F to 95°F—For each degree rise in temperature above 85°F, chicken could eat roughly 2-3% less feed. The condition affects significantly on egg size, number and shell quality.

96°F to 100°F—Intensity of heat stress exerts further influences on above mentioned effects. The wings may hang side wise loosely in relaxed posture. Emergency measures must be considered otherwise all chances are there for heat stroke and collapse of the birds.

101 °F and above—The temperature is often referred to as 'lethal' or killing temperature. The chickens pass into a state of shock culminating in death.

Physiological mechanisms by which chickens adjust rising temperature

1. In animal system, after feeding heat is produced during fermentation in the gastrointestinal tract and also during processing and use of food nutrients in the body. This heat is not wasted when the temperature is below the critical temperature, as it is used to keep the body warm. But under high environmental temperature, chickens have a problem in getting rid of the surplus heat. Therefore, they will eat less to avoid increment of physiological heat.
2. Due to absence of sweat glands, drinking excessive amounts of water is one way to keep their body cool.

3. Since movement increase body temperatures, birds at high environmental temperature will restrict their activity.

4. In a deep litter system, birds will often take a bath in their litter, which is generally cooler than their own body temperature.

5. At discomfort region of temperature (above 80°F), chickens open out their wings and begin to pant or mouth breathe. By doing so, birds give out large amount of moist warm air.

Effective managerial practices to combat heat stress among birds

A. Housing

1. The long axis of the house should run from east to west and the sides should face north to south to prevent direct sunshine falling in the house.

2. The house should be situated away from other buildings in order to facilitate free movement of air. Distance between 2 houses for the birds of the same age group should also be at least 20 meter to allow proper ventilation.

3. It is preferable to surround the house with tall trees, ideally canopy type shady trees.

4. High altitude of roofs is ordinarily 2.6 to 3.3 meter from foundation to the roof line is desirable io provide maximum ventilation.

5. Provide 1 meter overhang to cut the direct sun and rain into the house.

6. The thatched roof is suitable for hot areas particularly where rainfall is less. In such cases allowing pumpkin plants on the roof particularly during summer months is really a good proposition to keep the house cool. When the roof is build of asbestors apart from covering it with pumpkins, straws, coconut palms, or leaves etc. may also be spread to reduce roof heat.

7. White washing of roof with a good coat of lime or aluminium painting of roof will reduce the temperature by about 10°F as compared to ordinary darker coloured roof.

8. If possible, spreading of a layer of thermocole under the ceiling leaving an air gap between the insulation material and the ceiling will prove to be of great relief.

9. If necessary, use of fans, preferably of pedestal type at a time of maximum heating period will again be of much relief to the birds.

10. Similarly during the hottest part of the day spraying of water on the roof may be of some help.

11. Foggers may be used particularly when the temperature is too high (above 100°F), or birds appear to become distressed. Heavy panting will indicate the necessity of using foggers.

12. If foggers are not available putting up of curtains or gunnybags on the side from which hot winds are blowing and pouring water on these will help entry of cool breeze inside the house. Care should be taken to (i) keep the floor dry and (ii) not to put up curtains on all sides of the house as this will build up humidity in the shed with consequential bad results.

13. Overcrowing must be checked by increasing floor space.

14. Fermentation in the built up litter generate heat. Therefore the thickness of the litter in summer must be reduced to about 6 cm depth to get rid of excess heat. Raking of litter will prevent caking.

B. Water management

1. Birds drink water roughly about 2 litres for every kg. of feed at 70°F. For each degree of temperature rise above 75°F, birds will drink about 4% more water.
2. The normal intake of feed: water is 1:2. But this ratio rises to nearly 1:4 or even more when temperature exceeds 95°F.
3. Birds prefer cool water between 45°F to 80°F. Except for day old chicks, the temperature of drinking water for all categories of chickens should always be lower than the room temperature.
4. Provision of extra waters on deep litter is a must along with filling up these with cold water for 4-5 times a day.
5. Birds on cages should also get a continuous supply of fresh, cool water. Where there is a provision for automatic drinking devices, if necessary small ice pieces may be placed in drinking reservoirs.
6. When using water medication during severe summer heat, recommended concentration must be reduced as high amount of water consumption may increase excess of the normal levels, resulting in an overdose of the drug.

C. Feed and Nutrition

1. Ensure steps to feed birds in the early hours of the morning and late evening so that the broilers can consume feed while the air is comparatively cooler.
2. Provision of 10% more feeders inside the house may encourage the birds to consume little more feed.
3. Provision of wet mash during hotter parts of the day will result in higher intake. Wet mash should be made outside the house in a bucket instead of preparing it in the feeder. No wet mash should remain in the feeders overnight otherwise moulds may begin to grow and cause serious fungal infections.
4. Replacing carbohydrate calories suitably by fat calories will minimise extra heat generation inside gastrointestinal tract.
5. Daily ration should be enriched with a marginal increase of protein, minerals and vitamins simultaneously with a reduction of 10% energy.
6. Use of pelleted feed in the summer may be beneficial as pelleting increases feed consumption and improves metabolizable energy content of the diet. Pelleting also eliminates selective feeding and minimises load of microbes in poultry feed.

D. Medication and other managerial practices

1. Provision of glucose water (8 gm. glucose + 2 gm electrol in 100 ml. water) or 50 gm. cane sugar molasses per litre of water during noon time will keep the bird in comfortable position.

2. Vitamin C @ 10 mg. per bird and Geriforte @ 1 ml. per litre may be given with water.
3. It is advisable to assess the strain susceptibility of birds. Those greater prone to heat stroke should not be raised.
4. One should plan for lawns around the poultry house to reduce heat build up by radiation as well as to impart beauty of the farm.
5. In severe cases, birds may be dipped in cold water and left in open shady areas for drying.

CARE OF THE CHICKENS DURING MONSOON
(Summer monsoon)

In India summer monsoon is a season during which the wind blows from the south west during May to August characterized by heavy rains and from the north east during July to September with a primary cause of difference in air pressure due to changes in temperature over land and sea. Winter monsoons in India on the other hand are generally dry.

Poultry farms are always likely to be affected during summer monsoon unless proper precautionary measures are taken. In some parts of our coutnry during the season there are heavy rainfall, might lead to even cyclones whereas in other parts there may be scanty rainfall.

The following steps might help to keep the birds away from monsoon stress.

1. Maintenance of Poultry houses

Areas around the shed to the extent of 5 meters must be cleared and free from shrubs and grasses. For efficient drainage system the drains should be cleared. Leakage of roof must be corrected in time. If overhangs are not provided sufficiently, rain water may seep in. Necessary curtains of polythene may be provided without obstructing light. Care should also be taken to repair all *pucca* floor and to keep these dry as far as possible.

In case of litter, all care must be exercised to keep these dry by checking the possible leakage of rain water from the window and sides of the house. Occassional wrecking of litter and mixing of drying agents such as lime-powder, gammoxene 5%, ammonium sulphate etc. will maintain the dryness. Wet litter on the otherhand will be the breeding ground of coccidiosis, enterties, worm infestation etc. The use of bagasse should be done with caution as it may harbour *Aspergillus fumigatus*, a mould which penetrates the lung tissue and produces 'Brooders Pneumonia' in chicks.

2. Feed Storage

Prior to monsoon sufficient quantity of feed should be stored to cover the entire need during rainy season otherwise during transportation feed bags might get loaded with extra moisture from rain. Once purchased, feed bags should be stored on wooden planks one feet above the ground level as well as one feet from the side walls of the godown. If the inside humidity is high or there is any water leakage, the condition in any case will be inducing to heavy infestation of fungi and moulds. The most dreadful fungi affecting feeds like groundnut meal, maize, sunflower cake, seasame meal etc. is *Aspergillus flavus*. The toxins produced by this species is known as aflatoxins B_1, B_2, G_1 and G_2. The B_1 type is acutely toxic. The effect of feeding is reflected on poor growth, drop in egg production, low feed conversion, liver tumers and even mortality in layers and broilers. Though there is no fixed safe level of aflaloxin in all kinds of livestock feed, 0.05 ppm level in broilers and 0.1 ppm level in layers were found to be practically tolerable levels. Ducks and Turkeys are more susceptible to the toxin than chickens.

Storage of Shell-grit—Shell-grit becomes scarce in rainy season. Since it is a cheap ingredient and can be preserved for a long time, it will be a wise decision to store the material quite ahead of rainy season.

Storage of Fish-meal—After considering the total need, it is also advisable to procure good quality fish meal just before the rain starts. Otherwise the product may get oxidised when stored at high humidity at sellers godown. The addition of an antioxidant, *ethoxyquin* to the fish meal immediately following its manufacture will markedly preserve the original quality.

3. Improvement of water quality

It is but natural that in rainy season water from well, ponds, river or even from tap gets contaminated due to admixture of various microbes brought by percolation of muddy rain water through its environment.

Treatment of drinking water with alum followed by sedimentation for 24-hours will purify the water.

Another way of purifying water for drinking of birds may be done by mixing 2 gms. of bleaching powder containing 35% chlorine with 1000 litres of clean drinking water and ultimately exposing the treated water lor at least 3 hours before its actual use. Alternately 'Medichlor' may be added at the rate of 10 ml. in 100 litres of drinking water. The treated water should remain exposed for minimum 2-3 hours before being used.

4. Care of poultry excreta

When birds are housed in deep litter, it should always be kept dry. A conditioned or built-up litter contains about 25 percent moisture. The correct litter condition can be easily determined by taking a handful of litter and squeezing it lightly and then releasing it. The litter should neither form a cohesive ball nor it should fall apart. For maintenance of litter quality, it should be stirred at least once in a week. Wet litter, if any, should be replaced immediately with dry rice husk (not available in rainy season), grass cuttings, bagasse, wooden dust etc. Wet litter is related with the problems of coccidiosis as high moisture leads to sporulation.

When droppings are collected from battery type of brooders or laying cages should be exposed to spraying of disinfectants like Malathion, Sumithion or Baygon etc. Flies, mosquitoes and other insects proliferate during rainy season. Regular spraying of such disinfectants around the sheds will keep the disease level to a minimum.

PRESERVATION OF SURPLUS EGGS

There are some interesting methods very commonly found among the poultry keepers for preserving surplus eggs. The operation is very important in order to run a profitable poultry business. The methods are discussed below :

A. Home Preservation

1. **The water glass method**
   By this method eggs may be stored safely for as long as 6 months. During the months when eggs are plentiful, carefully select only clean, sound and unwashed eggs which are to be preserved.
   Sodium silicate or water-glass forms a viscous solution in water. When eggs are dipped in this solution, a coating of silica is formed over the shells and their pores are completely closed. For the solution, add commercial water-glass in boiled water @ 1 kg in 10 litres. Shake well with a rod. About 15 dozen eggs can be preserved in 10 litres of the solution.

2. **The lime water method**
   By this method also eggs can be preserved for nearly 6 months.
   Add 1 kilo of unslaked lime to 20 litres of water in an enamelled or glazed earthen vessel. Let the solution settle for 10 minutes. Then pour off the supernatant liquid which will constitute the lime water for the preservation of eggs. Sediments at the botton of the solution should never be used.

3. **Oil protected eggs**
   By this method eggs are dipped in warm oil generally in coconut oil having colourless, tasteless and in odorous qualities. Oiling should be made as soon as possible after the eggs are laid. In this way the pores of the shell are sealed which prevents evaporation and loss of carbon dioxide, thus maintains good internal quality and prevents weight loss.

4. **Thermostabilisation**
   This applies to the stabilisation of egg quality by heat. Eggs may be thermostabilised by immersing the shell eggs for 15 minutes in water at 54.4°C (130°F) or at 60°C (140°F) for 3 to 5 minutes and water are kept stirred. The process has got the following advantages : (i) Pasteurises the eggs (kills bacteria on the egg shell); (ii) Defertilises the eggs (kills the embryo); (iii) Stabilises the egg (improves the keeping quality).

B. Commercial Method of Preservation

1. **Cold storage (5 to 8 months)**
   The temperature of an egg-storage room should be maintained at + 0.5°C to − 0.5°C (31° to 33°F) being the temperature usually preferred. A relative humidity of 75 to 85 percent is necessary. Too much humidity favours the formation of moulds.

2. Frozen eggs

The freezing of the internal contents of eggs is now a common method of preservation specially in developed countries. The eggs are first candled and when they are broken out, the smell and appearance of the contents are noted for any possible defects. The yolk and the white may be frozen separately with addition of 5% glycerine. The egg contents are then frozen in a 30-40 lb., tin at a low temperature range of 10°F to 30°F below zero. The contents are then kept at a low temperature until required for use. In case the storage temperature is zero or below, the frozen eggs may be stored with little or no loss of flavour for 12 months or longer.

3. Dried eggs

Egg drying is now largely practised in place of freezing. Although the process is more expensive but there is a considerable saving in transport and less need for cold storage. The egg contents are dried at a temperature of 160°F and stored under 50°F to convert white, yolk or the whole egg into a fine powder. The whole egg is of use for bakery products, the yolk for flours and the albumen for confectionaries.

With the present day, low egg production and unsatisfactory marketing facilities, preservation and storing of eggs by freezing and drying cannot be of immediate interest to us under Indian conditions.

CONTROL OF BAD HABITS

Cannibalism

Occasionally hens, in attempting to lay too large an egg, will rupture the oviduct, or a part of the cloaca will protrude from the vent. Hens see this soft, red membrane and pick at it. The intestines sometimes may be pulled out before it is noticed by the poultry man. Cannibalism can also be caused by inheritance, by deficiencies in the ration, and by close confinement. Once hens get in the habit of picking at each other, it is difficult to stop them and heavy losses may result. The following method may be followed for preventing cannibalism :

1. Give the flock more room, or reduce the size of the flock by cullings.
2. Sprinkle fine salt, free of lumps, generously over the mash for 3-5 days.
3. Keep the chickens busy by hanging a pulled cabbage or other attractive material in such a position that the chickens have to jump up slightly to pick at it.
4. Cut off one-fourth to one-half of the upper beak, (Debeaking).
5. Avoid having too much light in the brooder house. Paint windows with an opaque, red poster paint when an outbreak occurs.
6. Feed brooders regularly. Mash should be in front of them at all times.
7. Provide good ventilation.
8. Cage the layers if possible.

Egg eating

This complaint usually originates with an egg being accidentally broken and the bird acquiring a taste for the contents, and later learning to break the egg herself. It may also be due to a desire for shell forming material lying around (Calcium, etc.) and therefore the following points may be of some use to control the vice :

1. Ample oyster shell or limestone grit should always be available.

2. Sufficient resting room should be provided, so that eggs are not accidentally broken.

3. Cut off one-fourth to one-half of upper beak with a sharp knife. The bird will not injure herself when she pecks at a hard substance, and the desire for egg-shell will be overcome by the time the beak has grown again. Until that time she should be given soft food.

Toe pecking

Toe pecking is more likely to occur with incubator chicks reared extensively. Yellow-legged chickens running in chopped straw sometime get a toe pecked by mistake, and blood is drawn which immediately attracts the others as a result the birds may be without a toe soon.

Another cause of this complaint is running chicks in damp litter, from which they step in the dry mash-trough, and this accumulates into a ball on the toe. The ball becomes so hard that when it is removed, frequently the nail is pulled off and blood comes out.

For such cases, the toe should be dipped in boric and zinc powder to stop the bleeding and before the chick is returned to the others the foot should be dipped in creosote, which not only acts as a disinfectant, but is unpalatable to them.

GRADING OF EGGS

Grading is the sorting out of eggs into different categories according to the interior quality and the individual weight of an egg. The practice brings more profit for the salesmen. This is due to the fact that eggs, which are cracked or of slightly lower grade if sent to distant markets most, if not all, of them will turn out to be a complete loss, but could probably fetch a concessional rate if sold locally. This additional income is further supplemented with the savings made in the packing and transport charges on such eggs. The consumers are also interested to know the quality of the products before paying.

Based on the quality of eggs, two grades Table 61 and according to size, four classes Table 62 have been adopted. Grading for internal quality is done by candling while for noting the weight of an individual egg there are various types of automatic devices in the market. The Agricultural Produce (Grading and Marking eggs) Rules, 1937, require that the mark on each egg shall consist of the word 'AGMARK' together with the grade designation placed centrally in a circle of not less than ½ inch diameter by means of a rubber stamp.

Table 61 Agmark standards for market table eggs

Grade	Weight (g)	Shell	Air cell	White	Yolk
A-Extra large	60 and above	Clean, unbroken and sound, shape normal.	Up to 4 mm in depth practically regular or better.	Clear, reasonably firm.	Fairly well centred, practically free from defects, outline indistinct.
A-Large	53-59				
A-Medmm	45-52				
A-Small	38-44				
B-Extra large	60 and above	Clean to moderately stained, sound and slightly abnormal.	8 mm in depth, may be free and slightly bubbly.	Clear, may be slightly weak.	May be slightly off-centered, outline slightly visible
B-large	53-59				
B-Medium	45-52				
B-Small	38-44				

Table 62 Standards For Weight Classification of Shell Eggs

S. No.	Size	Weight per egg (gms)	Weight per dozen eggs (gms)
(i)	Extra large	60 and above	715 and above
(ii)	Large	53 to 59	631 to 714
(iii)	Medium	45 to 52	535 to 630
(iv)	Small	38 to 44	456 to 534

A MODEL SCHEME FOR A LAYER OF 500 POULTRY BIRDS

(Price quoted are to be changed according to current market rate)

I. Fixed Capital

A. Building

i. Pucca Poultry house to accommodate 500 poultry birds @ 2.5 sq.ft. per bird with Aspholin (corrugated light roofing material) and pucca flooring @ Rs. 200.00 per sq.ft. (Total area 1250 sq.ft.)
(This house may be divided into four equal quarters. The chicks can be reared in a separate quarter of the layer house without additional investment for brooder house) — Rs. 2,50,000.00

ii. Store Room: 8 × 10 sq.ft. @ Rs.200.00 per sq.ft. — Rs. 16,000.00

iii. Electrical fittings and provision for supplying water — 20,000.00

Total (A) = Rs. 2,86,000.00

B. *Equipments*

i. Chick Brooder 6 Nos. at the rate of Rs.3000.00 each	Rs.	18,000.00
ii. Cost of equipments: feeder, waterer, laying nest etc.	Rs.	20,000.00
iii. Miscellaneous	Rs.	10,000.00

Total (B) = Rs.	**48,000.00**
Total Investment A + B = Rs.	**3,34,000.00**

II. Working Capital

For day old to 8 weeks old

a. Day old chicks 550 Nos. at the rate of Rs. 22.00 each (sexed)	Rs.	12,100.00
b. Feed consumption at the rate of 2 kg/bird at the rate of Rs. 2600.00 per quintal (Assuming 4% mortality, the present number of birds are 528), Total feed requirements : 10.56 qtl.	Rs.	27,456.00
c. Labour, electricity and medicine at the rate of Rs.20.00 per bird	Rs.	10,560.00
Total = Rs.	**50,116.00**

For growers 8-20 weeks old

a. Feed consumption at the rate of 7 kg/bird for 500 birds assuming 5% mortality @ Rs.2200.00 per quintal (Feed consumed 35 quintals)	Rs.	77,000.00
b. Labour: (Small flock at this stage can be taken care of by the farmer/his family members)	Rs.	-
c. Replacement of litter	Rs.	5,000.00
Total = Rs.	**82,000.00**

For layers from 20-72 weeks (end of laying stage)

a. Assuming 10% mortality and 10% cull, the present number stands to 400, Feed consumption at the rate of 40 kg/bird at the rate of Rs. 2500.00 per quintal. Total feed requirement = 16 qtl.	Rs.	40,000.00
b. Labour charges: 1 labour for 13 months at the rate of Rs. 5000.00 per month	Rs.	65,000.00
Total = Rs.	**1,05,000.00**

Total operating cost for 18 months = Rs. 2,37,116.00

Total costs:

1. Total operating cost	Rs.	2,37,116.00
2. Depreciation on building i.e., poultry house at the rate of Rs. 10% p.a. for 1½ years on Rs. 2,86,000.00	Rs.	42,900.00
3. Depreciation on equipments at the rate of Rs.10% p.a. for 1½ years on Rs. 48,000.00	Rs.	7,200.00
4. Interest on Capital @ 10% of Rs. 2,86,000.00	Rs.	28,600.00
5. Insurance of birds @ Rs.1.00 per bird	Rs.	500.00
Total = Rs.	**3,16,316.00**

Total Income of Receipt:

(i) Sale of 1,20,000 eggs at the rate of Rs.3.10 (Average production 300 eggs/bird)   Rs.   3,72,000.00

(ii) By sale of culls, 10% during laying stage i.e., for 40 birds @ Rs. 60.00   Rs.   2,400.00

(iii) By liquidating the flock at the end of first laying year. Number of birds 360 @ Rs.60.00 per bird (average)   Rs.   21,600.00

(iv) Income from manure assuming 18.20 kg/bird, say 10 tonnes at the rate of Rs.500.00 per tonne   Rs.   5,000.00

Total = Rs.   4,01,000.00

Summary of Accounts:

1. Total gross income   Rs.   4,01,000.00
2. Total costs involved   Rs.   3,16,316.00
3. Net Income from 500 layers   (Rs. 84,684.00 or say) Rs.   84,700.00
4. **Net Income per month**   **Rs.   4,705.00**

1. The Estimates for cost and returns given are only approximate and subject to variation from place to place and time to time.
2. If the poultry raiser takes loan from banks, he will be required to pay interest and/or a part of the capital loan after 7-8 months from the purchase of day old chicks out of his net profit,
3. It is profitable to run side by side one unit each of 1,000 layers and 1,000 broilers under the supervision of one labour only (Since one person can easily take care of 2,000 adult birds)

A MODEL SCHEME FOR A COMMERCIAL FARM OF 500 BORILERS

(Price quoted are to be changed according to current market rate)

A. Non-recurring expenditure:

1. Broiler house construction, assuming 1 sft. Per bird @ Rs. 200.00 per sft. (including water and electricity supply) total cost for 500 sft.   Rs.   1,00,000.00

2. *Equipments*:

(a) Brooders 2 nos. @ Rs. 3000.00 each   Rs.   6,000.00

(b) Chick size waterer and feeders   Rs.   1,000.00

(c) Hanging feeders (tub feeders) 20 numbers @ Rs.100.00 each   Rs.   2,000.00

(d) Waterer (linear, automatic) 3 nos. @ Rs. 250.00 each   Rs.   750.00

Total equipment = Rs.   9,750.00

B. Recurring expenditure

1. Cost of broiler chicks 500 broilers @ Rs. 25.00 each	Rs.	12,500.00
2. Feed cost to 6 weeks of age calculated at 3.4 kg per bird. Total feed consumed 1700 kg i.e. 17 qtl @ Rs.3000.00 per quintal. Cost of feed Rs. 51,000.00	Rs.	51,000.00
3. Medication and vaccination cost calculated @ Rs. 5.00 per bird	Rs.	2,500.00
4. Labour cost (For this small flock, for short period, care can be taken by the farmer/his family members)	Rs.	-
5. Misc. costs i.e. electricity, water, litter etc. from start to finish	Rs.	2,000.00
Total recurring expenditure = Rs.		**68,000.00**

C. Total costs:

1. Recurring Expenditure	Rs.	68,000.00
2. Depreciation on poultry house @ 10% per year (assuming 6 crops of broilers per year) depreciation per crop of broiler 1.67% on Rs. 1,00,000.00	Rs.	1,700.00
3. Depreciation on equipment @ 20% per year i.e. 3.34% per crop of broilers on Rs.9,750.00	Rs.	340.00
4. Insurance of birds @ Rs. 1.00 per bird	Rs.	500.00
Total costs = Rs.		**70,540.00**

D. Income of Receipts:

1. Sale of 500 broilers (assuming 2% extra chicks and 2% mortality to market time at 6 weeks of age) at an average live weight of 2.0 kg per bird. Total 1000 kgs @ Rs. 82.00 per kg live weight	Rs.	82,000.00
2. Sale of manure assuming 5 kgs per bird i.e. for 2500 kg/2.5 tonnes @ Rs.500.00 per tone	Rs.	1,250.00
Total gross income = Rs.		**83,250.00**

E. Summary of Accounts

Total gross income		Rs.	**83,250.00**
Total cost involved		Rs.	**70,540.00**
Net income per crop of 500 broilers	(Rs. 12,710.00 or say)	**Rs.**	**12,700.00**

Note:
1. If 6 crops of broilers are raised per year, then net income would be Rs.76,200.00 yearly or **Rs. 6,350.00** monthly
2. The profit may, however, vary depending largely upon the rate of weight grain, cost of feed and the price at which broilers are sold.
3. Broiler business is one of the quickest in returning investments, but continuously raising young stocks, calls for good experience.
4. If the farmer takes loan from bank, then he will have to pay the interest as per rate and that is to be added along with total costs.

POULTRY INSURANCE

Poultry (Chicken) farming has now been identified as a subsidiary occupation which has a vast scope for assured economic benefits and enhanced employment opportunities for the rural poor. Banks and other project authorities are now regularly financing small and marginal farmers in villages. Keeping this in view, the scheme of poultry insurance has been first introduced in this country for the poultry farmers by the General Insurance Corporation of India (GIC). The main objective of this poultry insurance is to give financial security to investors of poultry. At the present moment, insurance of poultry birds is on a very modest scale but all efforts are being made to expand and meet the growing insurance needs of poultry industry and now it covers the followings:

(i) Comprehensive cover for poultry farms
(ii) Epidemic poultry insurance through hatchery
(iii) Poultry insurance scheme for parent stock through hatcheries.

The main problem faced by insurers in selling poultry insurance is to collect premium at rates which are considered economic by poultry owners and would be adequate: (a) to meet losses that can be catastrophic at times; and (b) to take care of the element of hazard, since it is not possible to identify each bird separately in a fool proof manner and at an economic cost. The real financial and actuarial implications of poultry insurance can be known only through schemes, which are large enough to obtain representative experiences of the whole industry and at the same time small enough to keep the probable maximum loss within a certain prescribed limit.

In 1972, the insurance industry was nationalized. Some 126 companies were amalgamated into four to function under the direction of GIC. Which are: National Insurance Co. Ltd., New India Insurance Co. Ltd.; Oriental Insurance Co. Ltd.; and United India Insurance Co. Ltd.

I. Comprehensive cover for poultry farmers

1. **Scope of the agreement:** The agreement shall be observed by the constituent companies with regard to the rates, terms and conditions prescribed by this agreement to underwrite the poultry insurance business in India. The word "poultry" for this purpose refers to (a) layer birds, (b) broilers, (c) hatchery birds (breeding stock). Indigenous and non-descript birds will not be insured.

Note: (i) Exotic birds means whose parents are of foreign breed. This includes birds born in India as well as those born abroad.

(ii) A crossbred bird for the insurance purpose means, one of whose parents is of foreign breed.

2. **Applicability**

(a) The scheme is applicable to poultry farms consisting of all types of exotic and crossbred poultry birds in India.

(b) Since all the birds in a farm are covered, there is no need for identification. After issuing policy, if additional birds are introduced on the farm, immediate notice would be given to the insurer, otherwise, the claim will be repudiated.

(c) The scheme is applicable to poultry farms consisting of minimum
   (i) 500 layer birds
   (ii) 100 broilers per batch
   (iii) 2000 breeding birds in hatchery

(d) The poultry farmer is expected to maintain all the relevant records like feed register, flock record on day to day basis, daily stock register, mortality, culling, vaccination, feed consumption, production, debeaking, incidence of diseases, sales and purchase.

3. Age group

Layers
 (i) 1 to 72 week
 (ii) 21 to 72 week
 (iii) 1 to 20 week

Broilers
 (i) 1 to 6 week
 (ii) 1 to 8 week

4. Premium rates

It varies from time to time. So, the recent rates are to be collected by contacting respective insurance companies. However, for ready reference, the prevailing rate as collected from United India Insurance Company Ltd., Kalyani Branch, West Bengal is given below:

Birds	Age group	Non-scheme	Scheme
Layers	1 day to 72 week	5.50 %	0.85 %
	21 day to 72 week	3.50 %	0.85 %
	1 day to 20 week	3.20 %	0.85 %
Broilers	1 day to 6 week	1.20 %	0.25 %
	1 day to 8 week	1.50 %	0.25 %

* For all non-scheme groups 12.36% service tax is to be given and for scheme groups no service tax is required.

5. Valuation

In order to overcome the regional differences in input etc. cost, a multiplier formula is worked out to be applied to the prevailing feed cost and day old-chick cost should be added to arrive at week-wise valuation. Certain common and standard exclusions applied.

6. Insurance coverage

Standard policy wordings for poultry insurance are used by all insurance companies. The policy shall provide indemnity against death of birds due to accident including fire, lightning, flood, cyclone, famine, strike, riot and civil commotion or disease contracted or occurring during the period of insurance subject to the following exclusions:

194

(a) Malicious / willful injury, neglect
(b) Transit by any mode of transport
(c) Improper management (including overcrowding)
(d) Undergrowth, cannibalism, actions of predators like preying birds and carnivorous animals.
(e) Theft and clandestine sale of birds.
(f) Intentional slaughter of the birds except in cases where destruction is necessary to terminate incurable suffering on humane consideration on the basis of certificate issued by qualified veterinary surgeon or in cases where destruction is resorted to by order of lawfully constituted authority.
(g) Consequential loss however caused.
(h) Permanent and partial disablement of any nature.
(i) Loss of production.
(j) (i) Marek's disease, Ranikhet disease, Fowl pox and infectious Bronchitis. These diseases are covered by the policy if the birds are successfully inoculated against these diseases and the necessary veterinary certificates to that effect are supplied to the company. Coccidiosis and other diseases are covered only if preventive and curative measures are taken from time to time.
  (ii) Malnutrition
  (iii) Undergrowth
  (iv) Cannibalism
  (v) Loss due to hudding and / or pilling of birds.
  (vi) Avian Leucosis complex (A.L.C.)
(k) Salmonellosis covered subject to submission of clean certificate from competent Government Authorities immediately after testing.
(l) War, invasion, act of foreign enemy hostilities (whether war be declared or not), civil war, rebellion, revolution, insurrection, mutiny military or usurped power or any consequences thereof or attempt thereat.
(m) Accident of loss, destruction, damage or legal liability directly or indirectly caused by or contributed to by or arising from nuclear weapons.

7. **Veterinary Examination**
   (a) A veterinary certificate from a qualified veterinarian showing the following details is necessary for acceptance of risk.
     (i) Type of birds
     (ii) Age of birds
     (iii) Details regarding housing, lighting, ventilation, temperature, insulation, floor, feeds, water, sanitation etc.
     (iv) Vaccination and inoculation particulars
     (v) Debeaking
     (vi) Condition of health
     (vii) Type and source of feed
     (viii) Details of equipments
     (ix) Details of management / staff

      (x) Veterinary assistance
     (xi) Mortality rate with reasons for last 2 or 3 years
- (b) The insurer reserves the right to maintain his own check depute any representative for the purpose thereof.
- (c) Veterinary health examination fees should be borne by the Insurer.

8. Identification

- (a) All the birds would be covered on flock basis. No identification is necessary.
- (b) Insured must maintain at his own cost lot-wise records to show interalia (i) mortality, (ii) culling, (iii) feed consumption, (iv) incidence of diseases, (v) vaccination and medication, (vi) purchase and sales, (vii) daily Stock Register.

9. Important Policy Condition

- (a) The poultry farm should have veterinary facility.
- (b) The cages, if used must be maintained properly.
- (c) Proper house keeping
- (d) In the event of any outbreak, all healthy birds should be segregated and all precautions should be taken to arrest the spreading of the disease under advice to the insurance company immediately.
- (e) Proper balanced standard feed and clean water should be supplied to birds.
- (f) Proper flock record should be maintained on day to day basis.
- (g) Transfer of interest / ownership is not allowed.
- (h) In case of death / outbreak of epidemic, immediate notice within twelve hours should be given to the company. All birds should be segregated and produced to the representative of the company or to any person authorized by the company.
- (i) Debeaking and deworming should be carried out regularly and record to that effect should be maintained.

10. Blanket Policies

Blanket policies would be issued, subject to weekly declaration in the event of claim in favour of clients who maintain regular records to each unit / lot by which group of birds could be identified and in which all illness suffered, treatment provided and vaccinations carried out are recorded in the normal course of business. Additional premium at an agreed rate will be charged on prorata basis on receipt of declaration for the new stock, subject to veterinarian's certificate.

11. Procedure for claim settlement

- (a) **admissibility of the claim:** Claim under the policy would be admissible only if the mortality in the flock exceeds beyond the limits given below:

Types	Weeks	Mortality
Broilers	1 day old to 6 or 8 week	5% of the population in each lot
Layers	1 day old to 8 week	5% of the population in each lot
	9 to 72 week	3% of the population in each lot

Compensation towards loss of the birds will be made only for death of birds exceeding the mortality percentage given above.

(b) **Liability of the company:** The insured will be indemnified for 100% of the value of the bird at the time of death as per valuation table maintained by the insured company.

12. Claim procedure

In the event of death of birds immediate intimation should be given to the company and the insurer should be supplied with the following documents and required information.

(a) Duly completed claim form

(b) Death certificate from a veterinarian in the company's prescribed form

(c) Post-mortem report if required by the company.

13. Housing and equipments

A separate fire policy may be considered to grant cover for housing and equipments subject to the provision of fire tariff.

14. Companies may engage an independent veterinary surgeon or another investigator in special circumstances.

II. Epidemic poultry insurance scheme through hatchery

This scheme covers one day old chick supplied by hatcheries to commercial farms in India.

1. Applicability and age group

(a) An agreement will be entered into with the hatchery and insurance cover will be applicable to day old chicks from the hatchery itself for birds supplied to commercial farms.

(b) Insurance cover will commence from the time of despatch and will remain in operation for a period of 6/8 weeks in case of broilers and 72 weeks in case of layers.

2. Premium rate

It varies from time to time. So, it is advisable to collect the recent rates from the respective companies.

3. Insurance coverage

The policy shall provide indemnity to the extent of 80% of assessed amount to claim against death of birds during transit and at commercial farm to which the birds have been supplied. Epidemic diseases are excluded.

4. Claim settlement and procedure

(a) **Natural claim:** The claim will be settled with hatcheries and / or poultry farm depending upon the insurable interest at the time of loss.

(b) For admissibility of claim for catastrophic diseases, minimum 10% morality to any one or all the diseases specified in a period of 15 days is necessary.

(c) Losses at farm will be settled with the farmers directly. Farmers must report losses to the insurance company immediately within 48 hours of the outbreak of the disease.

(d) Hatchery doctors should check the farm whenever they visit in routine for appropriate management practices and submit their report to the hatchery with one copy to the farmer in the prescribed format.

(e) For settlement of claims, certification from the field veterinary doctor or hatchery doctor be made.

(f) Diagnostic material should be sent to any laboratory for confirmation of the disease. In case of mass mortality, the remaining birds should be sold after getting permission from company and the amount thus realized should be deducted from the claim amount.

III. Poultry insurance scheme for parent stock through hatcheries

The word parent stock for the purpose of this agreement refers to (a) Grand parent stock, (b) Parent stock, (c) Pure line stock which are exotic. Indigenous and non-descript birds will not be insured.

(1) *Age group:* 1 day to 72 weeks

(2) *Premium rate:* It varies from time to time. Current rates in vogue should be collected from respective companies.

(3) *Insurance coverage:* The policy shall provide indemnity against death of birds at the hatchery due to: (i) Fire, lightning, flood, cyclone, strike, riot and civil commotion, earthquake, storm, tempest, etc. (ii) Two epidemic diseases viz. Ranikhet and Gumboro.

(4) *Claim settlement and procedure:*
(a) In the event of death of birds immediate intimation should be given to the company and claim filed on the prescribed format.

(b) For admissibility of claim for catastrophic diseases, minimum 10% mortality due to any one or all the diseases specified in a period of 15 days is necessary. The claims with mortality less than 10% will not be admissible under the terms of the policy for any one incidence.

(c) In case of alarming death / outbreak of epidemic nature, immediate notice within 24 hours should be given to the company and all birds should be segregated and produced to the representative of the company for inspection to their very survival. Secondly, natural catastrophes such as floods and cyclones cause widespread destruction and therefore, insurance protection becomes essential. It is also necessary to augment income generation for poor families and protect their livelihood.

In conclusion, it may be mentioned that GIC is making continuous improvement in their existing policies to improve them still further with appropriate safeguards so that it becomes more attractive, simple and useful to marginal farmers and landless labourers. Towards, this end, various schemes are being regularly revised and new one being introduced. So, one should approach to concerned companies for the existing schemes at the time of insurance.

Poultry (Epidemic Disease) Insurance

This scheme is offered to a laying farm having a minimum flock strength of 10,000 birds and is not applicable to broilers. For hatchery birds, minimum flock strength must not be less than 1000 birds.

This cover is restricted to the following three epidemics only.

(i) Raniket, (ii) Fowl pox, (iii) Gumboro

For this scheme, minimum two epidemic diseases will have to be opted for and vaccination certificate from qualified veterinary surgeon or from the hatcheries (from where the birds have been purchased) is essential. For this purpose, if there is any cost that should be borne by the proposer. Before assumption of risk, a compulsory inspection of the risk by company's veterinary surgeon is generally suggested.

Age   :   8 to 72 weeks

Valuation :   As per market agreement of poultry insurance scheme

Premium   :   Should have to be collected from the insurance company

Claims are admissible only due to death of birds for the epidemic disease(s) as covered under the policy. To establish the outbreak of epidemic, a notice of death of at least 50 birds within 24 hours in case of hatcheries and 100 birds in case of commercial farms is necessary. Indemnity would be restricted to 90% of claim amount. For calculating indemnity, the number of birds died during 96 hours commencing from the time of outbreak of disease will be considered.

Duck Insurance

This scheme is applicable to farmers having 100 or more number of ducks. Pure graded or indigenous varieties of both migrating and non-migrating stocks can be covered if bank finance is involved. Otherwise the scheme is applicable only to non-migrating stock. The place of the migration of the bird, if any, should be intimated to the company by the financing bank regularly.

All the ducks in a farm should have to be covered, no selection is allowed.

Age: This insurance is akin to poultry insurance except the age group which is as follows:

(i) Day old to 52 week of age
(ii) 53rd to 104th week of age
(iii) 105th to 120th week of age

Value: The valuation table indicating the value of ducks over the ages should be submitted to the company, duly certified by a qualified veterinarian. The indemnity in the event of a claim is limited to certain percentage (to be informed from the Insurance Company) of the value of the bird at the time of death as per valuation table submitted.

Identification: Leg band identification should have to be strictly followed.

Premium rates: It varies from time to time. So, it is advisable to collect the recent rates from the respective insurance companies.

Insurance coverage: Death of ducks due to accident or disease contracted during the period of insurance with the following exclusions.

(i) Surgical operations other than that required due to accident or disease occurring during the period of cover.
(ii) Improper management
(iii) Famine
(iv) Transit by air or sea from foreign country to India or vice versa and transit by sea in India.
(v) Culling
(vi) Under growth
(vii) Intentional slaughter of ducks
(viii) Death during act of vaccination
(ix) Permanent and partial disablement of any nature
(x) Theft, clandestine sale or missing of the bird
(xi) Duck virus, Hepatitis, duck plague - If (a) vaccinations are done in proper time and (b) proper vaccination certificate(s) are produced to that effect, the risk is covered.
(xii) Helminthiasim – If proper deworming is done and suitable veterinary certificate to that effect is produced, the risk is covered.
(xiii) War, invasion, act of foreign enemy hostilities (whether war be declared or not) civil war, rebellion, revolution, insurrection, mutiny military or unsurped power or any consequences thereof or attempt threat.
(xiv) Accident, loss, destruction, damage or legal liability directly or indirectly caused by or contributed to by arising from nuclear weapons material.

Veterinary examination: Fee is payable depending on the number of ducks insured. If renewal is effected before the expiry date, no fresh veterinary certificate is required. The certificate should contain the type, age and identification of the ducks, vaccination, deworming and health of the birds besides the value of the duck at the time of insurance.

PROTECT POULTRY AGAINST COMMON DISEASES

Poultry keeping in the past was a hazard, because poultry keepers frequently sustained heavy loss due to some contagious diseases. Such calamities practically swept away the stock in a day's time and the poultry keepers were mere onlookers to these catastrophes. But, now-a-days, due to advancement of science and evolvement of new medicines and vaccines, schenario has been changed. Some of the important common diseases are discussed below:

(a) Ranikhet Disease (RD)
Also known as Newcastle disease-caused by virus. This is infectious, contagious and highly fatal disease and affects birds of all ages. It is transmitted directly from bird to bird through nasal or mouth discharges by air or by contaminated feed and litter.

Symptoms

(i) **In Chicks:** Coughing and rattling, gasping, trembling, lack of co-ordination, partial or complete paralysis of extremities, muscular tremor, abnormal movements, mortality rate is very high.

(ii) **In adults:** Respiratory problem, impaired appetite, nervous, sudden drop in egg production, soft shelled eggs and of poor quality, head may be twisted to the side, drawn back or down between the legs, chalky white diarrhoea and sometimes greenish diarrhoea.

Prevention

1. Ranikhet disease – F_1 strain or LASOTA strain for 5 to 7 days old chick.
2. Repeat F_1 vaccine at 5 to 8 weeks of age
3. Mukteshwar strain (R_2B) vaccine at the age of 9-10 weeks
4. A booster dose at 16 to 18 weeks.

Treatment

Not known. Minimize secondary complications by stimulating appetite with wet mashes, high level of antibiotic and vitamin mixture in drinking water.

(b) Fowl pox

Comparatively slow-spreading infection of chicken caused by a pox virus. Highly contagious and spreads by way of air, saliva, nasal washings, feather follicles and dropping of infected birds.

Symptoms

Pox lesions on comb, wattles, legs, loss of appetite, discharge from nostrils and accumulation of foamy material in the corner of the eyes; drop in egg production.

Prevention

To be vaccinated with fowl pox vaccine as per schedule.

Treatment

Treatment is not known but attempts should be made to stimulate appetite with wet mash and addition of antibiotic-vitamin mixture to drinking water. Using of good disinfectants during outbreak is beneficial.

(c) Marek's Disease

It is caused by herpes virus (MDV), it affects the nervous system, various visceral organs, eyes, skin and muscles.

Symptoms

Most of the affected birds will have some degree of paralysis; although chickens in acute form may not show this condition. As the paralysed birds are unable to reach feed and water they may die. Acute form generally affects younger age group (6-8 weeks); usually sudden death with high mortality. In mature birds, bilateral or unilateral paralysis of legs, wings or neck, marked loss of weight, difficult breathing, diarrhoea etc. may occur.

Prevention

Vaccination at day-old age protects birds through life time.

Treatment

Not known. Good sanitation and hygiene is essential to keep the mortality low.

(d) Gumboro Disease

It is also known as Infectious Bursal Disease (IBD) caused by IBD virus. It is highly contagious, transmitted through contaminated litter, feed, utensils and by the droppings of affected bird.

Symptoms

In chicks, diarrhoea, depression, in coordination, sudden and high rate of morbidity upto 100%. In adults, whitish watery diarrhoea, soiled vent feathers, loss of appetite, unsteady gait, listlessness, less mortality.

Prevention

Vaccination should be done at 14-15th day and at 7-8th weeks.

Treatment

Not known

(e) Infectious Bronchitis (IB)

It is caused by numerous strains of IB virus.

Symptoms

In chicks: Sudden onset and rapid spread of symptoms; sneezing, hoarse coughing, gasping, nasal discharge, wet eyes. Mortality in young chicks may be as high as 25%. No nervous symptoms are noted as in Ranikhet disease.

In adults: Sudden onset and rapid spread of symptoms; gasping and coughing; nasal discharge not usually observed; drop in egg production (10 to 50 percent), soft shelled eggs, low albumen quality.

Prevention

Vaccination for prevention as per schedule.

Treatment

No specific treatment. Overcrowding, if any should be taken care of. Good management practices and other housing conditions for flock comfort may improve the condition.

(f) Bird's flue

The other names of this disease are Avian Influenza, Fowl Plague or Avian flue. This is a viral disease and was first diagonesed at Italy in the year of 1978. Among various sub-types of this virus, under Orthomyxoviridoe H_5N_1 is particularly responsible for this bird flue in poultry. In India, it is first diagnosed in February 2006 and got special importance as it may contaminate human being also.

Symptoms

The affected birds will have watery discharges from nostrill and eyes, blackening of the comb, swelling of head and mouth region, drowsiness, loose faeces, anorexia and in extreme cases bleeding under skin and black patches on skin, sometimes moving in a circular way. Layers will stop laying, the respiratory tract may also be infected and a large number of birds may die at a time. The disease mainly spreads from the saliva, discharges from nostrils and eyes or faeces of the infected birds. Direct contact also helps in spreading the disease.

Treatment
Practically, there is no treatment for this disease as the Antivirus medicines like Seltamivir, Zanamivirar are costly and generally used for human being. So attempts should be taken to prevent spreading of the disease. No vaccine has yet been developed. The following control measures may be helpful.

  (i) Physical separation of healthy birds from ailing birds
  (ii) Minimizing the contact of poultry with feral and migratory birds
 (iii) Proper disposal of carcasses
 (iv) Creating a disease-free zone at international borders by de-population.
  (v) Banning importation of biologicals, reagents, livestock and their products from disease reporting countries and
 (vi) Periodical screening of poultry for maintaining the disease-free status.

(g) Infectious coryza
It is a bacterial disease caused by *Haemophilus gallinarum* and affects birds under 6 weeks of age, morality upto 80%. It is transmitted through recovered birds as carrier, contaminated feed and water, free flying birds, due to inclement weather and hyper vitaminosis-A.

Symptoms
Sneezing, coughing, gasping, difficult breathing, discharge from eyes and nostrils, swollen facial tissues and wattles, drop in feed consumption and egg production.

Prevention
Vaccinate with killed vaccine, wherever, necessary.

Treatment
Use of high level (100 – 400 ppm) antibiotics in feed and water give effective results. Long acting antibiotic injections are also effective.

(h) *E. Coli* infections
It is caused by a bacterium *Escherichia coli* (*E. Coli*), transmitted through drinking water and litter and is responsible for a number of diseases.

Symptoms
Droopiness, ruffled plumage, diarrhoea, low feed consumption and loss in weight, swelling of joints, wattle and comb.

Prevention
Sanitation, good litter management and supply of clean and chlorinated drinking water.

Treatment

Use of antibiotics in drinking water are somewhat effective.

(i) Pulloram (Bacillary white diarrhoea - BWD)

It is caused by *Salmonella pullorum*, transmitted through egg, recovered birds act as carriers, also contaminated feed and water.

Symptoms

In chicks: Chicks after hatching die suddenly (20 to 80%), ruffled feathers, drooping of wings, hudding together, less appetite, laboured breathing, brownish diarrhoea etc.

In adults: Dull, depression, paleness of comb, greenish and brownish diarrhoea, ruffled feathers etc.

Prevention

Hatchery and flock sanitation is most important.

Treatment

Affected birds should be given furazolidone, sulphate drugs and antibiotics in mash or drinking water. Sulphate treatment appears to be more effective than antibiotic. Treatment measures can reduce mortality and help in reducing the spread of the disease.

(j) Chronic Respiratory Disease (CRD)

It is caused primarily by *Mycoplasma gallisepticum* but often mixed up with other infections like IB and E. coli etc. It is transmitted from bird to bird, through eggs, nasal discharge, droppings, through visitor's hands, feet and clothes.

Symptoms

Sniffing, rattling, sneezing, nasal discharge, swollen sinuses, swollen eyes and other signs of respiratory distress; low feed consumption and egg production.

Prevention

Periodic testing for *mycoplasma* infection and dipping of hatching eggs in effective antibiotic solution prior to incubation can be followed as preventive measures. Rearing of birds on an all-in-all-out system is also effective.

Treatment

Treatment with antibiotic like tetracycline, erythromycin in feed or water is helpful. Strict isolation of the flock helps to avoid introduction of the disease.

(k) Coccidiosis

It is a disease of the intestinal tract, caused by a parasitic protozoa of which 9 recognised species of coccidia are responsible for affecting poultry. *Eimeria tenella* – Causes bloody or caecal coccidiosis. *E. nectarix, E. acervulina, E. praecox, E. mitis, E. brunetti, E. maxima, E. hagani, E. mivati*, all of them cause intestinal coccidiosis.

Transmission is done through injestion of oocyst in feed or drinking water, droppings, contaminated manure, rodents, pests, wild birds and shoes of visitors.

Prevention

It is not possible to prevent some infection from coccidia, however, good sanitation and dry litter may help in reducing the occurrence of the disease. Use of coccidiostat through feed is a normal practice to control the disease.

Treatment

Use of drugs, such as Amprolium, Nicarbazin, Nitrofurazone, Sulfaquinoxaline, Sulphadiazine, Sulphamezathine, Sulphamerazine etc. in feed or drinking water is quite effective in treatment of affected birds.

Caution

Treatment should not be continued for a long period. Laying birds acquire immunity before going into egg production. If a bird develops immunity to one species, it can still have disease outbreak by other species.

(l) Parasites

A. External parasites: Mainly mites and lice. Symptoms are irritation, reduced feed intake and body weight, drop in egg production, anaemic. Dust and spray the affected bird with Pestoban (1:10 ratio), Cypermethrin, Sodium fluoride or Melathion to reduce infection.

B. Internal parasites: Generally are of the three types:

(i) Tape worms: Caused by *Rallietina echinobothrida*; *R. tetragona* and other tapeworms. Symptoms are reduced feed intake, loss of weight; emaciation; diarrhoea and drop in egg production.

(ii) Roundworms: Caused by *Ascaridia galli*. Symptoms are, loss of weight, drop in egg production, emaciation etc.

(iii) Caecal worms: Caused by *Heterakis gallinae*. Symptoms are caeca inflamed and thickened, weakness, anaemia etc. Regular deworming programme should be followed. Piperazine compounds, mebendazole, Albendazole etc. for treating roundworms and Discestal and phenothiazine for tapeworms.

HEAT PROSTRATION

At low temperature in hill stations birds require more energy. At high temperatures above 85°F there is a gradual drop in feed consumption and productivity which can become a very serious factor and extremely dangerous to the birds at temperatures over 100°F. The chart below details the effect of temperature on poultry.

Inside temperature °F	Results
70°–80°	No danger
80°–85°	Slight reduction in feed consumption. No danger.
85°–90°	More drop in feed consumption.

90°–95°	Greatly reduced feed consumption. Heat prostration possible among layers.
95°–100°	Heat prostration likely.
100°	Extreme danger.

AUTOPSY FINDINGS

(Appearance after Death)

Appearance	Disease indicated
Bronze or greenish liver	Fowl typhoid
Bloody or cheesy plugs in caeca	Coccidiosis
Cheesy patches in mouth and throat	Fowl pox, Nutritional (Vitamin A deficiency).
Enlarged liver	Fowl cholera Fowl typhoid
Fissures or holes in gizzard lining	Gizzard erosion
Intestinal walls thickened	Worms Coccidiosis
Inflammation and thickening of peritoneum	Peritonitis
Nodule in gullet	Vitamin A deficiency
Plugging of air passage	Bronchitis, Fowl pox Infectious coryza
Small grey or yellow lesions on liver	Fowl typhoid.
Unabsorbed egg yolk	Improper brooding Pullorum disease
Worms in wind pipe	Tape worm

MINIMIZATION OF DISEASE INFECTION

With the present day system of high density rearing of poultry for increasing margin of profit per unit floor area, and high concentration of birds within a limited space, disease problems have assumed an alarming dimension. Outbreak of any disease impairs body function and adversely affect the growth, productivity and income from poultry farming.

So, most of the poultry farmers compromise with vaccination, but it cannot be a substitute for good management including sanitation and bio-security. Vaccination may protect the bird against a specific disease, but lack of bio-security, poor sanitation or faulty management can expose the birds to various health problems.

Cross infection from other stock may be due to ignorance and carelessness. Faulty hatchery management and poor flock sanitation may lead to egg-borne diseases like pullorum and fowl typhoid. Faulty brooding may predispose the chicks to brooder house pneumonia and increase chick mortality. Damp litter may be the cause of coccidiosis, aspergillosis and several other diseases. Poor ventilation in a poultry house may increase the concentration of toxic gases and help spread respiratory infections such as CRD, infectious bronchitis and infectious laryngotracheitis. Mouldy feed may cause mycotoxicosis or use of sub-standard diets may result in nutritional diseases. These examples indicate the importance of management and application of bio-security in the control of poultry diseases.

Good management can reduce disease infection. In most of the poultry farms disease problems arise due to:

(i) Infected stock brought in from outside
(ii) Contamination of hatchery, feed, equipment and premises
(iii) Cross infection from other stock due to poor sanitation, faulty management and lack of bio-security.

The fact that needs to be borne in mind is "a well hatched chick is half reared". On the other hand, even disease - free stock procured from a reputed hatchery can be infected subsequently due to lapses in management. Physical stresses like overcrowding, chilling, overheating, water deprivation, can lower the resistance of birds and make them prone to diseases. Clinical salmonellosis in chicks exposed to chilly environment is one such example.

A few management practices if properly followed may minimize the disease occurrence.

(i) **Segregation:** Sick birds must be separated from healthy stock. They should be separated and kept in isolation.

(ii) **Depopulation:** Birds even after recovering from diseases harbor disease-causing organisms and spread diseases through droppings, discharges etc. Disinfection of poultry houses, equipments prevents carry over infection from previous flocks. Therefore, an all-in-all-out system is always preferred, if possible.

(iii) **Proper bird density:** Maintenance of proper bird density is essential as over crowding causes stress and predisposes the flock to diseases.

(iv) **Old litter and feed should not be used:** To avoid some of the diseases like coccidiosis and other health problems, old litter and feed should never be used.

(v) **Hygienic removal of dead birds:** Dead birds should be removed as early as possible preferably by incineration and burying deeply with a thick layer of lime and away from the farm site to prevent spreading of diseases.

(vi) **Sanitation and disinfection:** Equipments, footwear etc. act carriers of infection. Thorough cleaning with proper disinfectant of the farm area and equipments used are essential for creating a disease free environment. Entry of visitors and vehicles should be restricted. Phenol compounds, chlorine and formaldehyde are effective disinfectants. After disinfection, sometimes insecticides are also used for controlling insects, beetles and ectoparasites which sometimes acts as carriers of pathogens.

(vii) **Preventive vaccination and medication:** Important infectious diseases like Marek's, Ranikhet and fowl pox in chicken can be prevented by building immunity through a sound vaccination programme as per recommended schedule. Along with vaccination, routine deworming and medication are also essential to relieve stress.

(viii) **Other health problems:** Some problems like cannibalism, feather peaking, heat prostration or nutritional diseases which are of purely managemental or nutritional may arise though these are not transmissible but may increase the susceptibility of the birds. So attention should have to be given to such problems to minimize disease prevention.

(ix) **Litter management:** Birds are mostly reared under deep litter system of management but wet and mouldy litter might be the cause of spreading coccidiosis and aspergillus. Smell of ammonia inside the poultry house (in deep litter) is a sign of poor management. Litter should be kept dry, addition of hydrated lime (5 kg for 10 sq. meter floor space) once in a while can improve litter condition. Seepage of water from drinking channels should be guarded.

(x) **Separate rearing of different aged birds:** Birds of different age groups should be reared separately to prevent infections of many diseases and parasites.

Table 63 Recommended vaccination schedule for layers and broilers

Age	Vaccine	Administration
LAYERS		
1 day	MD#	Subcutaneous
5-7 days	RD (F Strain)	Intranasal / Intraocular
14-15 days	Gumboro Disease (IBD)	Oral drops or Drinking water
5-6 weeks	RD (F Strain / Lasota)	Oral drops or Drinking water
7-8 weeks	Gumboro disease (IBD)*	Drinking water
9-10 weeks	RD (R_2B Strain)	Subcutaneous / Intramuscular
13-14 weeks	Infectious Bronchitis (IB)*	Oral drops or Drinking water
15-16 weeks	Fowl Pox**	Intramuscular
16-18 weeks	RD (R_2B Strain)	Subcutaneous / Intramuscular
BROILERS		
1 day	MD#	Subcutaneous
5-7 days	RD (F Strain)	Intranasal / Intraocular
14-15 days	Gumboro Disease (IBD)	Oral drops or Drinking water
21-28 days	RD (F Strain)	Drinking water

Generally given at hatchery; * Only in outbreak-prone areas;** May be given early in case of outbreak

Important:

• This schedule is only a guide. There are numerous vaccination programmes and types of vaccines. Vaccines should be selected on the basis of area and local disease situation.

- The advice of the local veterinarian and the recommendations of the vaccine manufacturers must be followed.
- Simultaneous vaccination with RD and IB vaccines is not advisable as birds may fail to develop a good immunity to one or both these diseases. Vaccines used in combination may place too severe a stress on chicks, increasing losses.
- Vaccines used in combination may cause an unduly severe reaction and may prevent the development of immunity. Vaccination against fowl pox and either infectious bronchitis or RD at the same time is not advisable. A combination of RD wing-web and fowl pox vaccines is particularly risky and not advisable.
- Vaccines against fowl cholera and tick fever may be administered in adult birds in areas where these diseases are endemic.
- MD = Marek's Disease; RD = Ranikhet Disease; IBD = Infectious Bursal Disease - also known as Gumboro; IB = Infectious Bronchitis.

Fresh Eggs are perishable ~~ Watch the temperature

Normal temperature of the hen.

Correct Temperature for incubation.

Danger Range
Eggs deteriorate very rapidly
In quality between 70° and 100°

Fertile Eggs start germination at 60

Avoid holding eggs above 60°

Suitable temperature for keeping eggs at farm, store or home.

Most favorable cold storage temperatures 20° to 30°.
Eggs freeze at 28°.

Keep a good reliable thermometer in your cellar or egg storage room.

It may help you in detecting the loss of egg quality.

FAHRENHEIT

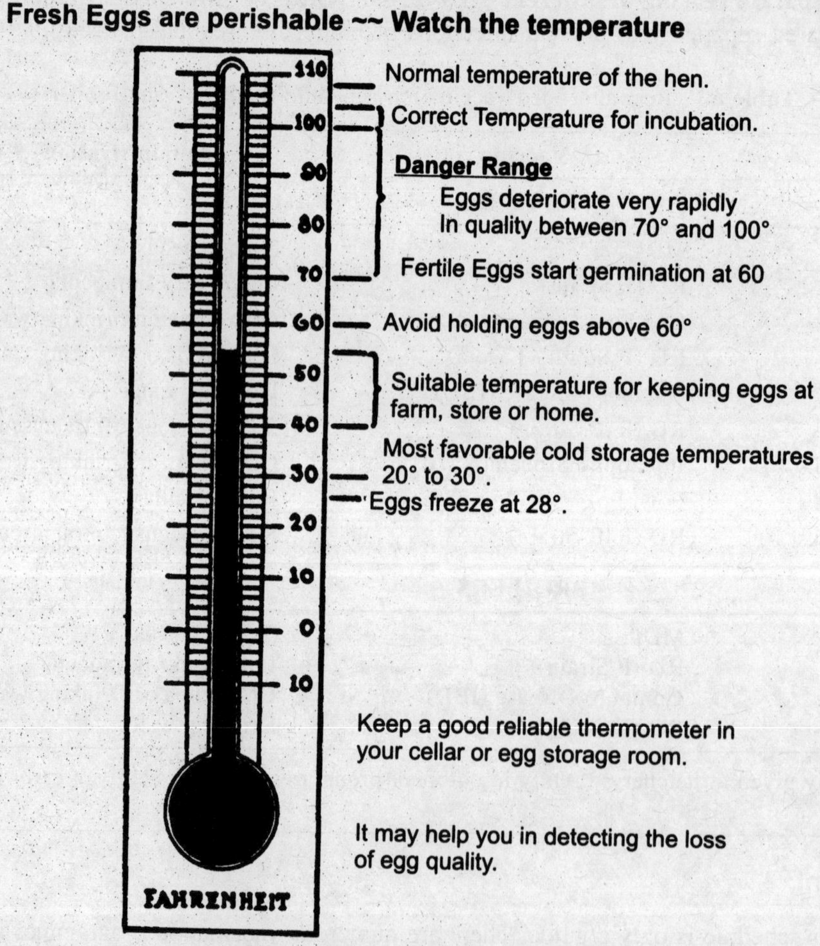

Figure 34 Egg and temperature

Table 64 Classes of Poultry

Bird-Class	Description
Chickens:	
• Rock Cornish game hen or Cornish game hen	A young, immature chicken (usually 5-7 weeks of age) weighing not more than 2 lb ready-to-cook weight, the progeny of a Cornish chicken or a Cornish chicken crossed with another breed of chicken
• Broiler or fryer	A young chicken (usually 6-8 weeks of age), of either sex, that is tender-meated with soft, pliable, smooth-textured skin and flexible breastbone cartilage
• Roaster	A young chicken (usually 3-5 months of age), of either sex, that is tender-meated with soft, pliable, smoothe-textured skin and breastbone cartilage that may be somewhat less flexible than that of a broiler or fryer
• Capon	A surgically unsexed male chicken (usually under 8 months of age) that is tender-meated with soft, pliable, smooth-textured skin
• Stag	A male chicken (usually under 10 months of age) with coarse skin, somewhat toughened and darkened flesh, and considerable hardening of the breastbone cartilage. Stags show a condition of fleshing and a degree of maturity intermediate between that of a roaster and a cock or rooster
• Hen or stewing chicken or fowl	A mature female chicken (usually more than 10 months of age) with meat less tender than that of a roaster, and nonflexible breastone tip
• Cock or rooster	A mature male chicken with coarse skin, toughened and darkened meat, and hardened breastbone tip
Turkeys:	
• Fryer-roaster turkey	A young, immature turkey (usually under 16 weeks of age), of either sex, that is tender-meated with soft, pliable, smooth-textured skin, and flexible breastbone cartilage
• Young hen turkey	A young female turkey (usually 5-7 months of age) that is tender-meated with soft, pliable, smooth-textured skin, and breastbone cartilage that is somewhat less flexible than in a fryer-roaster turkey
• Young tom turkey	A young male turkey (usually 5 7 months of age) that is tender-meated with soft, pliable, smooth-textured skin, and breastbone cartilage that is somewhat less flexible than in a fryer-roaster turkey
• Yearling hen turkey	A fully matured female turkey (usually under 15 months ot age) that is reasonably tender-meated and with reasonably smooth-textured skin
• Yearling tom turkey	A fully matured male turkey (usually under 15 months of age) that is reasonably tender-meated and with reasonably smooth-textured skin
• Mature turkey or old turkey (hen or tom)	An old turkey of either sex (usually in excess of 15 months of age) with coarse skin and toughened flesh

Table 64   (Continued)

Bird-Class	Description
Ducks:	
• Broiler duckling or fryer duckling	A young duck (usually under 8 weeks of age), of either sex, that is tendermeated and has a soft bill and soft windpipe
• Roaster duckling	A young duck (usually under 16 weeks of age), of either sex, that is tendermeated and has a bill that is not completely hardened and a windpipe that is easily dented
• Mature duck or old duck	A duck (usually over 6 months of age), of either sex, with toughened flesh, hardened bill, and hardened windpipe
Geese:	
• Young goose	Can be of either sex, is tender meated, and has a windpipe that is easily dented
• Mature goose or old goose	Can be of either sex, has toughened flesh, and hardened windpipe
Guineas:	
• Young guinea	Can be of either sex, is tender-meated, and has a flexible breastbone cartilage
• Mature guinea or old guinea	Can be of either sex, has toughened flesh, and a hardened breastbone
Pigeons:	
• Squab	Young, immature pigeon of either sex, and is extra tender-meated
• Pigeon	Mature pigeon of either sex, with coarse skin and toughened flesh

REARING OF LOW INPUT TECHNOLOGY BIRDS

Recently, two synthetic varieties have been developed by the Project Directorate on Poultry (PDP), Hyderabad under Indian Council of Agricultural Research (ICAR) for rearing in rural areas following back yard system of poultry rearing. Rearing of those birds are profitable in compare to deshi birds. As deshi birds are low producers and the size of the eggs are also quite small. On the other hand, rearing of the birds developed recently by project Directorate on Poultry, Hyderabad, India namely Vanaraja - a meat and egg type coloured bird (i.e. dual purpose) and Gramapriya - an egg producer are quite profitable. Characteristics of these birds are discussed below:

Vanaraja

In urban areas the per capita consumption of egg and chicken meat is ranged between 80-120 eggs and 2.25 – 3.50 kg, respectively against 5-20 eggs and 750 gm in rural areas. Further, these poultry products are expensive (10-40%) in rural tribal areas due to their non-availability. The backyards in rural/tribal areas are rich with "Natural food base" (fallen grains, insects, earthworms, kitchen waste, green grass etc.). These waste food materials can successfully be utilized by converting them into nutritionally balanced and delicious egg and chicken meat by adapting the rural poultry farming which can alleviate the protein hunger.

With these idea, a dual-purpose chicken variety i.e. Vanaraja has been developed which gives eggs and meat based on rearing and feeding practices. The main features of this bird are: (i) attractive-multi colour feather pattern, (ii) high general immune competence, (iii) low plane of nutrition, (iv) grow faster and lay more eggs than deshi hens and (v) colour of egg is brown like deshi hen.

In areas, where plants of natural feed resources are available, a small number of birds (10-20) can be reared for egg purpose under free-range conditions. If the local demand is for meat, they can be reared in large numbers under intensive / semi-intensive conditions by providing all inputs similar to commercial broilers. Typically, Vanaraja need to be reared under nursery upto 6 weeks and let them loose in open free range after 6 weeks of age.

I. Management under Nursery

Brooding is essential for these birds immediately after hatch to provide required temperature and protection from predators. Spread the newspaper on 2-3 inches litter in the brooder. Arrange the feeders and drinkers.

Brooding: Metal or wooden brooders can be used and generally electrical bulbs are used as source of heat. Heat source of 2 watts / chick is required. The movement of chicks can be restricted nearer the heat source with the help of chick guard. At higher temperature, birds will normally be away from the heat source.

Feeding: Under nursery management, balanced feed containing all nutrients, minerals and vitamins should have to be given. Feed should always be available to the birds. In nursery rearing, vanaraja chicks will require 2400 Kcal ME, 16% crude protein, 0.77% lysine, 0.36% methionine, 0.35% available phosphorus and 0.70% calcium. The diet may be prepared by locally available feed ingredients to minimize the feed cost but it must supply the above nutrients. Alternatively, commercial feeds may also be fed during initial 6 weeks of age.

Prevention against diseases: Vanaraja birds have better immune competence, but they need protection against Ranikhet disease and Fowl pox. Vaccination schedule as per Table 65 should be followed.

II. Management under Free Range

Under free range at 6 weeks of age, birds will generally attain 650-750 gm body weight (Table 66). These birds can be let out under backyard free-range conditions @ 10-20 birds/house depending on the areas and natural feed resources. During day hours the birds are let out foraging while at night they are kept in night shelter. The birds should be provided with clean drinking water before releasing in morning. After attaining the minimum body weight, the males can be sold at any time. Hens will lay upto 110 eggs per year under free range conditions.

Feeding: These birds under free range can easily pick up its feed from the backyards once it learns to scavenge in the fields. Requirement of extra feeds will depend on the free area available in the backyards. Normally, by scavenging the bird can meet up their protein requirement. Therefore, feeding the birds with cereals (bajra, ragi, jower, broken rice, rice polish, rice bran etc.) available is always helpful to get the production. The nature of extra feed depends on the purpose of rearing. For meat purpose, feeding the birds with commercial broiler/layer chick feed is suggested; for egg production, the birds will largely depend on feed available in free-range conditions. Care should be taken to restrict the weight of pullets (female) between 2.2 to 2.5 kg at 6.0 - 6.5 months of age. Excess body weight may hamper egg production. To minimize broken/thin shelled eggs supplementation of calcium is suggested (lime powder, shell grit, stone grit, etc. @ 3-4 gm/bird/day).

Disease prevention: Under free range system, the most important disease by which the birds are affected is Ranikhet disease, so vaccination is a must. Night shelter should have good ventilation, required light and protection from predators. Periodic cleaning of night shelter is necessary for controlling external parasites. To prevent internal parasitic infection, deworming at 2-3 months interval is required. Under free-range conditions, adult Vanaraja birds should be vaccinated against Ranikhet disease at 6 months interval preferably one should be before the onset of summer.

Table 65 Vaccination programme for Vanaraja and Gramapriya chicken

Age	Name of the Vaccine	Strain	Dose	Route
In the Hatchery:				
1st day	Marek's Disease	HVT	0.20 ml	SC injection
In the Nursery:				
5th day	Ranikhet Disease	Lasota	One drop	Eye drop
14th day	Infectious Bursal Disease	Georgia	One drop	Oral drop
21st day	Pox	Fowl pox	0.20 ml	IM/SC injection
28th day	Ranikhet Disease	Lasota	One drop	Eye drop
In the Field:				
9th week	Ranikhet*	R_2B	0.50 ml	SC injection
12th week	Pox*	Fowl pox	0.20 ml	SC injection

* Repeat these two vaccines at every 6 months interval

Table 66 Performance of Vanaraja and Gramapriya birds

	Vanaraja	Gramapriya
Body weight (g):		
Six weeks	650 – 750	400 – 500
At sexual maturity (restricted feeding)	2,000 – 2,200	1600 – 1800
Egg weight (gm):		
28 weeks	42 – 44	52 – 53
40 weeks	52 – 58	57 – 58
Age at first egg (days)	175 – 180	160 – 165
Egg production (number) upto 1½ years	100 – 110	200 – 230
Survivability % (upto 6 weeks)	**98**	**99**

Gramapriya

The average egg consumption in India is about 55 per person against 180 eggs required for a healthy human being. There is a great disparity in egg consumption among urban, semi urban and rural areas with lowest of 5 to 20 eggs in rural areas mainly due to non-availability of eggs. However, household backyards of rural/tribal regions are rich in natural feed base (fallen grains, insects, earthworms, kitchen waste, green grass etc.). These resources can be utilized by adopting backyard poultry farming by rearing chicken which lay more number of eggs.

For this purpose, Gramapriya, is best suited in rural areas which lay more number of eggs and have similarity with native chicken. These birds are highly resistance to diseases and can be reared upto 6 weeks of age in nurseries and then leaving in farmer's backyard for free range farming. The main features of this bird are: (i) multi colour feather pattern, (ii) moderate body weight, (iii) better egg production, (iv) produce brown shelled eggs.

I. Management under Nursery

Brooding is essential for Gramapriya during the initial 6 weeks of age, feeding and other management practices are similar to that of other layer chicks.

Brooding: Clean litter materials (chaffed paddy straw/saw dust/groundnut husk/paddy husk etc.) should be spread uniformly in the house at thickness of 2-3 inches. Spread the newspaper on the litter. The feeders and drinkers should be arranged alternatively. Heat source (electrical) of 2 watts/chick is adequate upto 4/6 weeks of age. At higher environmental temperatures, the birds will automatically move away from the heat source and if it is too cold, they will pile up nearer the heat source.

Feeding: Balanced feed fortified with required minerals, vitamins, antimicrobial and anticoccidial should be provided during the nursery period. Feed can be prepared using local feed ingredients (bajra, jowar, ragi, broken rice, maize, tapioca, sunflower cake, groundnut cake, sesame cake, maize gluten meal etc.) to achieve 2400 Kcal ME/kg, 18% CP, 0.85% lysine, 0.38% methionine, 0.70% calcium and 0.35% available phosphorus. Easy access to feed and clean drinking water should be assured.

Disease prevention

Protection against common diseases as provided in Table 65 should be followed. Providing anti-stress compound on the day of vaccination will ensure better immune response. For prevention of cannibalism, optimum level of trace minerals and salt (100 gm and 400 gm/100 kg of feed) should be provided.

II. Management under Free Range

Birds will attain 400 – 500 gm body weight (Table 66) at 6-7 weeks of age. These birds may be let loose under backyard free range conditions upto 10/20 birds/household depending on the area and natural feed base. During day time, the birds will be on foraging and at night they will be kept at night shelter. The birds should be provided with clean drinking water every day before releasing.

Feeding: The birds under these conditions can generally meet their protein requirement through scavenging but the possibility of energy deficiency is common. So, the birds are to be fed some cereals as available in the locality and this feeding should be done during evening. Care should be taken to restrict the weight of pullets between 1.6 to 1.8 kg at 6 to 6½ months of age (i.e. the age at sexual maturity). To minimize thin shelled eggs, supplementation of calcium is needed (lime powder / shell grit / stone grit etc.) @ 3-4 gm/bird/day. The males can be sold at any time after the desired weight or can be reared separately on balanced feed under intensive management for meat purpose.

Disease prevention: Repeat vaccinations against Ranikhet and Pox (Table 65) at 6 months intervals protect the birds from these diseases. Periodic deworming at 3-4 months intervals is essential for controlling internal parasites. Regular cleaning of night shelter with disinfectants is required to control external parasites.

DUCKS

In nature duck is a water bird. Man has domesticated the wild duck, and by selective breeding and removing it from its natural habitat, has produced strains which he uses for both meat and egg production.

The wild Mullard duck (*Anas boschas*) is the progenitor of all domestic duck with the exception ot the Muscovy which has been derived from the South American tree duck (*Cairina moschata*). The domesticated duck belongs to the genus *Anas* and species *platyrhynchos*.

Genetically duck belongs to the family *Anatidac*. As a class they are distinguished from other Anatidac by their small size, shorter neck, flatter body, shorter legs and broader bill. The male duck is known as drake while the female as duck. The young ones are known as ducklings.

Ducks must have been domesticated a long time since Romans referred to them as early as 2,000 years back. Also it is believed that commercial duck has been longer in China than in any other country. To-day among the leading duck producing countries of the world, Vietnam, Poland, Indonesia, Thailand, United States, Brazil, China, Bangladesh can be rated on decreasing order.

There are about 27.64 million ducks in India (18th Indian Livestock cemus 2007). Among the various states, West Bengal is having the highest duck population followed by Assam, Tamil Nadu, Kerala, Andhra Pradesh, Tripura, Jharkhand, Odisha, Mainpur and Bihar. However, they are also seen in all other states.

Duck constitutes about 10 per cent of the total poultry population, occupying second place to chicken in the production of table eggs in the country. Scientific duck raising was practically nonexistent in the country, except being tended to by the weaker and disorganised sections mostly in the Southern and Eastern coastal areas, North-eastern India and Jammu and Kashmir. Considering the greater scope tor duck farming as an effective tool for the socioeconomic development of rural masses, to provide leadership in research and training in respect of duck, a Central Duck Breeding Farm was established at Hessarghata during the Fifth Five Year Plan where a scientific breeding programme is being undertaken with imported Khaki Campbell ducks. The foundation and improved stocks are being supplied to different state duck farms, farmers and agricultural universities to augment duck development programmes in those states. Improved duck germ plasm is also being distributed at subsidised rates to improve the productivity of indigenous stock.

The production potential of desi duck is hardly 100-150 eggs per bird per year as against 250-300 eggs in khaki Campbell and Indian Runner.

Advantages of Duck Rearing Over Chicken

1. Ducks lay about 40-50 eggs more than chicken.
2. Duck eggs are 15-20 grams larger than chicken eggs.
3. Ducks require lesser attention than chicken.
4. Ducks by virtue of their feeding habits supplement a part of their feed requirement by foraging, and hence are economical to be raised as compared to chicken.
5. Ducks have a profitable life from commercial point of view as they also lay economically in second year, this reduces the cost of replacement.
6. Ducks are quite hardy, more easily brooded and are resistant to many avian diseases.
7. Marshy river side and wet land where chicken or other types of livestock will not flourish are excellent quarter for duck farming.

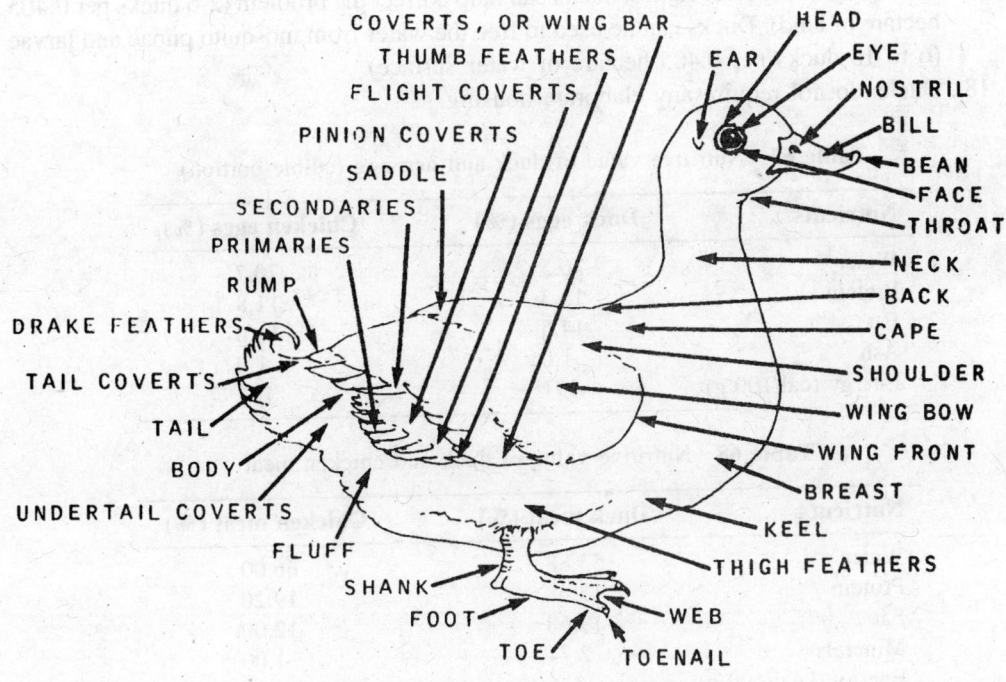

Figure 35 Parts of the male duck

8. Cannibalism and agnostic behaviour which is very common in chicken is not usually encountered with ducks.
9. Ducks lay more than 95 per cent of their eggs before 9.00 A.M. Thus data can be accurately recorded for breeding purposes without wastage of considerable amount of time and labour.
10. Ducks are quite intelligent and can be tamed easily. They can be trained to go to ponds and come back in the evening of their own.
11. Because of comparatively more heavy, duck eggs provide more nutrients per egg than chicken egg.
12. Ducks can live upto about 10 years but the effective laying period is about 4 years.
13. Ducks are suitable for integrated farming systems, such as duck cum fish farming where their droppings serve as feed to fish and some fish can be used as duck feed. (200-300 ducks per hectare of water area).
14. They are not so susceptible to disease and parasites in comparison to chickens. They are free from Leukosis, Marek's disease, Infectious Bronchitis and other respiratory troubles.
15. After hatching it is simpler to sex ducklings than chickens.
16. The down and small body feathers of the ducks are valuable as filler for pillows and as lining for comforters and winter clothing (one pekin duck produces about 100 gms. of down and small feathers)
17. Ducks are good exterminators of potato beetles, grass hoppers, snails and slugs. In areas plagued by liver flukes, ducks can help correct the problem (2-6 ducks per 0.405 hectare of land). Ducks can be used to free the water from mosquito pupae and larvae (6 to 10 ducks per 0.405 hectare of water surface).
18. Ducks do not require any elaborate housing.

Table 67 Nutritive value of duck and hen egg (edible portion)

Nutrients	Duck eggs (%)	Chicken eggs (%)
Water	70.5	70.7
Protein	13.3	11.8
Fat	14.5	11.0
Ash	1.0	1.0
Energy (cal/100 g)	191	163

Table 68 Nutritive value of duck and chicken meat

Nutrients	Duck meat (%)	Chicken meat (%)
Water	53.88	66.00
Protein	13.48	19.20
Fat	19.68	12.00
Minerals	2.74	1.00
Energy (kcal/100 g)	326	155

BREEDS OF DUCKS

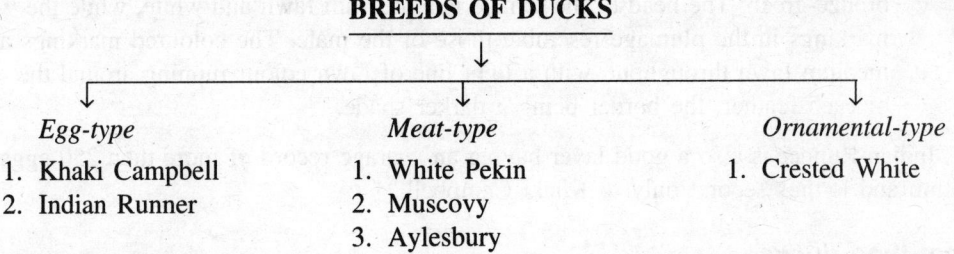

Egg-type	Meat-type	Ornamental-type
1. Khaki Campbell	1. White Pekin	1. Crested White
2. Indian Runner	2. Muscovy	
	3. Aylesbury	

Egg-type ducks

Ducks normally begin to lay at about 6 months of age, although Khaki Campbell come into lay 6 weeks earlier. Ducks of the improved laying breeds are for all practical purposes non-broody. For the purpose of fertilised egg, one drake for 5-6 ducks is normally allowed with slight increase in the number of drakes at the beginning and towards the end of the season, during which time the drakes are less active. Drakes should be placed with the ducks at least one month before fertile eggs are required. The belief that effective copulation can only take place in water is mistaken, although it is desirable that ducks should have access to water to keep themselves clean and nesting ducks are better able to keep their eggs at the correct humidity.

Khaki Campbell—The breed has been developed in England from a cross of Fawn and White Runner, and Mullard ducks. Drakes have brownish-bronze lower backs, tail coverts, head and necks— the rest of their plumage is khaki; they have green bills and dark-orange legs and toes. Ducks are of seal-brown heads and necks-the rest of their plumage is khaki; and they have greenish–black bills and brown legs and toes.

The adult drake weighs between 2.2 to 2.4 kg. While the female weighs between 2.0 to 2.2 kg and that of an egg is about 70 gms. Egg production have averaged close to 300 eggs per duck within a laying year.

Indian Runner received its name from its supposed introduction from East India. There are 3 standard varieties of Runner ducks:

(1) **The Fawn and White Runner:** The breed is fawn or grey and white, with a white neck and a line of white running upto the eyes and extending around the bill. The back and shoulders are fawn, and the upper part of the breast and wings are fawn, but the lower part is white. The breast is full; the body is long and narrow, sloping gradually into the neck, and is carried erect, with no indication of a keel, the body resembling somewhat that of a penguin in shape. The shanks and toes are orange red. The bill of the young drake is yellow, later becoming greenish yellow, while a young duck has a yellow bill spotted with green, which later becomes a dull green.

(2) **The White Runner** is pure white in all sections. The bill is yellow and the shanks and toes, are orange.

(3) **The Pencilled Variety** The head of the male is a dull bronze-green and white and the back has a soft, fawn ground, finely stippled with a slightly darker shade of fawn; the body and the upper section of the breast are medium fawn and the tail is a dull

bronze-green. The head of the female is a medium fawn and white, while the white markings in the plumage resemble those of the male. The coloured markings are a medium fawn throughout, with a light line of fawn colour running around the edge of each feather, the border being a darker shade.

Indian Runner is also a good layer having an average record of more than 250 eggs per annum and is thus second only to Khaki Campbell.

Meat-type ducks

Though duck meat is widely accepted among the non-vegetarians but still it is not so popular due to its non-availability. In comparison to hen, duck meat is slightly rich in fat (14.5 per cent) and total energy (190 Kcal/100 gm). The protein content is very close to hen and averages to about 13 per cent. White Pekin is the most popular meat-type duck in the world. Muscovy and Aylesbury are the next best types.

A sort of broiler type of ducks are reared at Kolluru lake area of Andhra Pradesh, specially for meat. They are similar to broiler chicken but, these are marketed at the age of about 6-8 months. The meat of such ducks is said to be more tasty besides, being more nutritive.

White Pekin: The breed originates from China. These are large white feathered birds. They have orange-yellow bills, reddish-yellow shanks and feet and yellow skin. Their eggs are tinted white which is considered less important than its capability to produce excellent quality meat. Birds of this breed are by virtue of nervous temperament, bad sitters and thus should be treated gently.

Muscovy: It is to be very much questioned if the Muscovy really a duck! It is more like a goose in more ways than one; for instance, it is a grazer and eats grasses in the same way as a goose. These are very strong and powerful in flight, yet very tame and friendly.

Unlike the drake of other breeds, the Muscovy male has no curl feathers in his tail. Unlike other females (ducks), the incubation period is 36 days; also the ducklings are not in first full feather until 16 weeks of age, whereas the ordinary duckling is in full feather at 12 weeks.

Another noteworthy point is that the drakes are very big, often weighing 4.5 kg., whereas the ducks are very small weighing about 3.0 kg. The breed is native to Brazil and very popular in Australia. When crossed with other breeds, it produces sterile duck, known as Mule ducks which produces satisfactory meat yield.

There are 2 standard varieties of Muscovy ducks, the white and the dark. The head and face of the Muscovy are partly bare, with red, rough, carunculated skin. It has a long, broad body, with greater breadth.

The white variety has pure white plumage, pale orange or yellow legs, and a pinkish, flesh-coloured beak. The dark variety has got a lustrous blue black, broken with some white breast, body and back.

The breed provides meat of excellent quality and taste, provided they are marketed before 17 weeks of age. They are also good sitters and will hatch and care for approximately 30 ducklings from the 40-45 eggs they produce annually.

Muscovies are armed with very long and sharp claws and are quite capable of opening one's wrist or hand unless it is firmly grasped by the wings.

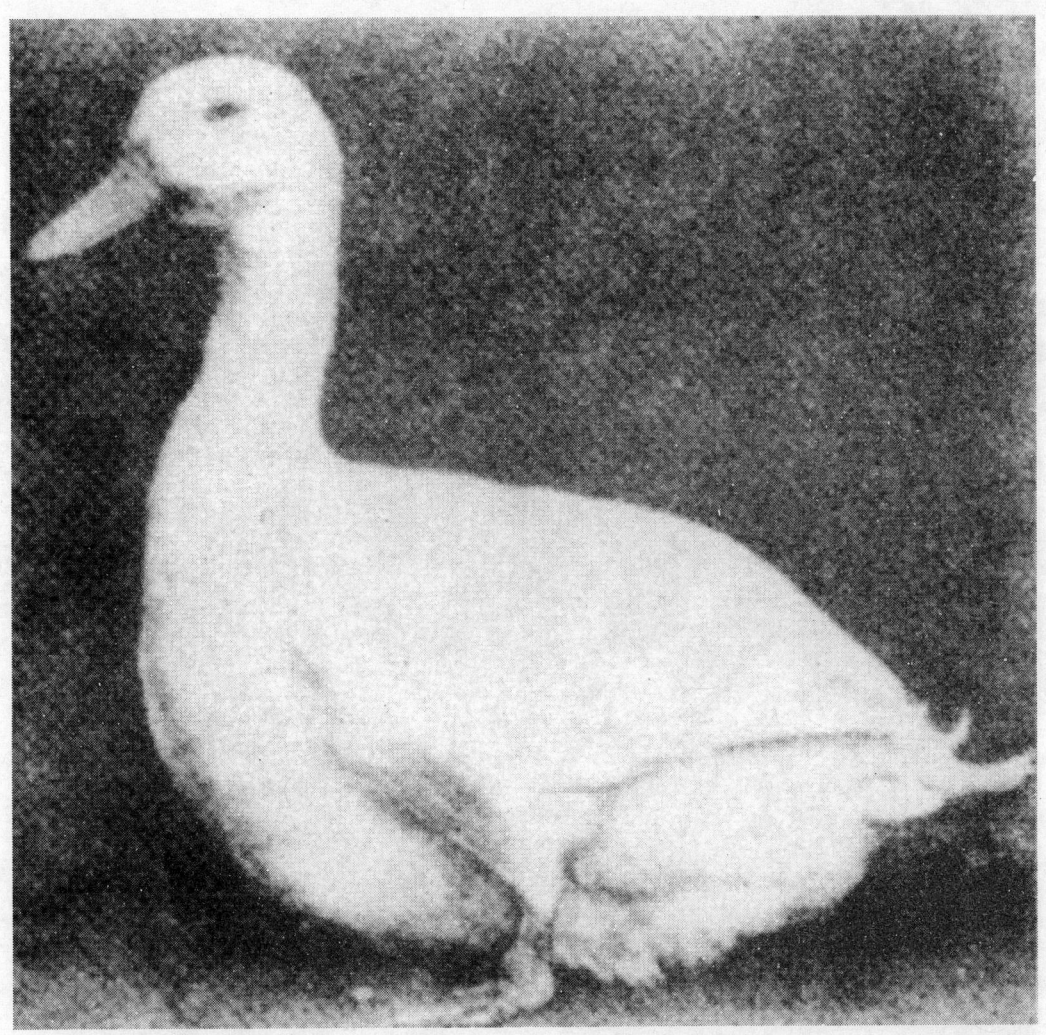

Plate 15.   Aylesbury Drake

220

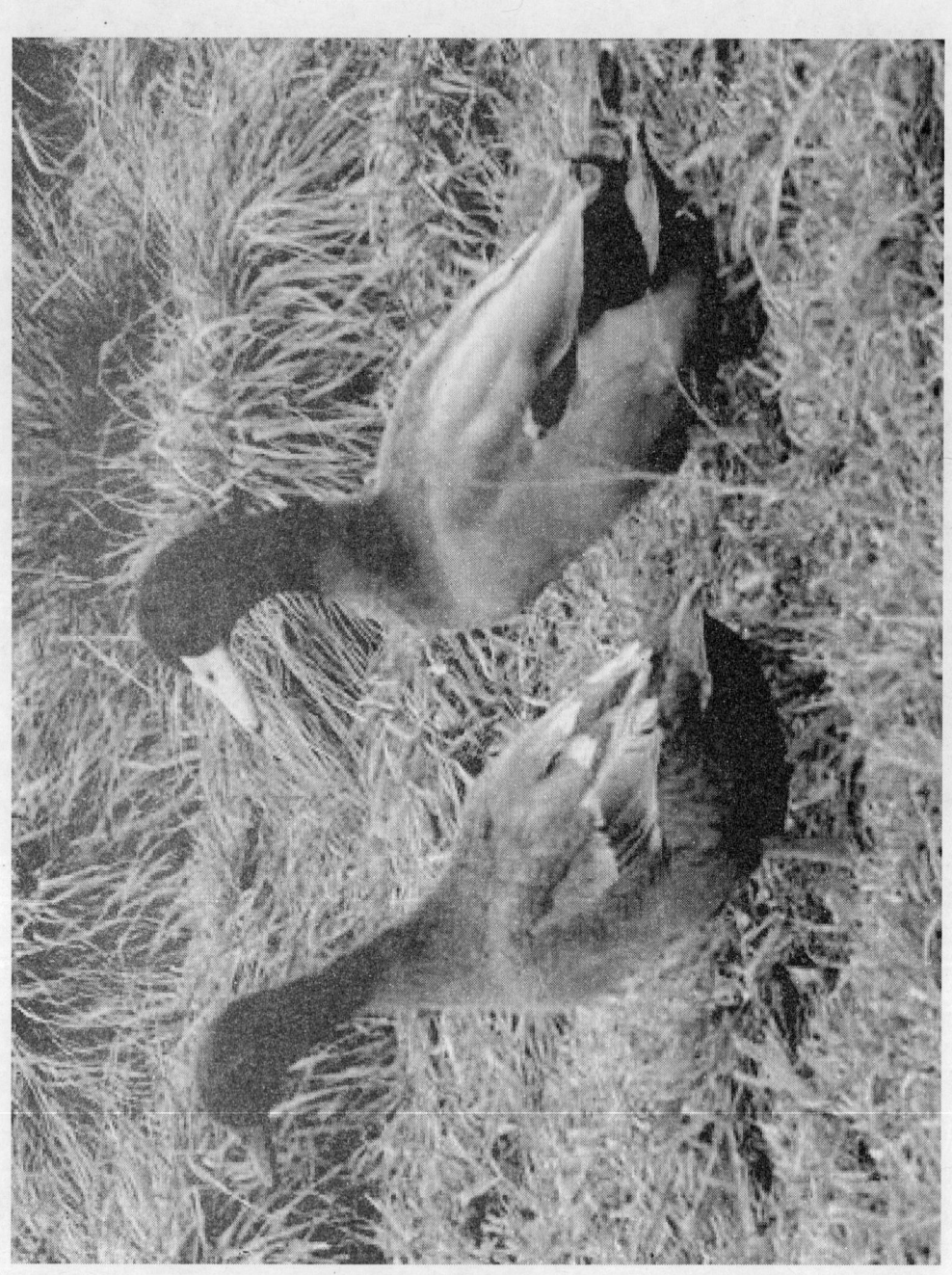

Plate 16. Khaki Campbells.

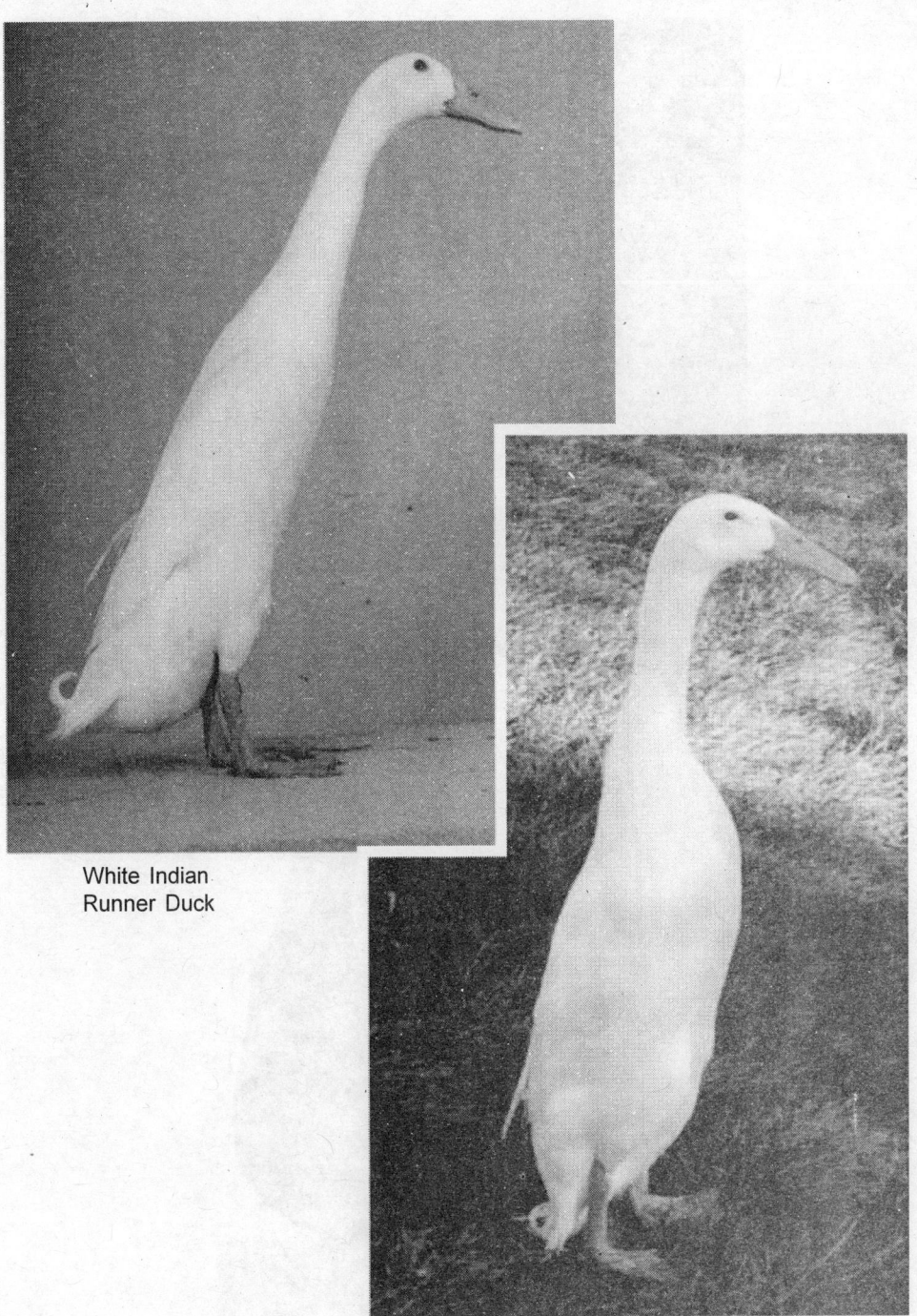

221

White Indian
Runner Duck

Plate 17.   Fawn Indian Runner Duck.

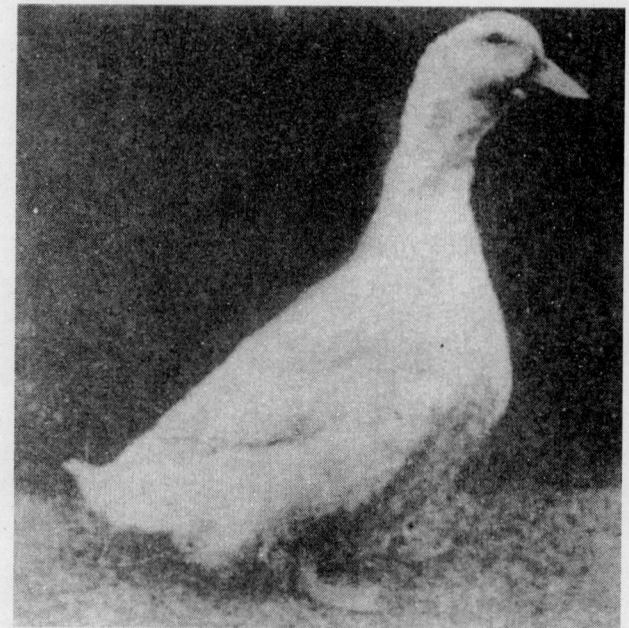

Plate 18.   Pekin Duck.

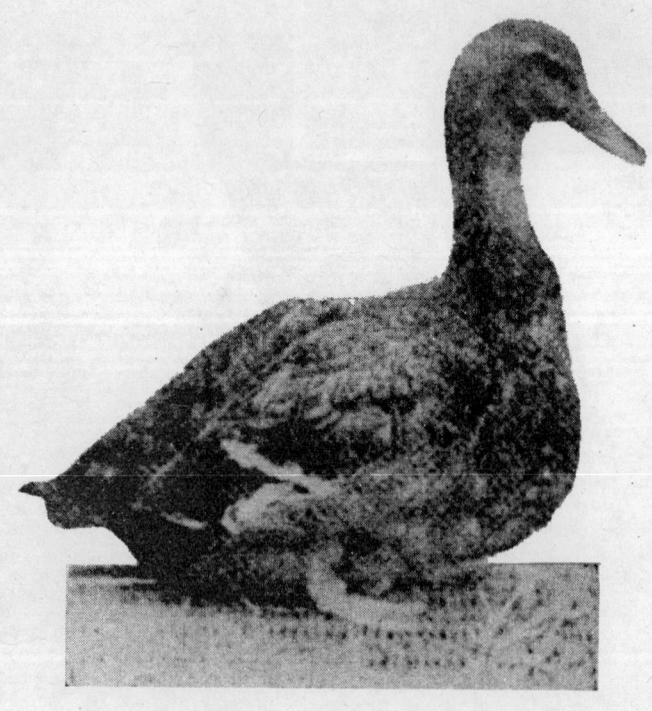

Plate 19.   Adult Rouen Duck.

Aylesbury: It has originated from Buckingham in U.K. The plumages are white, legs are short but sturdy and orange in colour. Due to its light bone and high percentage of creamy white flesh, the breed is regarded as delux table bird. It also produces excellent quality meat, and reaches market weight in 8 weeks. Eggs are tinted white.

Brooding

Any equipment that will brood chicks efficiently will also brood ducklings. The brooding period of Khaki Campbell ducklings is 3 to 4 weeks. For meat type ducklings such as Pekin, brooding for 2-3 weeks is sufficient. Providing hover space of 0.09 to 0.15 meter/bird from first to fourth week under the brooder should be sufficient. A temperature of 29°C to 32°C (84.2 to 89.6°F) is maintained during the first week. It is reduced by about 3°C (5°F) per week till it reaches 24°C (75°F) during the fourth week (Table 69).

Ducklings may be brooded on wire floor, litter or in batteries. A wire floor space of 0.046m2 (0.5 sq. ft.) per bird or solid floor space of an average of 0.093m2 (1 sq. ft.) per bird would be sufficient upto 2 weeks of age. The space requirement from first to 8th weeks of age is given in Table 70.

Table 69   Brooding temperatures

	Days 1-2	Days 3-7	Week 2
DUCKLINGS	29-32° C	26-29	23-26
	84.2-89.6° F	78.8-84.2	73.4-78.8

Table 70   Space allowances

	Age in weeks	Floor space sq ft/bird	Sq m/bird
DUCKS (fatteners, groups 40-50)	1-2	1.0	0.09
	2-3	1.5	0.13
	3-4	2.0	0.19
	4-5	2.5	0.23
	6-8	4.0	0.37

The forward edge of the upper bill is usually trimmed at the age of two weeks.

When small number of ducklings are brooded, the brooding is done with the help of a broody duck or hen as most breeds of duck are not good sitters. About 12-18 ducklings can be brooded by a large hen. For the first few days feed and water should be provided in the house. After 5-7 days, the hen along with the ducklings may be allowed to move within the restricted area. Young ducklings fall easy prey to wild birds. The entire brood should be protected from rain, cold winds, predatory birds, other animals and rodents. After 2-3 weeks no further mothering is necessary.

Rearing

After 4 weeks of age, birds are transferred to sheds of convenient size for their comfortable stay and growth. Ducklings can be reared in intensive, semi-intensive and range systems. In range system they need night shelter. They need a run for 16 weeks. Under intensive system, floor space of individual bird should be of $0.279m^2$ (3 sq. ft.) till it attains the age of 16 weeks. Under semi-intensive system, floor space for each bird at the rate of 0.186 to $0.279m^2$ (2.5 to 3 sq. ft.) per bird is allowed in night shelter and 0.929 to $1.394m^2$ (10-15 sq. ft.) as outside run till they attain an age of 16 weeks.

Usually ducklings are allowed to move to run at the end of 4 weeks. Water in the drinkers should be 12.5 to 15 cms. (5-6 inches) deep to allow the immersion of their heads. Partitions upto the height of 60-90 cm. (2-3 inches) inside the pens and outside runs are sufficient.

Under range system a flock of 2000 ducks can be reared per 0.405 hectare (one acre).

Adult Stock

Under intensive system, a floor space of 0.371 to 0.465 m^2 (4-5 square feet) per duck is essential, whereas in semi-intensive system, a floor space of 0.279 m^2 (3 sq. ft.) in the night shelter and 0.929 to 1.394 m^2 (10-15 sq. ft.) as outside run per bird would be adequate. For wet mash feeding in a 'V' shaped feeder allow 10-12.5 cm. (4-5 inches). For feeding *ad lib* in hoppers, a feeding space of 5 to 7.5 cm (2-3 inches) per duck would be sufficient.

Ducks do not need perches. Laying nests are essential for clean egg production. These can be compartments of 30 cm^2 with 35-37 cm height. For every 3 ducks 1 nest has to be provided. High egg laying strains of duck come into production at 16-18 weeks of age. Since 95-98 per cent of the eggs are laid before 9.00 A.M., layers should be kept confined until at least 9.00 A.M. Mating ratio of 1 male to 8 females in egg laying strains and only 4-5 females in meat strains gives satisfactory fertility.

Housing

Ducks do not require elaborate houses. In general, duck, prefers to stay outside day and night throughtout the year. In mild climates it is possible to raise the ducks without artificial shelter. A light fence of 4 feet high enclosing the yard is enough to stop most of the predators.

Ducks are fussier than chickens and will not tolerate or develop under battery conditions. As a result they are allowed houses with litter on solid floors and more space, natural day light, good ventilation and sometimes an outside yard. Straw makes a good bedding material. Peat moss, ground nut shells, or wood shavings can also be used. Litter should be added frequently and should be kept dry by providing plenty of sun shine and fresh air otherwise the whole atmosphere quickly become hot and smelly, causing the birds to do a partial moult and go out of production.

Wire floors seems to be costly and moreover are not liked by the breeders. The entire material may be of thatch material. For protection against thieves pucca houses comprising pillars and strong nettings may be thought of if funds permit for large commercial. Earth floors are generally better than wood or concrete. If the latter is used the litter should be deep enough for good insulation and should be changed when it becomes wet. A sandy soil is best.

Good ventilation is a must. The layers should go out of doors during day time throughout the year unless stormy. Water for swimming is not at all necessary, but a pool provides exercise, promotes health, keeps the eyes, bills and vents clean and gives lustre to the plumage. Water in drinkers should be sufficiently deep to allow the immersion of their heads and not themselves. If they can not do this, their eyes as said now, get scaly and crusty and in extreme cases blindness may follow.

Feeding

Ducks are the most efficient type of poultry to convert fallen grains of the fields, insect, plant materials and pond materials into edible meat and eggs.

Under intensive system of rearing ducks are fed diets like chickens to suit various age groups, viz., starter (0-2 weeks); growers (3-8 weeks and for 9-20 weeks or upto the point of lay); layers and breeders. Commercial feeds are available as mash, pellets or crumbs fed at *ad libitum* at least for first eight weeks and later on twice a day. Ducks prefer wet mash due to difficulties in swallowing. Pellet feeding though slightly costly, has distinct advantage of saving in amount of feed, labour convenience, no scouring and improvement in sanitary conditions. *Ducks should never have access to feed without drinking water.*

Ducklings should be fed as soon as they are removed from the incubator to the brooder, or immediately after they are received from the hatchery. Since ducklings do not readily learn to eat, it is necessary that extreme care should be given to them for the first few days to keep them from dying or starvation. If it is possible to put several chicks or ducklings that have already learned how to eat in the brooder with the new hatch, they will learn to eat quickly.

If it is not possible, it might be necessary to hand feed some of them for the first day or two. Ducklings grow at a very fast rate and therefore require a ration rich in all required nutrients.

Khaki Campbell duck consumes about 12.5 kg. of feed upto 20 weeks of age. Afterwards the consumption varies from 120-170 gm. per bird per day depending upon the rate of production and availability of greens.

The starter, grower and layer ration of laying type of duck should contain a protein percentage of 20, 15 and 18 respectively with a metabolizable energy of 2750, 2700 and 2650 kcal. per kg. of feed respectively. Some feed formulae are suggested in Table 74.

Feeds recommended for chicks are also suitable for ducklings. Day-old ducklings should be given coarse milled cereals moistened with milk or water as a first feed and then a proprietary mash or one with composition approximating to the following:

Milled cereal	35 parts
Fine cereal bran	30 parts
Fish or meat meal	20 parts
Extracted oil-cake meal	10 parts
Fine grit & minerals	5 parts

Table 71 Nutrients requirements of ducks

Nutrients	NRC(1971) Starting and growing	ARC (1975) Starting and growing	Level adopted at PRC	
			Starting and growing	Breeding
(1)	(2)	(3)	(4)	(5)
ME(Kcal/kg)		3,100.00	3,000.00	2,050.00
Crude protein (%)	17.00	23.00	22.00	18.00
Amino acids (g/kg)				
Arginine	–	8.4	11.8	5.5
Glycine + serine	–	11.3	11.3	–
Histidine	–	3.9	2.7	1.8
Isoleucine	–	6.9	6.4	6.0
Leucine	–	11.8	12.7	7.4
Lysine	–	8.9	8.9	8.2
Methionine	–	3.9	4.0	–
Methionine + cystine	–	7.4	7.4	5.2
Phenylalanine	–	6.9	–	–
Phenylalanine + tyrosine	–	12.8	12.8	9.0
Threonine	–	5.9	6.4	3.9
Tryptophan	–	1.7	2.0	1.8
Valine	–	7.9	8.2	6.0
Major minerals (%)				
Calcium	–	0.56	0.9	2.75
Available phosphorus	–	–	0.45	0.5
Total phosphorus	–	–	–	–
Minor minerals (mg/kg)				
Magnesium	–	500.00	500.00	300.00
Sodium	–	–	1500.00	1500.00
Chloride	–	–	–	–
Potassium	–	–	3000.00	–
Copper	–	–	3.5	3.5
Iodine	–	–	0.4	0.4
Iron	–	–	80.00	80.00
Manganese	–	–	100.00	100.00
Zinc	–	–	50.00	50.00
Selenium	–	–		
Vitamins (IU/kg)				
Vitamin A	–	–	2000.00	6000.00
Vitamin D$_3$	220.00	300.00	600.00	800.00
Vitamin E	–	–	25.00	25.00
Vitamins (mg/kg)				
Vitamin K	–	–	1.3	1.3
Thiamin	–	–	3.00	2.00
Riboflavin	4.00	4.00	4.00	4.00
Nicotinic acid	55.00	25.00	28.00	28.00

Table 71 (Continued)

Nutrients	NRC(1971) Starting and growing	ARC (1975) Starting and growing	Level adopted at PRC Starting and growing	Breeding
(1)	(2)	(3)	(4)	(5)
Pantothenic acid	1 1.00	1 1.00	10.00	10.00
Pyridoxine	2.6	2.5	2.5	5.00
Biotin	–	–	–	0.2
Folic acid	–	–	–	0.5
Vitamin B_{12}	–	–	–	0.01
Choline	–	–	1800.00	1100.00

Table 72 Suggested practical level of nutrients in feed for ducks

	Starter (0-2 weeks)	Grower (3-8 weeks 9-20 weeks)		Layer	Breeder
Metabolizable energy (Kcal/kg)	2750.00	2750.00	2700.00	2650.00	2650.00
Protein (%)	20.00	18.00	15.00	18.00	18.00
Minerals					
Calcium (%)	0.80	0.8	0.8	2.5	2.5
Phosphorus(%)	0.45	0.45.	0.45	0.45	0.45
Sodium (%)	0.15	0.15	0.15	0.15	0.15
Copper (mg/kg)	8.00	8.00	8.00	8.00	8.00
Iodine (mg/kg)	0.6	0.6	0.6	0.6	0.6
Iron (mg/kg)	80.00	80.00	80.00	80.00	80.00
Manganese (mg/kg)	100.00	100.00	100.00	100.00	100.00
Zinc (mg/kg)	60.00	60.00	60.00	60.00	60.00
Vitamins					
Biotin (mg/kg)	0.1	0.1	0.1	0.1	0.2
Choline (mg/kg)	1800.00	1,800.00	1100.00	1100.00	1100.00
Folic acid (mg/kg)	1.00	1.00	1.00	1.00	1.5
Niacin (mg/kg)	60.00	60.00	60.00	60.00	60.00
Pantothenic acid (mg/kg)	15.00	15.00	1 5.00	15.0.0	15.00
Pyridoxine (mg/kg)	6.00	6.00	6.00	6.00	9.00
Riboflavin (mg/kg)	5.00	5.00	5.00	5.00	8.00
Thaiamine (mg/kg)	4.00	4.00	4.00	2.00	2.00
Vitamin A (lU/kg)	4000.00	4000.00	4000.00	6000.00	8000.00
Vitamin B_{12} (mg/kg)	0.01	0.01	0.01	0.01	0.01
Vitamin D_3 (ICU/kg)	600.00	600.00	600.00	1000.00	1000.00
Vitamin E (mg/kg)	20.00	20.00	20.00	20.00	20.00
Vitamin K (mg/kg)	2.00	2.00	2.00	2.00	2.00

Table 73 Suggested levels of amino acids in feed for ducks

	Starter 0-2 weeks		Grower		Layer and breeder (from point of lay)	
	% protein	% diet	3-8 weeks % diet	9-20 weeks or up to point of of lay % diet	% protein	% diet
Arginine	5.9	1.18	1.06	0.89	3.1	0.56
Glycine and/or serine	3.0	0.60	0.54	0.45		
Histidine	1.4	0.28	0.25	0.21	1.0	0.18
Isoleucine	3.2	0.64	0.58	0.48	3.3	0.59
Leucine	6.4	1.28	1.15	0.96	4.1	0.74
Lysine	5.0	1.00	0.90	0.75	4.5	0.81
Methionine	1.9	0.38	0.34	0 29	1.5	0.27
Methionine + cystine	3.6	0.72	0.65	0.54	2.9	0.52
Phenylalanine	3.4	0.68	0.61	0.51	2.8	0.50
Phenylalanine + tyrosine	6.4	1.25	1.15	0.96	5.0	0.90
Threonine	3.2	0.64	0.58	0.48	2.2	0.40
Tryptophan	1.0	0.20	0.18	0.15	1.0	0.18
Valine	4.1	0.82	0.74	0.62	3.3	0.59
Protein		20.0	18.0	15.0		18.0

The mash should be dampened just sufficiently to make it 'crumble'. If it is too wet, much of it is lost through the sieving process to which it is subjected in the duck's bill. No more feed than can be eaten in about 10 minutes should be fed at any one time. Grit or sand and water should be available *ad lib.*

Adult ducks (Khaki Campbell) feed consumption normally varies from 120-200 gm. per day depending upon the rate of production and availability of greens. Feeds recommended for fowls are generally suitable for ducks.

Under semi-intensive system more use may be made of local feeds. One third of the meal ration may be replaced by cheaper vegetable feeds, household scrapes and fodders as available under local conditions.

Ducks on free range obtain most of their protein needs by foraging, from small fish, crustaceans and insects, thus resulting economy in evening meal.

Duck Handling

Ducks should be picked up by the neck, for the legs are broken rather easily. Since the windpipe of a duck is quite rigid, it may be carried by the neck without injury.

Table 74 Ration for ducks (in per cent)

Ingredients	Starter (0-2 weeks)		Grower				Layer and breeder	
			3-8 weeks		9-20 weeks			
	1	2	1	2	1	2	1	2
Maize	32.00	43.12	31.70	45.00	33.69	–	31.89	47.00
Sorghum	11.00	–	17.00	–	–	44.70	–	10.44
Rice polish	16.90	20.00	17.00	20.00	40.00	40.00	35.00	–
Rice bran	–	–	–	–	–	–	–	8.00
Wheat bran	–	5.00	–	9.00	10.00	–	–	–
Sal seed meal (deoiled)	5.00	–	5.00	–	–	–	–	–
G.N. Cake	11.00	–	9.00	–	–	–	–	11.00
Sunflower cake	11.00	7.00	9.00	5.00	5.00	–	11.50	11.00
Mustard cake	–	7.00	–	5.00	5.00	–	11.50	–
Maize gluten meal	–	7.00	–	5.00	–	–	–	–
Sesame cake	–	–	–	–	–	–	–	–
Fish meal	12.00	10.00	10.00	10.00	5.00	6.00	4.00	–
Meat meal	–	–	–	–	–	–	–	–
Bone meal	0.70	0.50	0.90	0.60	0.70	1.00	0.75	0.75
Common salt	0.24	0.25	0.24	0.24	0.20	0.19	0.25	0.22
Limestone	–	–	–	–	0.30	–	5.00	4.10
Choline chloride	0.05	0.02	0.05	0.05	–	–	–	–
Minerals and vitamins	0.11	0.11	0.11	0.11	0.11	0.11	0.11	0.11

1. If good quality fish meal is available, the quantity of fish meal can be reduced.
2. Mineral mixture/100 kg diet: $FeSO_4$ 20 g; $MnSO_4$ 40 g; $ZnSO_4$ 25g; $CuSO_4$ 1.5 g; and KI 100 mg.
3. Vitamin mixture/100 kg diet: Vitamin-A 800,000 I.U.; Vitamin-D100,000 IU; Riboflavin 400 mg; Folic acid 100 mg and Niacin 5 g.

Duck Sex-distinguishing

(a) **Sexing of day-old ducklings:** Recently much interest has developed in the matter of sexing day-old ducklings. In comparison to chicks, the early determination of sex in ducks is easy and very accurate, its practical value is limited. Ducklings of the meat breeds are usually hatched for market purposes and no differentiation made in sex. Hatcherymen specializing in day-old ducklings of the laying breeds may find it practical to offer only female ducklings to customers who desire to start flocks for egg production.

At hatching, the cloaca is often full of greenish excreta. Some people find it more pleasant to sex the ducklings at a few days old. However, the procedure is as follows:

(i) Take hold of the duckling's toil between the first finger and thumb of the left hand so that its breast is upwards and away from you and its head hangs down.

(ii) Then stretch the cloaca longitudinally by bending the duckling gently "but firmly over the first finger and holding its body there with the middle, third and little fingers (Figure 36).

(iii) Now stretch the cloaca transversely and so force out the copulatory organ, if it is there, by closing the thumb and first finger of the left hand, placing them while closed on the cloaca and then parting them slowly. It is important that the thumb and first finger are kept together until they are placed on the cloaca because before they are parted, they must catch the edge of the cloaca and exert sufficient tension to force out the copulatory organ. This organ looks like a pinkish root tip and its presence denotes a drakelet. No such organ is seen in the cloaca of a ducklet.

Geese can also be sexed in the same way.

(b) **Distinguishing sex afterwards:** The female ducks do the loud quacking. The drakes have a softer voice. Voice differences appear when ducks are 6-9 weeks old. Later the drakes develop curled tail feathers. After a duck lays for some time, part of the colour fades from the bill which changes from an orange to light yellow.

Incubating Duck Eggs

Duck eggs have the reputation of being rather difficult to hatch. This is not so, especially if one bears in mind that they are not just another type of hen eggs, and that are to be dealt with waterfowl instead of roosting fowl and make good use of the subtle difference.

As with hen eggs, much of success in incubation depends on how they are selected and prepared prior to setting in the incubator. Before discussing the actual incubation period, it is therefore useful to dwell a moment on what to do or what not to do beforehand.

Storing and selecting duck eggs: The shells of duck eggs have much larger pores than hen eggs. For this reason, hatching eggs should not be stored for too long before setting them in the incubators. First of all, the eggs tend to "dry out" more quickly, specially when the atmosphere is rather dry; and also on account of these large pores, harmful bacteria can be drawn in more easily. This "sucking in" of bacteria is most likely to happen immediately after the egg is laid. The temperature of the egg when laid is 37.8°C (100°F), and its content immediately contracts on account of the usually much lower ambient temperature which causes the airspace to be formed at that moment.

Nature has provided the eggs with quite formidable defences against outside bacteria, but if there are too many of them the battle could be lost. The conclusion is, therefore, not to store hatching eggs too long and collect them in as clean a condition as possible.

Hatching eggs should be set within seven days of their being laid. Cleanliness can be promoted by changing the litter in the duck houses frequently and by making the ducks lay in nest boxes. These nest boxes should all be at ground level and in position about one month before the ducks are expected to start laying. If the boxes are introduced when the ducks have already commenced laying, they will not use them and drop their eggs anywhere. Ducks lay 99 per cent of their eggs between 6 and 9 in the morning. For the commercial egg producer, this has the advantage that when the birds are let out in the morning on streams or paddy fields, nearly all eggs are safely in hand.

For hatching eggs, this has an additional and very important advantage. Eggs laid in low temperatures hatch much better than those laid in high temperatures. More important still,

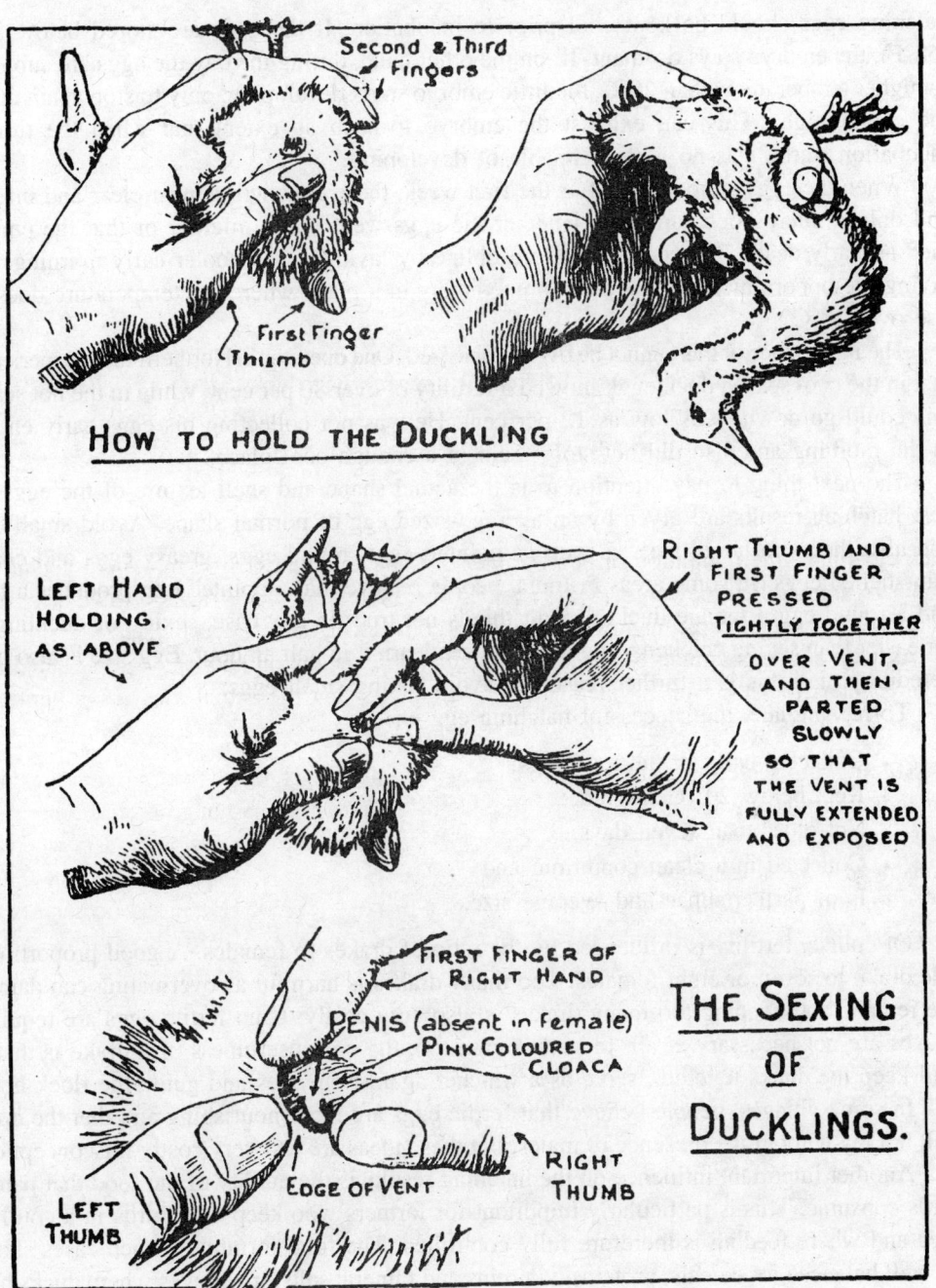

Second & Third Fingers

First Finger

Thumb

HOW TO HOLD THE DUCKLING

LEFT HAND HOLDING. AS. ABOVE

RIGHT THUMB AND FIRST FINGER PRESSED TIGHTLY TOGETHER

OVER VENT, AND THEN PARTED SLOWLY SO THAT THE VENT IS FULLY EXTENDED AND EXPOSED

FIRST FINGER OF RIGHT HAND

PENIS (absent in female)

PINK COLOURED CLOACA

RIGHT THUMB

EDGE OF VENT

LEFT THUMB

THE SEXING OF DUCKLINGS.

Figure 36

hatching eggs should be kept cool prior to incubation. If the eggs are stored below 20°C (68°F), the embryo stays dormant. If, on the other hand, during the day the eggs are subjected to higher temperatures than 20°C, the little embryo starts developing, only to stop again during the cooler night. This can exhaust the embryo to such an extent that when the time of incubation starts, it is no longer capable of developing.

When the eggs are candled after the first week, these eggs will appear clear and infertile and only a microscope can show whether the eggs were really infertile or that the embryo died an early death. The ducks therefore oblige by laying in the cooler early morning, thus giving the opportunity to store them immediately in a place where the temperature does not rise over 20°C.

The importance of this cannot be overemphasized. One operator in Northern India experienced that in the cool season duck eggs showed a fertility of over 80 per cent, while in the hot season this could go down to as low as 12 per cent. He was not collecting his eggs early enough in the morning and also did not store them in a enough cool place.

The next thing to pay attention to is the actual shape and shell texture of the egg. The best hatching results are given by an average-sized egg of normal shape. Avoid small eggs and also the extra large ones, as well as pointed eggs, round eggs, greasy eggs and chalky thin-shelled eggs. In some areas in India, people believe that a pointed egg produces a male and a round egg a female duckling, but this is not true. In any case, sexing of ducklings is far easier than sexing chickens, and anybody can learn it in half an hour. Egg size is also quite hereditary, and this is a further reason to avoid setting small eggs.

To recapitulate, the successful hatching egg is:

- Collected early in the mornings;
- Kept below 20° Centigrade;
- Not older than seven days;
- Collected in a clean condition; and
- Is of perfect shpae and average size.

Of course, fertility is influenced by the ratio of drakes to females. A good proportion is one drake to seven or eight females. Too many drakes is harmful as overmating can damage the female, and keeping too many drakes is also very costly. If no fertile eggs are required, drakes are not necessary at all. In such a case too, the only usefulness of a drake is that he will keep the ducks together, serve as a watcher against enemies and guide the flock home.

In some villages, people believe that fertlie eggs are more nourishing and that the ducks will not lay without the presence of males, but these ideas are just very costly misconceptions.

Another important influence on the hatching results is the quality of the food that parent-birds consume. This is particularly important for farmers who keep their birds in a confined area and where feeding is therefore fully controlled. The food formula in such cases should be well balanced for cereals, proteins, vitamins and mineral salts. In villages where ducks have access to a sufficient land and water area, the ducks will stand a good chance of balancing their food intake themselves.

Mechanical incubation: Modern mechanical incubation started in Europe and America at the turn of this century. Since then, many types of incubators have come on the market with a steady stream of improvements and refinements. These machines are nearly always designed for hen eggs and are not necessarily suitable for duck eggs. There are roughly three types of mechanical incubators:

(1) Flat type, still air incubators, usually with small capacity for 50 to 500 eggs.
(2) Cabinet incubators from 600 to 10,000 eggs.
(3) Walk-in incubators where the operator works inside the machine. This type is very economical for floor space—67,500 eggs can be accommodated in a space of 205 square feet.

Only the first two types of machine are suitable for duck eggs without getting involved in too many complications. The reason is that while hen eggs do well with an even temperature through the incubation process, duck eggs should be cooled daily for short periods with the exception of the first three days. There are two ways of doing this. Either the trays can be taken outside the incubator for air cooling, or the eggs can be sprayed with luke-warm water while the air stirring equipment is turned off.

Most hatcheries in Europe favour the latter method. A disinfectant either chlore or quarto Ammonium based, should be added to the water. This not only disinfects the eggs but also the incubator itself.

A Dutchman, Dr. R. S. Kaltofen has done extensive tests with spraying duck eggs during the incubation period. He found, for example, that duck eggs which were sprayed daily from the third day onwards, produced an average 6 per cent more ducklings than eggs which were sprayed only once per week. Even more remarkable, he also found that the weight loss of the sprayed eggs during the incubation period was greater than the eggs which were not sprayed. There is also no delay in the total incubation period due to spraying and regular candling of the eggs at different stages and it shows a much healthier and more vigorous development of the embryo.

It would seem that by spraying duck eggs one is just imitating nature. In the wild, most ducks will choose their nesting place near a stream or pond and take a dip once or twice a day. In that way the eggs will be dampened the moment the bird returns and continues hatching, so that the idea is not so novel after all.

When using Hat still-air incubators, the rules of the manufacturers should be followed as closely as possible–with two exceptions. The recommended incubation temperature for duck eggs should be one-quarter of one degree Fahrenheit lower, and when the ducklings start pipping, the temperature should be one degree Fahrenheit lower than during the first 26 days, while the humidity should be boosted to 85° relative humidity. All flat type still-air incubators suitable for hen eggs, will also hatch duck eggs successfully.

In the case of cabinet incubators however, this is not the case. In the first place, duck eggs must have a separate hatching compartment. Most cabinets are designed for multistage loading. In other words, up to one quarter of the setting capacity is loaded once a week and at the 25th day the first setting is removed to the hatching compartment. Due to the very high relative humidity required during these last three days the development of the airspace in the eggs set in the second and third week would be hindered in development if they came in contact with this very humid air. During the first 25 days, the humidity should not exceed approximately 60° in order to allow the airspace to grow to one-third of the egg by the 25th day. Therefore, a separate hatcher is essential for duck eggs when cabinets are used.

234

Secondly, the design of the air moving equipment and the air ducts in case of duck eggs is more critical than in the case of hen eggs so that even when is used a cabinet machine with a separate hatcher, not all types designed for hen eggs will give maximum results for duck eggs.

Some makes of cabinet incubators use air paddles or air stirrers while others use propeller type equipment to distribute the air in the cabinets. All paddle type incubators which are successful for hen eggs will also be successful for duck eggs, while only some machines equipped with propellers will be suitable for duck eggs.

Like hen eggs, duck eggs should be placed in cabinet machines with the round end uppermost. When the pointed end is uppermost this will result in malpositioning of the embryo and consequently a great many dead-in-shell birds. Modern cabinet incubators are usually equipped with automatic gear which ensures hourly turning during the first 25 days. In the hatching stage, namely the 25th to 28th day, no turning should be done. If hand turning is practised, the eggs should be turned at least five times in 24 hours. Some manufacturers claim that turning every hour as compared to five times in 24 hours gives 6 per cent better results.

These are the most important points where incubating and hatching duck eggs differ from the better-known problems with hen eggs.

Common Duck Diseases

Ducks appear to excel all other domestic poultry in their resistance to common avian diseases, but they do suffer from duck plague, duck virus hepatitis and some other diseases. The list of common diseases presented here is far from complete. It should not be used as a substitute for accurate diagnosis by veterinarians.

Duck Plague

Serious outbreaks of duck plague also known as duck virus enteritis can cause 80-90% mortality in flocks of all ages.

This highly contagious disease strikes swiftly without warning.

Symptoms:

1. Listless with drooping wings, ruffled feathers.
2. Swollen and moist eyes with sticky discharge.
3. Laboured breathing and loss of appetite with increased thirst.
4. Watery greenish yellow diarrohea sometimes mixed with blood
5. Swollen and protruding penis.
6. In laying females, haemorrhages can be observed in the deformed discoloured ovarian follicles.

Prevention and Control:

The birds can be protected by Duck Plague Vaccine, available in the country, given at the age of 8 weeks.

Duck Cholera

Highly infectious disease caused by bacterial organism *Pasteurella multocida* in ducks over 4 weeks of age.

Symptoms:

1. Loss of appetite along with increased thirst.
2. High body temperature.
3. Initial diarrhoea followed by mucoid droppings.

Prevention and Control:

1. Vaccinate the birds with duck cholera vaccine first at the age of 4 weeks and again at 16 weeks. Vaccine is available in the country.
2. Sulphonamides and antibiotics are effective in controlling the disease and reducing mortality.
3. Since the organisms of this highly infectious disease live for long periods in tissue of dead birds, be sure to burn such cases.

Aflatoxicosis

Ducks are very susceptible to aflatoxin content of the feed. The minimum toxic dose for ducks is 0.03 mg. per kg. in feed. Ducklings are more susceptible.

It is a condition caused by aflatoxin produced by the mould *Aspergillus flavus* in the feed stuffs such as groundnut, maize, rice polish etc.

Symptoms:

1. Lower doses produce chronic effects such as poor intake, poor growth, falling of feathers, lethargy, unthriftiness, lameness.
2. On higher dose, it produces liver lesions, ataxia followed by convulsion and death.

Prevention & Control:

Feeding of mouldy feeds should be avoided. Feeds should be checked for aflatoxin particularly during and after rainy season.

Botulism

The disease occurs in young and adult stock. It is caused by the bacterium *Clostridium botulinum*, which grows in decaying plant and animal material.

Symptoms:

1. Birds lose control of their neck muscle and usually drown if swimming water is available.

2. Dullness, ruffled feathers, lameness, drooping wings, laboured breathing, coma and death.

Prevention and Control:

1. C-type antitoxin may be given to the affected birds.
2. Removal of dead birds and rotting vegetation, plus maintenance of cleanliness including surroundings, will prevent this disease.

Ducks can live upto about 10-15 years but the effective laying period is about 3-4 years. Schedule of vaccination of ducks is presented in Table 75.

Table 75 Vaccination schedule

Vaccine	Age (weeks)	Dose	Route
1. Duck cholera	3-4	1 ml	Subcutaneous (Ducklings)
(Pasteurellosis)		2 ml	After 1 month of above vaccination (adults)
2. Duck plague	8-10	1 ml	Subcutaneous (adults)

QUAILS

Japanese quail (*Coturnix coturnix japonica*) also known as Coturnix quail, Pharoah's quail, Eastern quail and in Hindi as *bater*. Coturnix are widely distributed in Europe, Africa-and Asia, where they are regarded as migratory species. Apparently coturnix were either domesticated in Japan about the 11th century or brought to Japan from China about that time. They were first raised as pets and singing birds, but by 1900 Coturnix in Japan had become widely used for meat and egg production. By virtue of high acceptability of quail meat and eggs, it has occupied a prominent position in many other countries like Hongkong, Singapore, Malaysia, France etc.

In India quails were first introduced at Central Avian Research Iastitute by Dr. B. Panda, Founder Director (CARI) in 1974. Thereafter various research centers of the country including some Agricultural Universities namely, Andhra Pradesh Agricultural University, Hyderabad; Bidhanchandra Krishi Viswavidyalaya, West Bengal etc. were actively engaged in finding economic aspects of rearing the species. Private organisations like AVM hatcheries and Poultry Breeding Research Centre at Tamil Nadu can now be rated as one of the biggest commercial quailary in the country. This new avian species, unknown in India a decade back, has now spread across the length and breadth of our country.

The few facts which make quail raising an economical proposition are as follows:

1. Fast growth rate, mature in about six weeks. The body weight of adult male quail will be about 140 gms. While the females are slightly heavier, weighing 150 to 180 gms. Growth rate is about 3½ times as fast as domestic fowl.

2. Very early sexual maturity. By about 50 days of age, the females are usually in full egg production.
3. High rate of egg production. With proper care, quail hens should lay 260 eggs in their first year of lay.
4. Short generation interval. Its ability to produce three to four generations per year has made it possible to use it as laboratory animal.
5. Small incubation period of only 17 days.
6. Fitness for high density rearing as they require less floor, feeder and water space in comparison to chicken and ducks.
7. No need for vaccination as the species is fairly resistant to many common chicken diseases.
8. Quick return on low investment.

Table 76 Comparison of important traits of quail and chicken

Trait	Quail	Chicken
Egg size (weight)	10 g	58 g
Weight of day-old chick	6 g	35 g
Age of production of first egg	40-42 days	126-140 days
Feed efficiency (kg/dozen of eggs)	1.70-2.10	1.80-2.50
Protein per cent of egg	13.3	11.8
Protein per cent of meat	25-26	19-20
Incubation period	14 days	21 days
Hen-housed egg production	260-275	280-310
FCR	3.3-3.8	1.9-2.2
Live weight (boilers)	140-150 g	1250-1400 g
Dressing percentage	68-72	73-75

Varieties of Japanese Quail

Japanese quail comes under the class Axes, order *Calliformes*, genus Coturnix, species Coturnix and subspecies, *Japonica*, hence named *Coturnix coturnix Japonica*.

There are five varieties of Japanese quails namely, (1) Pharach (wild type): It has got a mixture of feather colours with black and various shades having predominency of brown colour. In male the face and throat is rusty brown, the upper breast is cinamon. In female, the face, throat and upper breast are light cinamon with black while the lower breast is tan. (2) British Range: A dark feather coloured variety of quail in which the male and feamles are similarly pigmented. (3) English White: A white feathered variety of quail with dark eyes. Few black spots are not uncommon. (4) Manchurian Golden: Birds are of golden to wheat straw coloured. (5) Tuxedo: It is a bi-colour variety of quail. The ventral surface including neck and face is white and the remaining part is black to that of Pharach type.

Reproduction

Domesticated quails reproduce in all seasons of the year when they attain their age between 10-20 weeks. The females proceed, like machines, to lay an egg every 16 to 24 hours for 8 to 12 months. Eggs should be collected for hatching 4 days after the introduction of males (one male: three females) and till the 3rd day after the sexes are separated. The average egg weighs about 10 gms. This is about 8 per cent of the body weight of quail hen as against 3 and 1 per cent for chicken and turkey respectively. Each hen appears to lay eggs with a characteristic shell pattern or colour. Some strains lay only white eggs. Young chicks weigh from 6 to 7 gms. When hatched, are brownish with yellow stripes. Fertility decreases markedly with older birds. The albumen to yolk ratio is 61:39. Percentage of yolk is more and that of albumen is less in quail than in chicken eggs.

Sexual development of domestic quail is photic controlled. Keeping birds in continuous dark results in almost complete inhibition of sexual behaviour and egg production, whereas keeping birds in continuous light results in a very high rate of egg production during the first year, with production coming to a halt by the end of the second year.

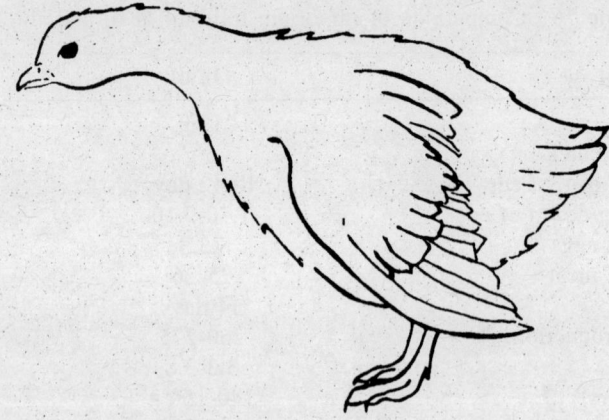

Figure 37   Male Japanese quail courting. The male approaches the female, walking stiff-legged on his toes, feathers erect, and the neck extended horizontally

Chickens lay about 75 per cent of their eggs in the morning whereas the coturnix by nearly 75 per cent of daily total production between 3 to 6 P.M. and the balance of 20-25% at night.

Coturnix come to production at about 6 weeks of age. Fifty per cent production level is generally achieved at the age of 7-8 weeks, while peak (over 80%) is attained after 10 weeks of age. A wide range of sexual maturity (35-40 days) in commercial quail flock is reported by many workers. Under ideal conditions they produce about 250 to 300 eggs per year. Second year production is 48% of first year's production in quails as against 65% in case of chickens.

Incubation and Hatching

Successful quail propagation begins during pre-incubation period. Eggs should be collected several times a day and should be handled with great care as these are very susceptible to shell damage. Before storage hatching eggs must be exposed to formaldehyde gas for about'20 minutes and then preservation is made at a temperature of 15.5°C having 80% humidity for 7-10 days. A household refrigerator is not satisfactory as it is too cold. Domesticated Japanese quail have lost the broodiness trait; hence, eggs must be incubated under a hen or artificially.

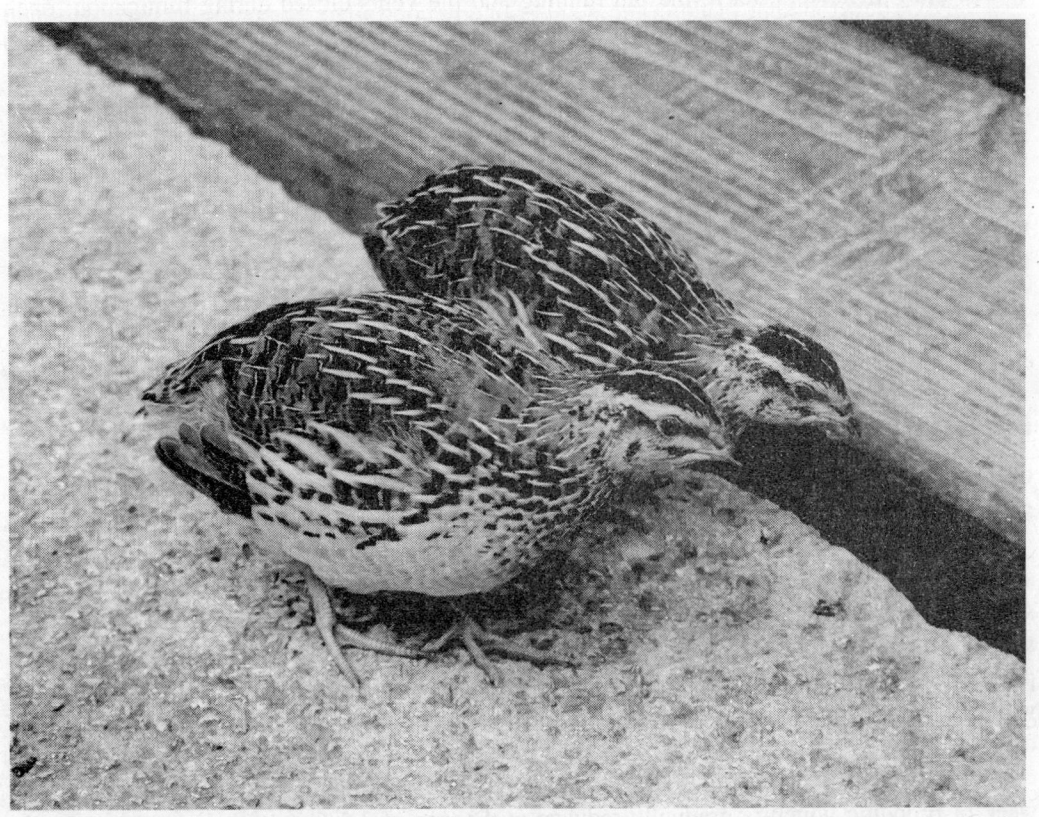

Plate 20　A Pair of Quail

The incubator used for chickens may be used for quail hatching but setting trays need to be modified to hold the small sized eggs in position. A dirty incubator or hatchery area is a major source of contamination and disease. By the help of a quaternary ammonium compound or commercial disinfectants the hatching units should be thoroughly washed and disinfected. Only clean eggs should be set which had an exposure of fumigators. Alternatively they can be fumigated within 12 hours after being placed inside the incubator.

For fumigation 25 gms of potassium permanganate in an earthen ware or enamelware is taken and then 35 ml. of formaldehyde for each cubic meter of incubator space is added. In forced draft incubators, leave the fan running and the vents closed during fumigation; open vents after 20 minutes. Humidity at this stage should be high with a temperature between 20 to 30°C.

Incubation period varies between 17 to 18 days depending on the strain and procedures adopted. Eggs should be placed large end up in the setting trays. Forced-draft incubators are maintained at a temperature of 37.5° ± 0.3°C (99.5° ± 0.5°F) with a relative humidity of 60 percent (wet bulb reading 30° + 0.5°C (86° ±1.0°F) upto 14th day of incubation. Egg turning rate should be once for every 2-4 hours. On 14th day or earlier transferring of eggs to hatching trays should be followed which also marks the end of further turning. A separate hatcher should be operated at 37.2°C (99°F) with a relative humidity of 70%. The hatcher should remain strictly closed for the entire hatching process till the quail chicks are removed on the 17th or 18th day of incubation.

Brooding and Rearing

Quails are comparatively more delicate than chickens and need better care during the first 2 weeks of their life. Thereafter they become harder.

Although both battery and floor system of brooding and rearing can be employed with satisfactory-results, but battery brooding upto 3 weeks of age gives better result due to small size of the chicks. Like chickens, the floor should preferably be covered with wood shavings and sand upto a height of 5-10 cm (2 to 4 inches). Of course, for the first week corrugated paper should be placed on top of the floor to provide better foothold. If chicks are raised in wire cages, or batteries, the wire floor also must be covered with hard paper for the first week or so.

Newly hatched chicks require desirable temperature of about 35°C (95°F) during the first week of brooding which is gradually reduced at the rate of 3.5°C per week untill the chicks are fully feathered at about 4 weeks. The best guide for adjusting the temperature is chick behaviour. When the temperature is further required to be high, chicks will crowd near the source of heat and vice versa. The feeder and water space requirement during this period are 2-3 cm and 1-1.5 cm respectively. Floor, feeder and water spaces should be increased with advance in age.

Feather picking or other forms of cannibalism may occur when Japanese quails are kept on wire. Beak trimming may be necessary as early as 2 weeks of age and may be done by using nail cutters.

Depending upon the type of chicks and the season 150 to 180 cm^2 space should be provided in the batteries and between 200-250 cm^2 per chick when grown on the floor under litter system.

Young birds can be transferred from brooder to cages or floor around the fourth week.

Housing and Equipment

When the birds are raised for commercial egg or meat production, small pair cages are suitable. For cage or pen construction, 1.25 cm welded wire mesh is recommended. Adult quails will live and produce efficiently with an area of 130 cm^2 of floor space per bird. Often, in community pens, they will not build a nest but will hide their eggs in the litter. For this reason cages are always preferred to litter system. A cage of 12.7 × 20.3 cm. (5 × 8 inches) is sufficient for a pair of layers. Regarding feeder space, an adult quail will need 1.25 to 2.5 cm of feeder space.

Males and females should be separated as soon as possible and grown separately. Continuous lighting is necessary for the first 48 hours. After this the females should have a total of 14-18 hours of light a day to maintain maximum egg production and fertility. Males not required for breeding, or any quail being grown for meat production, can be given only about 8 hours of low intensity light a day for depressing sexual maturity and increasing faster fattening.

Feeding

Like that of chickens, quails are also classified as starter (0-3 weeks), grower (4-5 weeks) and layer or breeder (6 weeks onward) depending upon their growth rate and reproduction performance. For the first three to four weeks, quails should be fed a diet containing approxiamately 27% protein and about 2,750 kcal/kg ME; growers are fed diets having 24% protein containing same amount of metabolizable energy while the protein content is further reduced to 22% for layers and breeders having ME value of 2,650 kcal/kg. of the feed. Daily feed consumption is around 25–30 gm per day/quail.

Quails being simple stomached species require all essential amino acids like that of chicks along with essential fatty acids, 21 essential mineral elements and 13 vitamins other than ascorbic acid (Vit. C), which the body can synthesise. Supply of fresh water for 24 hrs. is a must.

A standard ration for starter, grower or for breeding quail may not be available commercially. In that case, good quality broiler chick mash diets are recommended. The dietary requirements of birds nearing maturity are similar except that calcium and phosphorus levels must be increased. Shell grit or ground limestone can be added to the diets after 5 weeks of age or may be provided as a free choice. The requirements and practical rations as recommended by CARI for quails are given in Tables 77, 78 and 79.

Quail Diseases

Although the Japanese quail is a hardy bird compared to other poultry species but are very sensitive to sudden environmental changes particularly during the first 2 weeks of their life. In general, they do not require to be vaccinated or deworming. Sanitation is the best preventive measure, including the control of rats, mice and flies. However, administering any routine antibiotic through drinking water for initial 3 days sand anticoccidials for 12-15 days, helps in controlling mortality and enhancing weight gain.

Table 77 Suggested practical level of nutrients in feed for Japanese quail

Nutrients	Starter 0-3 weeks	Grower 4-5 weeks	Layer/breeder adult (6 weaks and above)
Metabolizable energy (Kcal/kg)	2,750	2,750	2,650
Protein (% diet)	27	24	22
Minerals			
Calcium (% diet)	1	0.8	3
Phosphorus (% diet)	0.45	0.45	0.45
Sodium (% diet)	0.2	0.2	0.2
Copper (mg/kg diet)	8	8	8
Iodine (mg/kg diet)	0.6	0.6	0.6
Iron (mg/kg diet)	100	100	100
Manganese (mg/kg diet)	120	120	120
Zinc (mg/kg diet)	80	80	80
Vitamins			
Vitamin A (lU/kg diet)	10,000	10,000	10,000
Vitamin D_3 (ICU/kg diet)	1,250	1,250	1,250
Vitamin E (IU/kgdiet)	50	50	50
Vitamin K_1 (mg/kg diet)	3	3	3
Vitamin B_{12} (mg/kg diet)	0.005	0.005	0.005
Thiamine (mg/kg diet)	4	4	4
Riboflavin (mg/kg diet)	6	6	6
Niacin (mg/kg diet)	60	60	60
Pantothenic acid (mg/kg diet)	50	50	50
Pyridoxine (mg/kg diet)	6	6	6
Biotin (mg/kg diet)	0.2	0.2	0.2
Folic acid (mg/kg diet)	1	1	1
Choline (mg/kg diet)	3,000	3,000	3,000
Amino acids			
Arginine (% diet)	1.57	1.39	0.99
Glycine (% diet)	1.44	1.28	–
Histidine (% diet)	0.54	0.48	0.37
Isoleucine (% diet)	1.08	0.96	0.88
Leucine (% diet)	1.89	1.68	1.43
Lysine (% diet)	1.4	1.24	0.73
Methionine (% diet)	0.41	0.36	0.33
Methionine + cystine (% diet)	0.76	0.67	0.62
Phenylalanine (% diet)	0.97	0.86	0.64
Phenylalanine + tyrosine (% diet)	1.81	1.61	1.17
Threonine (% diet)	1	0.89	0.64
Tryptophan (% diet)	0.27	0.24	0.18
Valine (% diet)	1.19	1.06	0.88

Panda, B; Mohapatra, S.C. 1989. Poultry production, published by Indian Council of Agricultural Research, New Delhi.

Table 78 Suggested levels of amino acids for Japanese quail

Amino acids	Starting and growing quail*		Breeding quail	
	% protein	% diet	% protein	% diet
Arginine	5.8	1.57	4.5	0.99
Glycine	5.2	1.44		
Histidine	2.0	0.54	1.7	0.37
Isoleucine	4.0	1.08	4.0	0.88
Leucine	7.0	1.89	6.5	1.43
Lysine	5.2	1.40	3.3	0.73
Methionine	1.5	1.41	1.5	0.33
Methionine + cystine	2.8	0.76	2.8	0.62
Phenylalanine	3.6	0.97	2.9	0.64
Phenylalanine + tyrosine	6.7	1.81	5.3	1.17
Threonine	3.7	1.00	2.9	0.64
Tryptophan	1.0	0.27	0.8	0.18
Valine	4.4	1.19	4.0	0.88
Protein		27		22

*Froin 3 to 5 weeks of age, protein content can be reduced to 20-22 per cent; accordingly amino acid levels also can be reduced.

Table 79 Recommended feed formulae for Japanese quail (in per cent)

Ingredients	Starter mash		Grower mash		Layer/Breeder mash	
Mixing percent	0-3 weeks		4-5 weeks		6 weeks and above	
Maize (yellow)	33.5	45.5	30.5	40.5	36.5	46.5
Rice polish / Jowar	10.0	-	10.0	-	10.0	-
DORB/Wheat bran	-	-	7.0	7.0	6.0	8.0
GNC (43% protein)	12.0	5.0	10.0	12.0	10.0	7.0
Soyabean meal (45% protein)	15.0	20.0	12.0	10.0	12.0	14.0
Sunflower cake (37.50% protein)	12.0	15.0	14.0	15.0	10.0	10.0
Fish meal (44% protein)	8.0	12.0	7.0	7.0	7.0	6.0
Meat Meal	7.0	-	7.0	6.0	6.0	6.0
Mineral mixture	2.5	2.5	2.5	2.5	2.5	2.5
Total	**100.0**	**100.0**	**100.0**	**100.0**	**100.0**	**100.0**

TURKEY

Turkey is the original inhabitant of North America and they were first domesticated in Europe. The scientific name is *Meleagris gallopaveo*. Turkey birds in India have gained some popularity in recent years and are mainly reared for meat purposes. Raising of turkey as meat bird is advantageous due to the following reasons:

(i) Turkey provides excellent meat and has a better meat to bone ratio than the broiler.

(ii) Small turkey reaches 2.25 to 3.20 kg at about 11 weeks under commercial conditions.

(iii) Medium strain of turkey gain body weight up to 5.46 - 6.35 kg at 16 weeks of age.

(iv) Breeder and catering turkey strain will attain 13.6 kg and more in 25 weeks of age.

(v) They are as efficient as chicken in the utilization of feed for growth to any attainable weight.

(vi) Turkey meat is delicious and nutritious. The protein content is higher and fat % is less. It contains sufficient amount of minerals particularly calcium, potassium, magnesium, iron, zinc etc. and vitamins like niacin, vitamin B_6 and B_{12}. The cholesterol content of turkey meat is also lower.

(vii) Generally turkeys are marketed for meat purpose at the age of 16 weeks. At this age, the average weight of males (Toms) become 7.5 kg and that of females (hens) are about 5.5 kg. Feed efficiency ratio of broiler turkey is 2.7 to 2.8 and the dressing percentage is 80-87%.

Other characteristics of Turkey are as follows:

(i) The nutritive value of turkey egg is like that of chicken and it is also delicious. The turkey egg weighs about 85 gm and average body weight of day old turkey is about 50 gm.

(ii) Turkey hen generally starts laying at about 30 weeks of age. They can lay 80-100 eggs in a year if proper feed and management is provided. About 70% of the eggs are laid during afternoon hours. One end of the egg is tapering and the shell is also very hard having different coloured spots.

(iii) For fertilized egg, one tom is required per five turkey hen. Both male and female turkeys attain maturity at 30 weeks of age and after one year they are not generally used for breeding purpose. It has been reported that male turkeys are not able to function properly under natural matings. Artificial insemininination, therefore, is being commonly used to obtain desired fertility levels. Because of reduced fertility, turkey toms are rarely used after first year.

(iv) Incubation period of turkey egg is 28 days; the required temperature of incubator is 37.5 °C and the relative humidity at setter is 60-65% and at hatcher it is 85-90%.

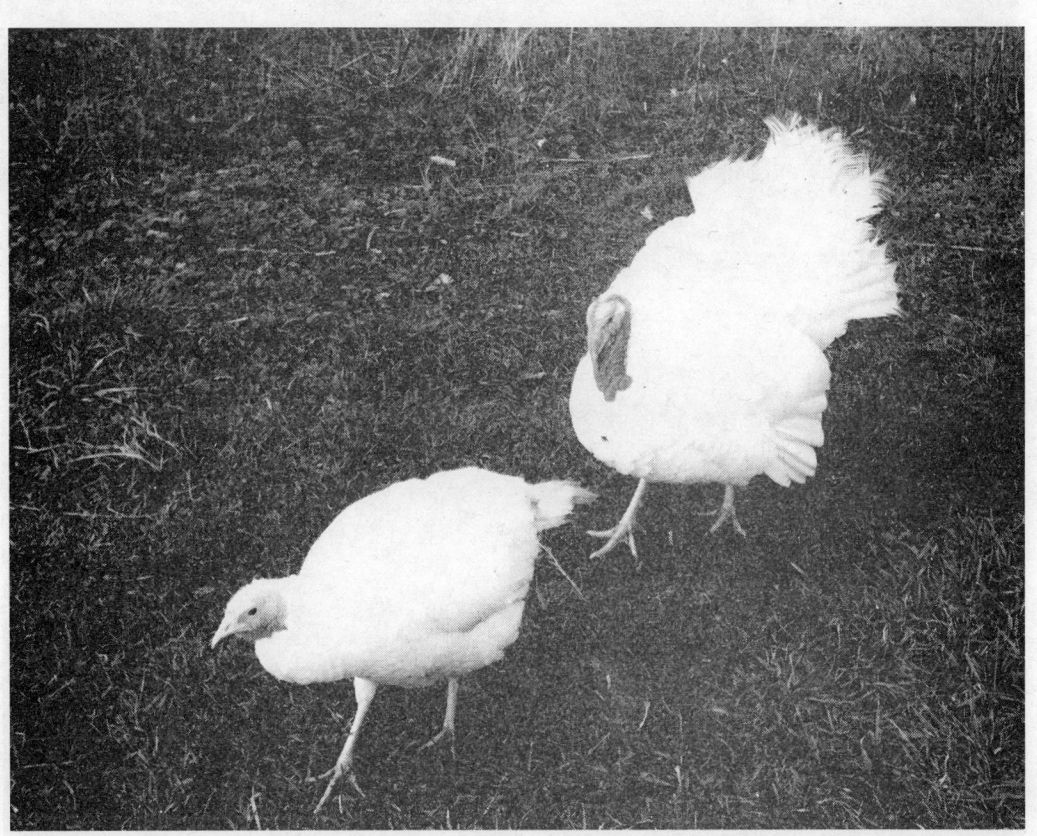

Plate 21   A Pair of Turkey

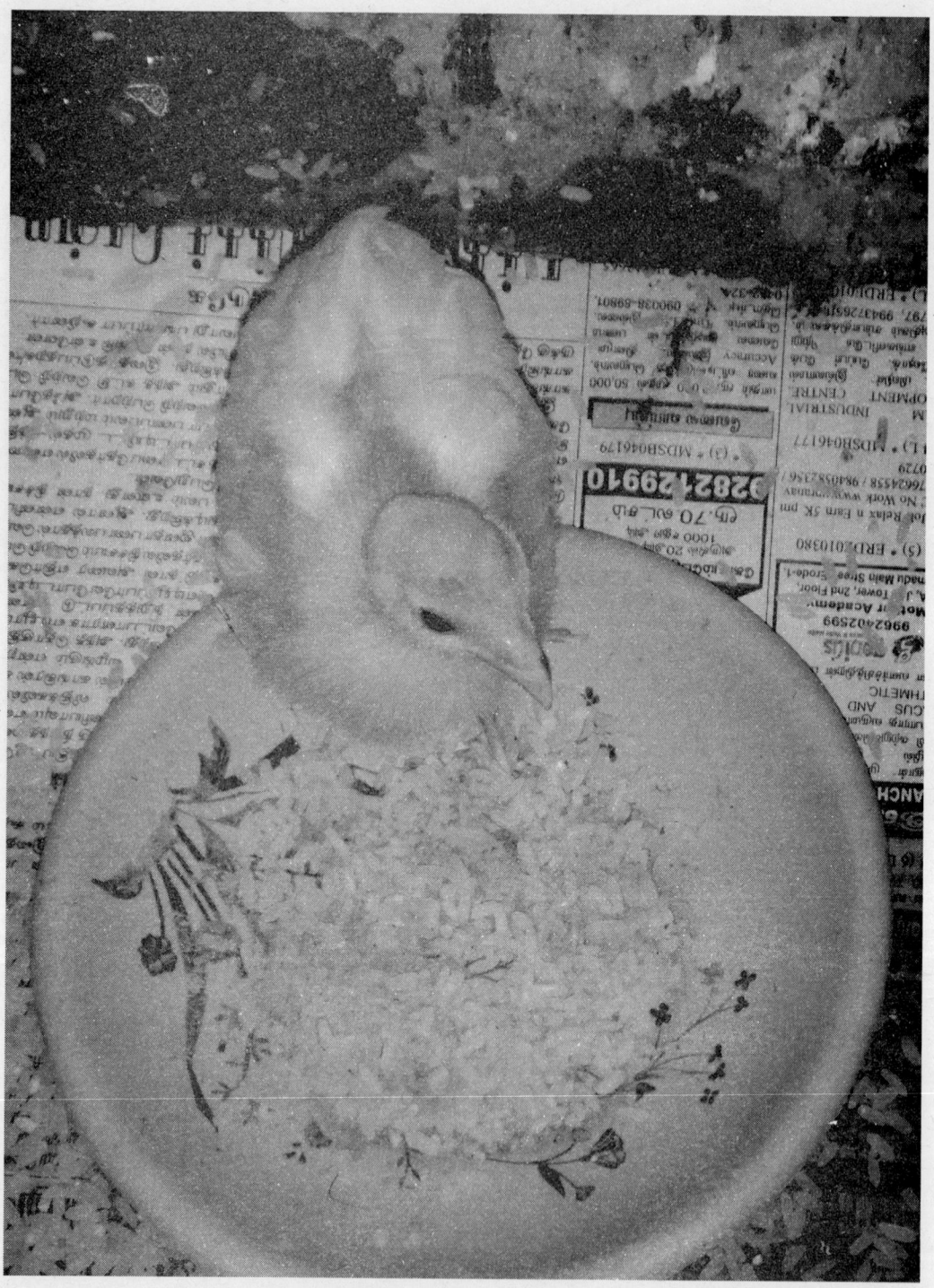

Plate 22 Feeding of Turkey Chick

Varieties

As per American standard for poultry, there are seven varieties of turkey and these are Bronze, Narragansett, Bourbon Red, White Holland, Black, Slate and Beltsville Small White. At present, the three most popular varieties are Broad Breasted white (BBW); Broad Breasted Bronze (BBB) and Beltsville Small White (BSW). In India the preferred variety is BBW i.e. the white one.

Rearing

Turkeys can be very well grown on range. But it requires clean fields on which poultry or turkeys have not been reared for previous two years. In range system, for night shelter 3-4 sft space will be required per bird and 200-250 adult turkeys can be reared in one acre of land. The land should be fenced around 3-3.5 m high for protecting them from predators. Feeders and waterers should be kept under roof to provide protection from animals, wild birds, climate and predators. Birds should be rotated from one range to another frequently. Under range system, the floor space is reduced to almost one-third.

In intensive rearing, adequate floor area and ample fresh air should be provided for growing birds. This method is similar to deep litter method of poultry rearing but the requirement of floor space; feeding and watering space is more (Table 80) as it is a fast-growing bird.

Table 80 Space requirement for turkey

Age (weeks)	Floor space (sft)	Space for feeders (cm)	Space for waterers (cm)
0-4	1.25	2.5	1.5
4-16	2.50	5.0	2.5
16-29	4.00	6.5	2.5
Breedable turkey	5.00	7.5	2.5

The length of the house should be on East-West basis and the breadth might be 9 m at maximum and the height should be 2.6 to 3.3 m. Initially, the litter should be about 2" thickness and then it should be slowly increased up to 3"–4".

Cage system of rearing is not much popular except in small flocks or for research work.

Brooding

Generally, brooding should be done upto 4 weeks of age, but in winter season this may be extended upto 5-6 weeks. Brooding temperature should be 95 °F at first week and then it should be lowered by 5 °F at every week. For the first few days, the turkey chicks may not be interested in feed or water probably due to panicky as they are usually nervous and also due to poor vision. So to avoid fasting, a solution of 100 ml milk mixing with one liter of water along with one boiled egg per 10 chicks may be fed upto 15 days of age. To attract them towards the feed trough and water container, some coloured marbles may be kept.

Feeding

Readymade turkey feeds are not available in the market. The ingredients which are used for preparation of feed for chicken may be used in definite proportions for preparation of turkey feed (Table 81) also. However, the demand for some of the nutrients, particularly energy, protein, minerals and vitamins are higher in turkey, because of its faster growth. Turkey requires practically higher quantities of vitamins - A, D niacin and choline. The practical level of nutrients in the diet of turkeys are presented in Table 82. Whereas average body weight, feed consumption and feed efficiency of Broad Breasted Bronze (BBB) turkey has been given in Table 83.

Table 81 Feed compositions of turkey (in percent)

Ingredients	For young	For growing
Maize crushed	42	49
Soyabean meal	40	26
Sunflower meal	8	8
Fish meal	5	13
Dicalcium phosphate	2	2
Lime	1	1
Mineral mixture	2	1

In addition, 10 gm of vitamin AB_2D_3, 150 gm choline chloride, 20 gm vitamin B-Complex and100 gm micro-nutrients should be mixed per100 kg of feed.

Health Management

Vaccination

Routine vaccination should be given for Ranikhet and Fowl pox diseases and in case of need, fowl cholera vaccine may also be given. Vaccination schedule is given below:

Ranikhet vaccine (F_1)	- 7 days of age
Ranikhet vaccine (Lassota)	- 28 days of age
Fowl pox	- 42 days of age
Ranikhet vaccine (R_2B)	- 56 days of age
Ranikhet vaccine (R_2B)	- 25 weeks of age
Fowl cholera vaccine	- 8-10 weeks of age

Deworming

In range system of management, deworming for each turkey is essential. Good results are obtained if turkeys are dewormed first at 16 weeks of age followed by 3 months interval. Turkeys are generally infected with roundworms and in that case piperazine citrate acts as a good dewormer.

Table 82 Practical level of nutrients in the diet of turkeys

Nutrients	Starting (0-6 weeks)	Growing (weeks) 6-12	Growing (weeks) 12-18	Pre-breeding (18 weeks to 4 weeks before laying)	Laying/breeding
ME (k cal/kg)	3000	2850	2850	2750	2700
CP (%)	28	24	16	14	15
Minerals					
Calcium (%)	0.9	1.0	0.8	0.8	2.75
Phosphorus (%)	0.45	0.5	0.4	0.4	0.5
Magnesium (mg/kg)	360	360	360	360	300
Sodium (mg/kg)	1750	1750	1750	1750	1750
Potassium (mg/kg)	4400	4400	4400	4400	4400
Copper (mg/kg)	4.2	4.2	4.2	4.2	3.5
Iodine (mg/kg)	0.48	0.48	0.48	0.48	0.4
Iron (mg/kg)	96	96	96	96	80
Manganese (mg/kg)	120	120	120	120	100
Zinc (mg/kg)	60	60	60	60	50
Selenium (mg/kg)	0.12	0.15	0.15	0.15	–
Vitamins					
Vit.-A (IU/kg)	12000	12000	12000	12000	12000
Vit.-D (IU/kg)	1800	1800	1800	1800	1500
Vit.-E (IU/kg)	36	36	36	36	36
Vit.-K (mg/kg)	4.8	4.8	4.8	4.8	4.0
Thiamine (mg/kg)	4.8	4.8	4.8	4.8	4.0
Riboflavin (mg/kg)	12	12	12	12	10
Nicotinic acid (mg/kg)	60	60	60	60	50
Pantothenic acid (mg/kg)	19.2	19.2	19.2	19.2	16
Pyridoxine (mg/kg)	6	6	6	6	5
Biotin (mg/kg)	0.12	0.12	0.12	0.12	0.1
Folic acid (mg/kg)	2.4	2.4	2.4	2.4	2
Vit.-B_{12} (mg/kg)	0.024	0.024	0.024	0.024	0.02
Choline (mg/kg)	1760	–	–	–	1350

Table 83 Average weight, feed consumption and feed efficiency in Turkey

Age (weeks)	Average weight (kg) Hens	Average weight (kg) Toms	Total cumulative feed required (kg) Hens	Total cumulative feed required (kg) Toms	Cumulative feed efficiency Hens	Cumulative feed efficiency Toms
1st	0.12	0.12	0.08	0.09	0.67	0.67
2nd	0.24	0.27	0.24	0.27	1.00	1.00
3rd	0.40	0.45	0.49	0.54	1.20	1.20
4th	0.63	0.72	0.81	0.95	1.30	1.30
5th	0.86	1.09	1.27	1.54	1.50	1.40
6th	1.13	1.45	1.85	2.18	1.60	1.50
7th	1.49	1.90	2.54	3.04	1.70	1.60

Table 83   (Continued)

Age (weeks)	Average weight (kg)		Total cumulative feed required (kg)		Cumulative feed efficiency	
	Hens	Toms	Hens	Toms	Hens	Toms
8th	1.90	2.36	3.49	3.99	1.80	1.70
9th	2.35	2.90	4.72	5.49	2.00	1.90
10th	2.86	3.49	6.26	7.35	2.20	2.10
11th	3.40	4.08	7.76	9.34	2.30	2.30
12th	3.85	4.72	9.25	11.34	2.40	2.40
13th	4.25	5.35	10.66	13.38	2.50	2.50
14th	4.72	5.98	12.24	15.56	2.60	2.50
15th	5.12	6.67	13.83	17.69	2.70	2.60
16th	5.53	7.26	15.69	19.86	2.80	2.70
17th	5.89	7.85	17.55	21.99	3.00	2.80
18th	6.21	8.43	19.41	23.99	3.10	2.80
19th	6.53	9.03	21.27	26.08	3.34	2.90
20th	6.75	9.62	23.13	28.26	3.40	2.90

EMU

Emu farming in India is in primitive stage and the activity is rapidly increasing in size and number, expanding into many states and this expansion is likely to continue in coming years.

Features: Emu (*Dromaius novachollandiae*) is a large flightless bird from Australia. It is the 3rd biggest bird in the world after ostrich and cassowary. It belongs to the order Ratite and adaptable to varied climatic conditions. Emu is reared commercially in many parts of the world, viz. United States, Australia, China, etc. for their meat, oil, skin, feathers which are of high economic value.

Emu has long neck, relatively small naked head, three toes and body covered with feather. Mature birds have bare blue neck and mottled body feathers. Body weight of adult birds is generally around 45-60 kg with a height of about 6 ft. Legs are covered with scaly skin adaptable to hard and dry soil. Female is the larger of the two especially during the breeding season when the male may fast. Birds can be maintained as a flock or pair. Emu are omnivorous and eat leaves, vegetables, fruits, insects, worms etc. Though they are originally wild, they are tamed, docile and are easily manageable.

Indian Scenario

In India, emu farming started in 1996 with import of live birds from USA. Vijaya Ratites, a company first undertook the activity on a commercial basis and later the entire farm was sold to Flightless Birds of India (FBI) in 1997. FBI is the only foundation farm and the total strength of birds in the country are derived either from the birds imported by them or from their progeny. Most of the present day farms are rearing the birds for breeding and multiplication purpose. Uptil now, no farm has started organized and regular slaughter. Only problem birds are maintained separately and slaughtered at the age of 14 to 18 months. The registered associations in the country for emu farmers are: India Emu Association with its head quarter at Hyderabad; Emu Farmers Welfare Association, at Vijayawada; Maha Emu Association and Indian Emu Association. As per Indian Emu Association, there are about 360 farmers and the population of the birds is around 1.65 lakh.

Housing

(i) **Brooding Stage (up to 3 months)**
The young ones are retained in the hatcher for a day or two after hatching to ensure absorption of yolk and drying and then shifted to brooder house. As the birds are hatched out in winter, the younger ones require hot temperature which is provided mostly by electrical brooders. In the first week, a temperature of 90°F is to be furnished and it is to be reduced to 85°F which is to be maintained during 2nd and 3rd week. In India, the brooder house is either a brooder shed where the birds are confined by way of chick guards or divided into small pens to accommodate 50 to 75 birds in each pen upto 3 months of age after which the birds are shifted to grower pens.

(ii) **Grower stage (3 months to 18/24 months)**
30 to 50 birds are mostly housed per pen in colony pens. Two inch GI chain linked wire mesh fencing is provided, the pens are either square or circular in shape. For free movement of birds, the minimum width of the pen is usually kept at 40 ft and length ranging from 100 to 120 ft. Generally 80 to 90 sq. ft. of space is provided per bird. Feeders are hung to the fencing or feeds posts and water is given in troughs which are distributed evenly in the pen. One feeder is sufficient for 5 to 7 birds.

(iii) **Breeder stage**
At present, almost all the birds produced and retained in the farm are reared for breeding purpose. At about 18 month's age, the birds are shifted from grower pens to breeder pens. In India, either flock or pen mating is being practiced. In flock mating, group of birds ranging from 4 to 25 pairs are housed in each pen depending on the floor space. About 100 to 120 sq. ft. of floor space is provided per bird. In pen mating, a pair of birds is housed in separate pens of 15 ft × 15 ft size.

Where the floor is cemented / paved, it is mud flooring in grower and breeder houses. Usually, chain linked wire mesh is used for fencing. Cement poles / wooden posts (10 to 12 feet apart) are used as supporting material. Usually 2′ × 2′ GI mesh is used upto 6 to 8 feet height. One acre can house about 100 adult birds (breeders).

Feeding

Balanced diet is essential for proper growth and reproduction of Emu birds. Birds do not require any feed on the 1st day of hatch as the yolk is sufficient to take care of nutrients. From 2nd/3rd day onwards, the birds are fed starter ration upto 14 weeks of age, thereafter grower

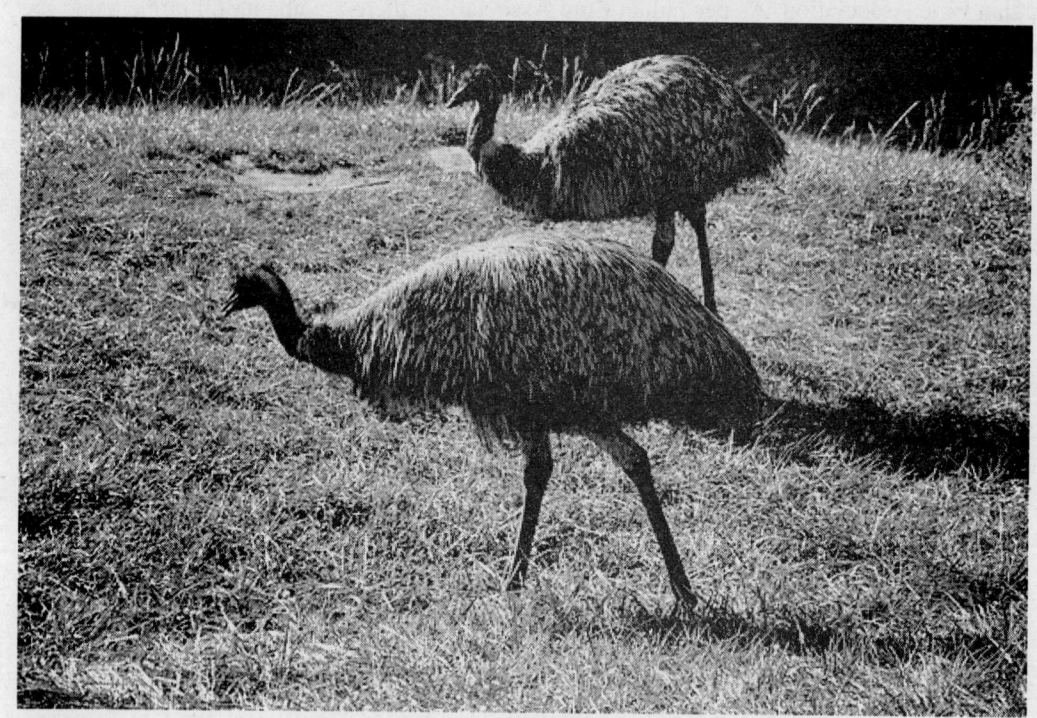

Plate 23   A Pair of EMU

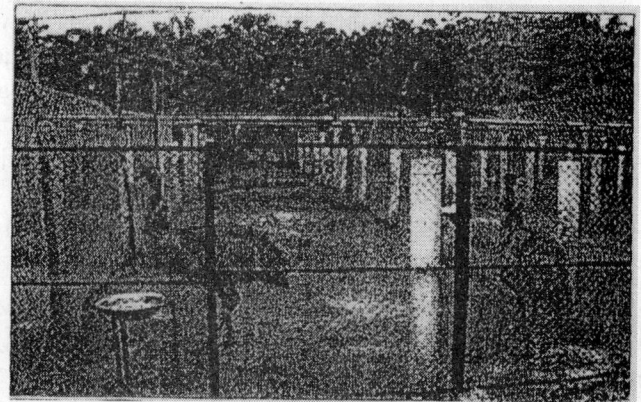

Plate 24 Rearing of EMU

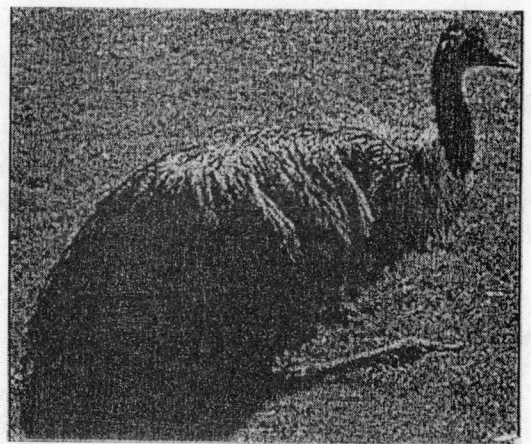

Plate 25 An adult female EMU

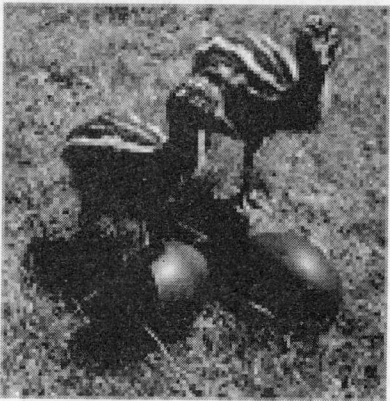

Plate 26 Newly hatched EMU chicks

ration - I from 15 to 34 weeks of age and then grower ration - 2 from 35 weeks to maturity. Breeder ration is fed a month before breeding. The feed consumption which starts at 35 to 40 gm per bird per day increases as the bird gains weight and becomes 1 kg per bird per day by the time the bird attains maturity. Average feed consumption upto 10months would be about 600 gm per bird per day and thereafter 1000 gm per bird per day. Commonly used feed ingredients are maize, soybean meal, de-oiled rice bran, sunflower meal, etc. The nutrient requirements as standardized by the Poultry Science Department, APAU, Hyderabad upto 20 weeks are as under:

| Upto 8 weeks | - 20% CP | - 2800 KCal ME |
| Upto 9 to 20 weeks | - 18% CP | - 2600 KCal ME |

For adult birds, the following standards are adopted:

21 weeks to maturity	- 16% CP	- 2600 KCal ME
Breeders	- 20% CP	- 2600 KCal ME
Maintenance	- 15% CP	- 2400 KCal ME

Vegetables like cabbages, tomatoes, fruits like papaya and mangoes, forages like lucerne meal can be fed during maintenance period.

Feeding is generally done either *ad-libitum* or with known quantities in two installments (morning and evening). Using of pellets reduce wastage of feed and vitamin and mineral imbalances. Feed consumption is reduced by 40 to 60% during breeding period. To supply adequate nutrients, feed rich in CP and ME is to be supplied during this period. FCR of emu is 5:1.

Breeder stock management

The birds attain sexual maturity by 18-24 months of age. The breeding season of emu birds is from October to February / March, the cooler parts of the year. The birds hatched out in January to March will be ready for breeding only in October of third year. The female birds attain maturity at 18 months and male birds at 24 month of age. However, as the breeding season is confined to a part of the year, the birds have to wait till the breeding season in the following year for mating and laying of eggs.

In breeding season, mating takes place once in 3 to 4 days. With one mating, the female bird can lay 3 to 4 eggs. The egg laying interval is about 72 hours. The male, after mating, goes into brooding stage. If eggs are available, this brood stage lasts for the incubation period of 52 days. Otherwise, it will last for a week to 10 days. Hence, in pen mating where only a pair is housed, mating takes place at an interval of 10 to 15 days, whereas in flock mating, another male bird courts and mates with the female bird. Thus, in a season, two male birds met with one female.

Eggs are usually laid in the evenings. An emu hen lays about 10 to 15 days during first year cycle. The egg weight is about 400 to 600 gm and the colour is deep blue. In subsequent years, the egg production will reach 30 to 40 eggs. Thus, the average egg production in a farm will be about 25 eggs per female. Hatching of eggs should be preferably done within 3 days of laying for increased hatchability. Incubation period of emu egg is 52 days, of which 48 days are in the setter and on 49th day they are shifted to hatcher. Hatching parameters as required are as follows:

Dry bulb temperature	: 97 to 97.5 0F
Wet bulb temperature	: 78 to 80 0F
Relative Humidity	: 30 - 40%
Turnings	: Hourly

After hatching, the chicks are kept in the hatcher for a day or two till the yolk absorbed and they get dry. Day old chicks weigh about 370 - 450 gm.

Products

Fertile eggs, meat, oil, skin and feathers are products of emu farming. The peculiar nature of emu is that the fat will be accumulated as a layer on the back instead of in the muscles, thereby the extraction of oil is much easier and the meat will be devoid of fat. On an average, a bird of 14-18 months, yields about 5-6 kg of fat which gives about 4 litres of oil, 2 sq. ft. of leather and about 16 to 18 kg of meat. Older birds yield more oil and meat depending on their body weight. Emu meat contains low fat and emu oil is reported to have medicinal properties. Oleic acid, the monounsaturated fatty acid is the major fatty acid in emu oil. It also contains omega 3 and 6 fatty acids which lowers blood cholesterol. Emu oil reportedly is effective against arthritis. In western countries it is also used in cosmetics.

Skins are being processed and made into certain products like handbags, shoes, etc. The dressing percentage ranges from 50-57% and the life span is 25-35 years.

OSTRICH

Due to low calorie, ostrich meat ranks highest among health foods in terms of health value due to "Zero" percentage fat, low cholesterol and calories, rich protein and iron. Ostriches were originally farmed exclusively for their exquisite feathers but now ostriches are commercially reared for meat, leather, oil and other by products.

Advantages of ostrich farming

1. Along with other animals the bird can be reared in paddock.
2. The bird can thrive in extreme temperature and fellow lands.
3. The bird can sustain in irrigated as well as rainfed farming conditions
4. Practically, there are no waste products in the bird.
5. An ostrich produces not less than 40 chicks annually that reach marketing age after only 407 days from conception (42 days incubation + 365 days of age) and yield 1,800 kg of meat, 50 m^2 of leather and 36 kg of feathers each year.
6. The net weight of meat represents 50 percent of live weight in ostriches, a percentage much higher than that of farm animals.

7. Female ostrich can continue annual production for upto 40 years of age.

Limitations

1. High capital investments for setting up a farm.
2. Marketing facility for its meat and by-products are to be created.
3. Birds are susceptible to some of the avian disorders particularly for New-Castle disease.

General Features

Ostrich is the world's largest living, flightless giant belonging to the Ratite (flightless/running birds) family. The scientific name is *Struthio camelus*. Camels means it is somewhat similar to camel like prominent eyes, eyelashes, large size and tolerance to desert conditions. Due to large body size and small wing they are not capable of flying. Adult males stand 2.4 m tall and can weigh upto 100 kg; the hen is slightly lower. The birds have long neck, small head, large eyes, short broad beak, long bare legs and two toes. They can run upto 70 km per hour with their long strong legs with strides of upto 8 m and are used for defence. Neck and thigh muscles are without feather and well developed. Ostriches can live upto 60-70 years.

Ostriches control heat loss during cold weather by covering its thighs with its wings and creates a gentle breeze by lifting and moving its wings during hot weather. The feathers are excellent insulators, minimizing heat gain from direct solar radiation, as well as reducing heat loss during cold desert nights. Heat can also be lost by panting due to well developed air-sac system.

Behaviour

Ostriches are completely diurnal birds. They move about for most of the daytime except when dust bathing, resting or nesting. They remain seated during dust and virtually inactive throughout the night unless disturbed. Wild ostrich is sexually mature at four to five yeas of age while domesticated ones mature at two to three years; female matures slightly earlier than male. Mature male ostriches attain black and white plumage while females and immature birds have much duller colouring, with grayish-brown plumage. During breeding season, cock's plumage became brighter. Male and female chicks look alike and their sex can only be identified by examining sexual organs as the penis of the male is tiny and easily confused with the clitoris of the female. By about seven to eight months of age, sex can be determined as during urination and defecation, the penis emerges out. Full distinction between sexes can be made at about two years of age by observing colour of feathers.

Ostriches are seasonal breeders. The mating season generally lasts from six to eight months every year, it can vary with latitude and altitude. The breeding season mostly depends on food availability, bird's condition, weather etc. Male ostriches are polygamous and can mate with more than one female. In the wild, the cock stays with one/two or even more hens. On the other hand, domesticated ostriches are kept in pairs (one male and one female) or in trios (one male and two females) for breeding season. The female starts to lay fertile eggs shortly after mating. Eggs are laid in alternate days in clutches of 20 to 24 eggs. High

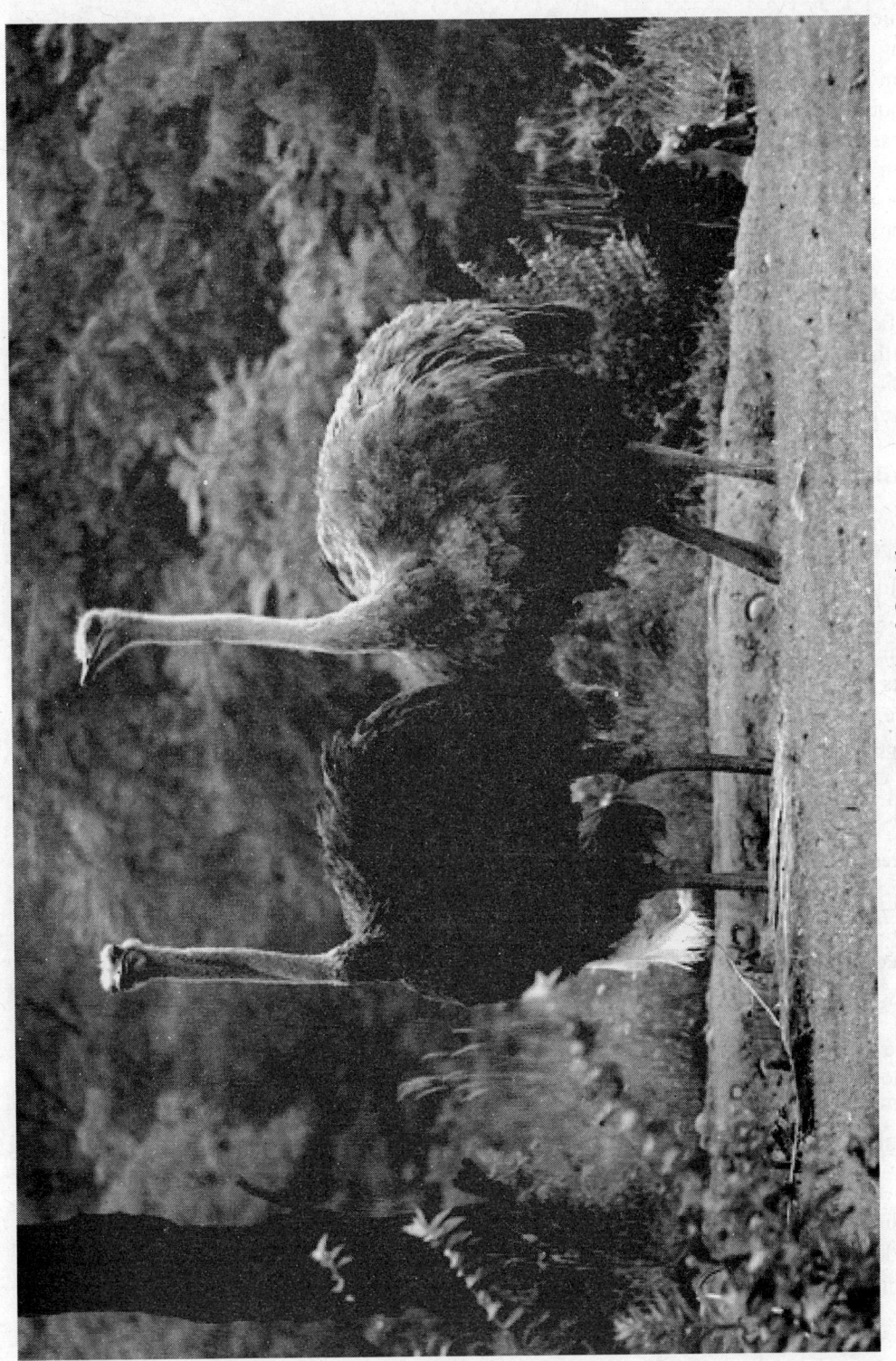

257

Plate 27   A Pair of Ostrich

producing females can lay between 80 to 100 eggs during breeding season. The hen stops laying for a period of 7 to 10 days after which she starts a new clutch. Eggs are laid in a common nest on the ground with other females laying their eggs in the same nest. If the eggs are not removed, the females start incubating during day time while the male incubate from dusk to dawn. The ostrich lays the largest egg of any living bird measuring 17 to 19 cm in length, 14 to 15 cm in width with a volume of about 1.4 litres and weighing upto 1900 gm, white to yellowish white in colour and the hard surface is pitted with superficial pores of various sizes and shapes. Incubation period is 42 days; eggs can be hatched naturally or artificially. If natural hatching is done, the female will not lay eggs until the chicks have reached 4 to 5 weeks of age, thus there will be economical loss. So artificial hatching is beneficial. So eggs should be collected daily for 2 times and stored for not more than 7 days with their broad end up at 16 - 18°C. Eggs can be set at the incubator (0 - 38 days) at 97.3 - 97.5°F and at 25% relative humidity and later shifted to hatcher (39 to 42 days) at 97-97.1°F and relative humidity 40% (these eggs require very low relative humidity).

Feeding

Ostriches roam about freely and feed off all natural feed including lucerne, maize, soya and wheat etc. They can walk at least 20 kms for the purpose of foraging food under wild conditions. Fresh and clean water should be supplied at all the times as they can drink upto 9 liters of water per day. The feed to weight gain ratio of ostrich is 2:1 during first few months and this may raise to 3.5:1 during their normal development for processing at 9 months. The chicks do not feed for first few days as they utilize nutrients of their yolk sac during this time. Hence, they should be trained with other feeding chicks to avoid starvation. Nutrient composition of feed given during different age groups should be as per Table 84.

Table 84 Nutrient composition of feed given during different age groups

Nutrient	Chick starter (0-6 m)	Grower (6-18 m)	Maintenance (> 18 m)	Laying
CP %	21-22	16-17	14-15	20-21
ME (kcal/kg)	2700	2800	2400	2300
Ca%	1.20	1.20	> 30	> 30
P%	0.60	0.60	1.50	1.50
Lysine (%)	0.70	0.70	0.70	1.20
Methionine (%)	0.30	0.30	0.30	0.45

Housing

Birds are usually reared in large paddocks. However, the birds require limited area for brooding of chicks. The birds are reared indoors for first two months thereafter they are provided with night shelter along with day grazing and after 6 months, outdoor provision is recommended. Space requirements as birds grow is given in Table 85.

Table 85 Space requirement for an ostrich farm

Age	Indoor	Outdoor
1–21 days	Building 0.5 sq. m/bird	According to climate 3.5 sq. m/bird
22– 90 days	Building 1.00 sq.m/bird	Required 10 sq.m/bird; minimum 50 sq.m
90–300 days	Open shelter 1 sq.m/bird	100 sq.m/bird (slaughtering) minimum space 1000 sq.m
Breeders / selection; 12 months and older	Open shelter 5 sq.m/bird	500-800 sq.m/bird; minimum space 1000 sq.m

Note: (a) The open shelter should after protection on 3 sides with a door on the 4th side. The opening will be minimum 1.50 m in wide. The shelter will be minimum 2.50 m high.

(b) The fence will be minimum 1.50 m high for birds and breeders (according to farm and objectives) with a post for every 4 meters.

However, recently the intensive system is also becoming popular because of adoption of scientific technologies, reduced selection, nutritional innovations, health regimes and extensive disease surveillance.

Products

Meat: The healthy red meat of ostrich is an alternative to traditional red and white meat due to its low fat, low calorie, low cholesterol and high protein content and by its similar taste and texture to veal and beef depending on the age of their slaughtering. A recent United States Department of Agriculture (USDA) publication compared nutritive value of chicken and beef with that of ostrich meat is given in Table 86.

Table 86 Nutritive value of ostrich meat compared with beef and chicken

Per 100 g raw meat	Ostrich	Beef	Chicken
Protein (g)	21.9	20.0	21.4
Fat (g)	1.0	15.6	2.6
Cholesterol (mg)	63	86	74
Energy (cal)	114	276	163
Calcium (mg)	5.2	9.0	13.0

The study indicates that ostrich meat contains less fat, and particularly less cholesterol, than other types of meat. Lately, with greater consumer awareness of problems of high cholesterol levels in blood and possible probability of heart attack, demand for ostrich meat in international markets has been growing. Latest report shows that current ostrich meat production is not enough to meet the increasing demand.

Hide

Ostrich skin (hide) is considered to be the most luxurious leathers, and is placed at par with crocodile and snake skin. Exquisite ostrich leather is the strongest commercially available leather in the world. It is also used in the manufacture of shoes, bags, purses and jackets.

Feathers and oil

Ostrich feathers are used for cleaning machinery and equipment as well as for decorations and in brush and fashion industry. Best quality feathers are obtained from arid regions of the world. In addition to meat, skin and feathers; ostriches are being explored for medical and medicinal purposes. Ostrich oil is a well recognized product of cosmetic industry.

Prospects

An ostrich chick requires good care, a balanced diet containing all essential nutrients in optimal quantities, and right temperature must be maintained during brooding upto the age of four months. If proper care is taken during this early period and sales of ostrich products, ostrich farming can certainly be financially rewarding.

LITERATURE CITED

Annual Report **2011-12**. Department of Animal Husbandry Daring and Fisheries, Ministry of Agriculture; Govt. of India.

Barman, R.S.D.; Singh, D.K.; Jha, D.K.; Mahto Dinesh and Anjay **2014**. Present status and future prospects of Indian Poultry Industry. Pashudhan; March 2014, **Vol: 40** Issue: 03.

Bureau of Indian Standards **2007**. Indian Standard - Poultry Feeds - Specification (IS 1374:2007) Manak Bhavan, 9 Bahadurshah Zafar Marg, New Delhi - 110 002.

Ensminger, M.E. **1992**. Poultry Science. Published by International Book Distributing Co. (Publishing Division). Chaman Studio Building. 2nd Floor, Charbagh, Lucknow - 226004, UP.

Ghosh, Nilotpal **2013**. "Unnat Prathay Pashupalan-o-Pashu-Chikitasa" Bengali Version. 2nd Edition, Reprinted, Published by Kalyani Publisher I/I - Rajinder Nagar, Ludhiana-141008.

Gupta, P.S. **1994**. Indian Poultry Industry Yearbook. Tenth Annual Edition. Editor & Publisher. S.P. Gupta A-25 Priyadarshini Vihar, Delhi - 110 092.

India **2012**. A Reference Annual; Compiled by Research, Reference and Training Division - Published by Publications Division, Ministry of Information and Broadcasting. Government of India.

Indian Council of Agricultural Research **2013**. Handbook of Animal Husbandry, 4th Revised and Enlarged Edition. Krishi Anusandhan Bhavan, New Delhi-110012.

Jadhav, N.V. and Siddiqui, M.F. **2007**. Handbook of Poultry Production and Management. 2nd Edition Published by Japee Brothers, Medical Publishers (P) Ltd., New Delhi.

Leeson, S. and Summers, J.D. **1993**. Commercial Poultry Nutrition. First Indian Reprint. Published by International Book Distributing Co. Chaman Studio Building, 2nd Floor, Charbagh, Lucknow-226004, U.P., India.

Nesheim, M.C.; Austic, R.E. and Card, L.E. **1979**. Poultry Production. Indian Edition, Published by K.M. Varghese Company, Post Box:7119, Bombay-400031.

Prasad, J. **2000**. Poultry Production and Management. Published by Kalyani Publishers. B-I-1292 Rajinder Nagar, Ludhiana-141008.

Project Director; Directorate on Poultry **2013**. Leaflets on Vanaraja and Gramapriya - Published by Project Directorate on Poultry; Rajendra Nagar, Hyderabad - 500030.

Reddy, D.V. **2009**. Applied Nutrition: Livestock, Poultry, Pets, Rabbits and Laboratory Animals. 2nd Edition. Published by Oxford and IBH Publishing Co. Pvt. Ltd. New Delhi.

Sastry, N.S.R.; Thomas, C.K. **2011**. Livestock Production Management. Reprinted: 2011, Kalyani Publishers, Ludhiana-141008.

Singh, R.A. **2009**. Poultry Production. 3rd Edition Published by Kalyani Publishers B-I/1292 Rajinder Nagar, Ludhiana-141008.

Sreenivasaiah, P.V. **2006**. Scientific Poultry Production - A Unique Encyclopedia. Third Revised and Enlarged Edition. Published by International Book Distributing Co.; Chaman Studio Building, 2nd Floor Charbagh, Lucknow-226004, U.P., India.

Sulaiman, E. and Vijayachandran Pillai **2005**. Working of Poultry Industry in India. Published by J.V. Publishing House, Jodhpur - 342001, Rajasthan.

Vasanthi, B. **2008**. Ostrich Farm. Pasudhan, Nov. 2008; Vol: 34 Issue 11.

Verma, D.N. **1999**. Livestock Production Management in Tropic. Published by Kalyani Publishers. B-I-1292 Rajinder Nagar, Ludhiana - 141008.

GLOSSARY

ABATTOIR   A slaughterhouse

ACTIVE IMMUNITY   Immunity or resistance to disease that has been acquired by host response to a disease agent. It can be acquired by having a disease and recovering or by vaccination.

ACUTE   A disease which has a short and relatively severe course.

ADDITIVE   An ingredient or substance added to a basic feed mix, usually in small quantities for the purpose of fortifying with certain stimulants and/or medicines. Need not add any nutrient.

ALLERGY   A severe reaction, or sensitivity, which occurs in some individuals following the introduction of certain antigens into their bodies.

AMBIENT TEMPERATURE   The prevailing or surrounding temperature

ANEMIA   A condition in which the blood is deficient in quantity or quality (lack of haemoglobin content or in number of red blood cells), characterised by paleness of skin and mucous membranes and loss of energy.

ANIMAL PROTEIN FACTOR (APF)   The term formerly used to refer to an unidentified growth factor essential for poultry and swine and present in protein feeds of animal origin. It is same as vitamin B_{12}.

ANTHELMINTIC (Vermifuge)   A product which removes worm parasites.

ANTIBIOTIC   A chemical substance, produced by molds or bacteria, which has the ability to inhibit the growth of, or to destroy, other microorganisms.

ANTIBODY   A substance that opposes the action of another substance.

ANTIDIURETIC HORMONE (ADH)   A pituitary gland hormone that controls the reabsorption of water by the kidney.

ANTIGEN   A foreign substance which, when introduced into the body, stimulates formation of protective antibodies.

ANTIMETABOLITE   A substance bearing a close structural resemblance to one required for normal physiological functioning which exerts its effect by replacing or interfering with the utilisation of the essential metabolite.

ANTIOXIDANT   A compound that prevents oxidative rancidity of polyunsaturated fats. Prevents rancidity in feeds and foods.

ANTISEPTIC   A compound that inhibits the growth of microorganisms, and which is usually applied to skin.

ANTISERUM   A serum containing a specific antibody used to treat a specific disease.

ANTITOXIN   A specific kind of antibody that will neutralise toxin.

ATROPHY   Wasting away or dimunition in size.

AUTOPSY   Inspection, and partial dissection, of a dead body to determine the cause of death.

BACTERICIDE   A product which kills bacteria.

BACTERIN   Killed suspension of bacterial organisms used as an immunising agent.

BACTERIOSTAT   A product which retards bacterial growth.

BALANCED RATION   The daily food allowance of livestock or fowl, mixed to include suitable proportions of the nutrients required for normal health, growth, production, reproduction and well-being.

BASAL DIET   A diet common to all groups of experimental animals to which the experimental substance(s) is added.

BRAILING   A technique used to prevent birds from flying. This may be accomplished by tying one wing in a closed position with a bandage type material. For more permanent results primary flight feathers on one wing may be clipped, the distal wing section may be removed or the tendon to that section may be severed.

BREATHING RATE   Normal for poultry ranges from 15 to 36 per minute.

BREED   Birds having a common origin with specific characteristics, such as body shape, that distinguish them from other groups within the same species.

BREED TRUE   To have the ability to transmit a characteristic uniformly to offspring.

BROAD-SPECTRUM ANTIBIOTIC   An antibiotic which attacks both Gram-positive and Gram-negative bacteria, and which may also show activity against other disease agents.

BROILER   A young bird of either sex, up to six to eight weeks of age and weighing 1½ to 2½ kilogrammes, usually of the meat-type breeds. The term is used inerchangeably with the term fryer

BROODER   A heat source for the period of growth from day of hatch to approximately five weeks of age. The heat source generally has a large reflector (hover) under which the birds may gather and where the heat is captured.

BROODING   The period of growth in the life of a young bird where it must be provided a source of heat in addition to that generated by its own body.

BROODY   The condition of a hen when she is prepared to sit on eggs for the purpose of incubation and when she becomes receptive to caring for the young. Both physiological and psychological changes have taken place in the hen's body and she ceases to lay eggs during this period.

BROOD ANIMAL   An animal reserved for breeding and raising young.

CANDLING   The process of examining an intact egg to determine interior quality, shell soundness, or stage of embryonic development. This is accomplished in a dark room by holding the egg in front of a strong beam of light and reciprocally turning the egg.

CANNIBALISM The habit of one animal pecking at or eating on another animal, such as a fowl pecking at or eating on another fowl.

CAPON   Castrated male chicken, chickens are usually caponised (castrated) between three and four weeks of age.

CAPONETTES   Male, chickens that have had their reproductive organs (testes) made useless by the injection of estrogenic hormones (stiibesterol). The testes of these animals decrease in size, and the secretion of testosterone is inhibited which in turn results in a regression of the secondary sex characteristics (comb, wattles, earlobes, mating instinct, and crowing).

CARCASS   The body of a dead animal.

CARCINOGEN   Any cancer producing substance or agent.

CURBUNCLE   The red and blue fleshy unfeathered area of skin on the upper region of the neck of a turkey.

CARRIER   An apparently healthy animal that harbors disease organisms and is capable of transmitting them to susceptible animals.

CATALYST   Any substance which speeds up the rate of a chemical reaction without being destroyed or inactivated in the process. Enzymes are catalysts.

CATARRHAL   Describes an inflammatory condition of the mucous membranes characterised by an increased flow of mucous.

CEREAL   A plant in the grass family (Graminae), the seeds of which are used for human food and animal feed; e.g., maize, rice, wheat.

CHICK   A young chicken, pheasant, or other gamebird from one day to about five to six weeks of age, either male or female.

CHOLECYSTOKININ   An intestinal hormone that stimulates gallbladder contraction and pancreatic enzyme release, but inhibits gastric acid secretion when the stomach is actively secreting.

CHRONIC   A disease of long duration.

COCCIDIOSTAT   A drug incorporated in feed at low levels and fed continuously to prevent coccidiosis.

COCK   Mature male chicken (rooster).

COCKEREL   A young male chicken from day of hatch to approximately one year of age.

COMB   A fleshy outgrowth on the top of the head of a chicken, generally red in colour and of various types and shapes.

COMBUSTION The combination of substances with oxygen accompanied by the liberation of heat.

CONFINEMENT   Practice of rearing birds completely housed so that they spend their total time indoors.

CONGENITAL   Malformation existing at birth, acquired during development in the uterus and not through heredity.

CONGESTION   Excessive accumulation of blood in a part.

CONTAGIOUS   An infectious disease that may be transmitted readily from one individual to another.

CULTURE   The propagation of microorganisms, or of living tissue cells, in special media conducive to their growth.

CRIMPED   Rolled between corrugated rollars. The grain to which this term refers may be tempered or conditioned before crimping, and may be cooled afterwards.

CRUMBLE   A physical condition of feed prepared at the mill by pelleting of the mixed ingredients and then crushing the pellet to a consistency coarser than mash.

CULLING   The process of eliminating nonproductive or undesirable animals.

CYANOSIS   Bluish discoloration of the skin, particularly the comb and wattles in birds.

CYTOPLASM   Protoplasm of a cell otuside the nucleus.

DEBEAKING   (Beak Trimming) Trimming of the beak involving removal of the upper one-third to one-half of the mandible in growing and mature birds or about one-fourth of both mandibles in day-old chicks and poults, to prevent cannibalism.

DEBILITATING   Weakening.

DECORTICATION   Removal of the bark hull, husk or shell from a plant, seed, or root.

DEW DROP WATERER   Equipment for providing drinking water to birds in cages, basically consisting of a pipe with a ball-bearing-type valve activated by the bird as it pecks at the valve, releasing drops of water.

DISEASE   Any departure from a normal stage of health.

DISINFECTANT   A product which, at certain concentrations, will kill on contact a wide range of disease organisms.

DIURETIC   An agent that increases the flow of urine.

DRY MATTER   That part of a feed which is not water. It is computed by determining the percentage of water and substracting the water content from 100 per cent.

DOWN   Soft fluffy type of feather located under the contour feathers and serving the bird as an insulating material.

DRAKE   Mature male duck.

DUBBING   Comb removal, usually in single comb type birds; may sometimes include removal of wattles. This is usually performed in young bird's from day of hatch to five or six weeks by the use of a scissor, with minimal bleeding if trimmed close to head. In older birds the operation should not be performed due to more serious hemorrhage potential.

DUCK   Mature female duck.

DUCKLING Young duck, either sex, from day of hatch to about six weeks of age.

DYSPNEA Laboured or difficult breathing.

EARLOBE A rounded, sometimes pigmented area of skin below the external ear canal of chickens.

EDEMA Presence of abnormal amounts of fluid in tissues.

EGG EATING A habit which, once it gets started, is difficult to contain in flock houses and usually is associated with overcrowding or thin-shelled eggs. Birds will eat their own eggs and those of other hens when eggs become broken in the nest or on the floor and will even proceed to break the shells and eat eggs once the habit is started.

EGG DIPPING The process of submerging eggs in an antibiotic solution under specific conditions of time and temperature. The purpose is to reduce or eliminate certain microorganisms on or within the egg.

ELASTIN The main protein in elastic fibres of connective tissues.

EMACIATED A severe loss of weight.

ENCEPHALOMALACIA A condition characterised by softening of the brain in young poultry, caused by a deficiency of vitamin E in the diet.

ENDOCRINE Pertaining to glands that produce secretions that pass directly into blood or lymph. Hormones are secreted by endocrine glands.

ENZOOTIC A disease confined to a certain locality.

ERGOSTEROL A plant sterol, that, when activated by ultraviolet rays becomes vitamin D_2.

ETHER EXTRACT The fatty substances of foods or other materials that are soluble in ether.

ETIOLOGY Study of the cause of disease.

EXCRETA Excreted material; waste matter.

EXUDATE A fluid oozing from tissue.

EXUDATIVE DIATHESIS Symptom of vitamin E deficiency of poultry. It is characterised by an accumulation of fluid in subcutaneous fatty tissue.

FECUNDITY The ability of an individual to produce egg or sperms regularly.

FILTERABLE VIRUS An organism so small that it is capable of passing through filters which will retain the ordinary bacteria

FOWL Any bird, but more commonly refers to the larger ones.

FUNGI Certain vegetable organisms such as molds, mushrooms, and toadstools.

GANDER Mature male goose.

GENE The smallest unit, or particle, of inheritance-a portion of a DNA molecule. Genes occur in pairs located on chromosomes in the nucleus of every cell.

GOOSE   Mature female goose.

GOSSLING   Young goose, either sex, from day of hatch to about eight to ten weeks of age.

GRAM-NEGATIVE BACTERIA   Those bacterial species which are decolourised by acetone or alcohol.

GRAM-POSITIVE BACTERIA   Those bacterial species which retain a crystal-violet colour even when exposed to alcohol or acetone.

GROSS   A change in tissue which can be seen with the naked eye.

GYNANDROMORPH   Both male and female plumage on the same bird; a sex mosaic, one side (right) having male characteristics and plumage and the other side (left) having female characteristics and plumage.

HAEMATOCRIT   The percentage of erythrocytes to total blood volume.

HATCHER   A machine or that portion of the incubator that is used for the last two or three days of incubation and hatching of the eggs. No turning of the eggs is required and the eggs are allowed to hatch in flat bottom trays.

HATCHING   The process by which the fully developed faetus (chicks) leaves the protected environment of the egg and emerges into the world, birth.

HEMATOCRIT   Concentration of red blood cells in a given amount of blood.

HEMORRHAGE   Escape of blood from vessels; bleeding.

HOMOTHERM   An organism that produces its own heat and maintains a constant body temperature.

HYPERSENSITIVITY   A state in which the body reacts to a foreign agent more strongly than normal.

HYPOXIA   A condition in which a physiologically inadequate amount of oxygen is available to tissues.

IMMUNE   Resistant to a particular disease.

IMMUNITY   Condition of being immune.

INCUBATOR   A machine developed to provide the proper environment for the development of the fertile egg and embryo into a chick or poult.

INFECTION   Invasion of the tissue by pathogenic organisms resulting in a disease state.

INFECTIOUS   A disease produced by living organisms.

INFLAMMATION   Response of tissues to an injury or other irritant.

INGESTION   The taking in of food and drink.

INTERSTITIAL FLUID   The fluid between the cells or body parts.

INTRACELLULAR FLUID   The fluid within a cell.

INTRADERMAL Into, or between, the layers of the skin.

INTRAMUSCULAR   Within the substance of a muscle.

268

INTRAPERITONEAL   Within the peritoneal cavity.

INTRAUTERINE   Within the uterus.

INTRAVENOUS   Within the vein or veins.

IN VITRO   Occurring in a test tube.

IN VIVO   Occurring in the living body.

ISOTOPE A different form of a given element. Isotopes have the same atomic number but different mass numbers.

"ITIS"   Suffix denoting an inflammatory state, such as enteritis-an inflammation of the intestines.

LAYING   The expulsion of an egg. The term is commonly associated with hens in active egg production.

LEG BAND   Aluminum or plastic bands that may be placed around the shanks of birds for the purpose of identification. The bands can be obtained in various colours and may be numbered.

LESION   Visible change in size, shape, colour, or structure of an organ.

LINE BREEDING   A form of inbreeding in which an attempt is made to concentrate the inheritance of some ancestor in the pedigree.

LISTLESS   Indifferent to surroundings.

LITTER   The accumulation of materials used for bedding farm animals. Also, the pigs farrowed by a sow or the pups whelped by a bitch at one delivery period.

LIVESTOCK   Domestic farm animals kept for productive purposes (meat, milk, work and wool); include dairy and beef cattle, buffaloes, sheep, goats and horses.

LIQUID PROTEIN SUPPLEMENTS   Protein products which usually contain molasses and urea, with added vitamins and trace minerals. Used only in ruminant feeding.

LYMPHOCYTE   A variety of white blood corpuscles that originate from the lymph glands.

LYOPHILISATION   The evaporation of water from a frozen product with the aid of high vacuum. Also called freeze-drying.

LYSIN   Antibody that causes the death and dissolution of bacteria, blood corpuscles and other cellular elements.

MALNUTRITION   Any disorder of nutrition. Commonly used to indicate a state of inadequate nutrition.

MAMMAL   Any animal that suckles or provides milk for its young.

MARSUPIAL   One of a class of mammals characterised by the possession of an abdominal pouch in which the young are carried for some time after birth.

MASH   A form of a complete feed that is finely ground and mixed so that birds cannot easily seperate out ingredients; each mouthful provides a well-balanced diet.

MECONIUM The first excreta of a new born animal.

MEDIUM-SPECTRUM ANTIBIOTIC An antibitoic which attacks a limited number of Gram-positive and Gram-negative bacteria.

METABOLIC Pertaining to the nature of metabolism.

METABOLISM Refers to all the changes which take place in the nutrients after they are absorbed from the digestive tract including (1) the building-up processes in which the absorbed nutrients are used in the formation or repair of body tissues, and (2) the breaking-down processes in which nutrients are oxidized for the production of heat and work.

MICROCURIE The amount of radioactive material that has the same intensity of radiation as one-millionth of a gram of radium.

MICROINGREDIENTS Any ration component, such as minerals, vitamins, antibiotics and drugs, normally measured in milligrams or micrograms per kg.

MICROORGANISM Any organism of microscopic size, applied especially to bacteria and protozoa.

MICROSCOPIC Invisible to the naked eye. Visible only by the aid of a microscope.

MINERAL SUPPLEMENT A rich source of one or more of the inorganic elements needed to perform certain essential functions.

MOLT (MOLTING) The shedding and replacing of feathers.

MORBIDITY Sick rate.

MORPHOGENESIS The origin and evolution of morphological characters (form and structure). The establishment of shape and patterns.

MORTALITY Death rate.

MUSCULAR DYSTROPHY A progressive disorder, marked by atrophy and stiffness of the muscles.

MYOGLOBIN Muscle haemoglobin.

NARROW-SPECTRUM ANTIBIOTIC An antibiotic whose activity is restricted to either Gram-negative or Gram-positive bacteria. For example, penicillin is active primarily against Gram-positive organisms, whereas Streptomycin attacks only Gram-negative organism.

NECROSIS Death or drying of local tissue.

NECROPSY An examination of the internal organs of a dead body to determine the apparent cause of death. Also called autopsy, postmortem.

NEOPLASM Abnormal growth such as a tumor.

NEURITIS An inflammatory or degenerative condition of the nerves.

NITROGEN BALANCE The state in a normal adult in which the nitrogen excreted equals the nitrogen intake in the form of food.

NUTRIENT A substance (element or ingredient) that nourishes the metabolic processes of the body.

NUTRITURE   Nourishment.

ORAL   Given by mouth

ORTS   The leftover feed which an animal refuses to eat.

OVOTESTIS   Development of tissue on the inner right dorsal wall of the female fowl, which normally only has one functional ovary on the left side. If the left ovary is destroyed, the right side may develop this organ.

OSMOSIS   The passage (diffusion) of a solvent through a membrane from a dilute solution into a more concentrated one.

OVULATION   The maturation and release of an ovum.

PARASITE   An animal form that lives on or within a bird to its detriment.

PARENTERAL   As applied to drug or vaccine administration, to inject subcutaneously, intramuscularly.

PATHOGENIC   Disease-producing.

PATHOLOGICAL   Diseased, or due to disease.

PECTORAL   Pertaining to the breast.

PEDIGREE   A list of animal's ancestors.

PELLET   A form of a complete feed that is compacted and extruded to about 1/8 inch in diameter and ¼ inch long, usually fed to mature poultry.

PERISTALSIS   The rythmic contractions and movements of the alimentary canal.

PEROSIS   A disease of chicks marked by bone deformities and associated with deficiency of certain dietary factors, such as biotin, choline, folic acid, or manganese. Also called *slipped tendon or hock disease.*

PINIONING   Amputating the last joint of one wing.

POSTMORTEM   Examination after death.

POTENTIATION   Process used to increase blood levels of specific antibiotics generally by temporarily decreasing dietary calcium intake.

POULARDE   A bird that has had the ovary removed or destroyed and as a result acquires male-type plumage. This may occur at the time of molt, and if the ovary is reactivated the cock-like bird could lay eggs.

POULT   An immature turkey. After the sex can be determined, the turkey is called a young tom (male) or young hen (female).

PREDISPOSE   To confer a tendency toward disease.

PREPARTUM   Occurring before birth of the offspring. Before parturition.

PREPOTENT   Designating an animal that transmits its own characters to its progeny to a marked or highly uniform degree.

PROPHYLAXIS   Preventive treatment against disease.

PROSTAGLANDIN A large group of chemically related 20-carbon hydroxy fatty acids with variable physiological effects in the body.

PROTOZOA One-celled animals which reproduce by splitting in half; found largely in water, and include many parasitic forms.

PULLET A female chicken less than a year old. Generally the term is applied through the first laying year.

PULSE RATE Normal for poultry ranges from 200 to 400 per minute.

PURIFIED DIET A mixture of the known essential dietary nutrients in a pure form that is fed to experimental animals in nutrition studies.

RANCID A term used to describe fats that have undergone partial decomposition.

RATION The food allowed to an animal for 24 hours. A balanced ration provides all the nutrients required to nourish an animal for 24 hours.

ROASTER A young chicken (meat type); weight more than 1.5 kg.

ROOST A resting or lodging place for fowls.

ROOSTER (COCK) An adult male chicken.

SDA (SPECIFIC DYNAMIC ACTION) The increased production of heat by the body as a result of a stimulus to metabolic activity caused by ingesting food.

SEPTICEMIA Blood poisoning, which results from the presence of toxins or poisons of microorganisms in the blood.

SETTING HEN A broody hen in the act of incubating eggs.

SEX CHROMOSOMES One pair of chromosomes in an individual that determines the sex of that individual. In mammals, the female is XX and male is XY. The X chromosome is considerably longer and carries more genes than the Y chromosomes.

SEX-INFLUENCED TRAITS Such traits are due to genes carried on autosomes; however, the gene is dominant in males and recessive in females. For example, the gene for baldness, Ba, in humans is a sex-influenced gene. Its allele is Bn, for nonbaldness phenotype.

SOILAGE Freshly cut green forage feed to animals in confinement. Also called green chop.

SPORATIVE A disease outbreak occurring here and there; not widely diffused.

SPORE Bacteria or fungi capable of resisting unfavourable environmental conditions.

STRESS Factor tending to lower resistance of an animal to disease, such as chilling, moving etc.

SUBCUTANEOUS Under the skin.

SUCCULENCE A condition of plants characterised by juiciness, freshness, and tenderness, making them appetising to animals.

TEMPERATURE   Normal for popultry is 106°F, with a range of 105° to 107° F.

THROMBIN   An enzyme that induces clotting by converting fibrinogen to fibrin.

THROMBOCYTE   A blood platelet thought to be part of the blood clotting mechanism.

TOXAEMIA   A condition produced by the presence of poisons (toxins) in the blood.

ULCER   A lesion or erosion of the mucus membrane, such as gastric ulcer of stomach.

UNIPARUS   Producing only one egg or one offspring at a time.

UNSATURATED FATTY ACIDS   Any one of several fatty acids, containing one or more double bonds, such as oleic, linoleic, linolenic, and arachidonic acids.

VACCINE   A suspension of attenuated or killed microorganisms (bacteria virus or rickettsiae) administered for the prevention, amelioration (improvement), or treatment of infectious diseases.

VASECTOMY   The surgical removal of part or all of the vas deferens. This renders a male sterile without affecting his libido.

VFA (Volatile fatty acids)   Commonly used in reference to acetic, propionic and butyric acids produced in the rumen of cattle, goats, sheep and buffaloes, in the caecum of sheep, the caecum and colon of swine, the colon of the horse and the caecum of the rabbit.

VIRUS   The smallest living microorganism, not visible under ordinary microscope, which lives parasitically upon plants and animals and sometimes causes disease.

WEANING   The stopping of young animals, from suckling their mothers at young age.

WING BAND Aluminium or plastic bands that are placed in the wing web area of the bird at day one of age. These may be.of various colours and may be numbered.

ZOONOSES (Plural of zoonosis)   Those diseases and infectious that are naturally transmitted between vertebrate animals and humans.

ZYGOTE   A diploid cell produced by the union of haploid male and female gametes.

INDEX